ADULT T CELL LEUKEMIA
AND RELATED DISEASES

GANN Monograph on Cancer Research

The Japanese Cancer Association supports two series of publications. GANN is an official organ of the Association, and is published bimonthly. The "GANN Monograph on Cancer Research" series consists of collected contributions on current topics in cancer problems and allied research fields. This semiannual series was initiated in 1966 by the late Dr. Tomizo Yoshida (1903–1973), and is now published jointly by Japan Scientific Societies Press, Tokyo / Plenum Press, New York and London. The publication of this monograph owes much to the financial support given by the late Professor Kazushige Higuchi of Jikei University.

The planning to publish a monograph is made by the Board of Executive Directors of the Japanese Cancer Association, with the final approval of the Board of Directors. It is hoped that the series will serve as an important source of information in cancer research.

Japanese Cancer Association

JAPANESE CANCER ASSOCIATION
GANN Monograph on Cancer Research No.28

ADULT T CELL LEUKEMIA AND RELATED DISEASES

MASAO HANAOKA
Edited by   KIYOSHI TAKATSUKI
MASANORI SHIMOYAMA

JAPAN SCIENTIFIC SOCIETIES PRESS, Tokyo
PLENUM PRESS, New York and London

© Japan Scientific Societies Press, 1982

Softcover reprint of the hardcover 1st edition 1982

December 1982

ISBN-13:978-1-4615-8338-7   e-ISBN-13:978-1-4615-8336-3
DOI: 10.1007/978-1-4615-8336-3

Distributed in all areas outside Japan and Asia between Pakistan and Korea by Plenum Press, New York and London.

PREFACE

Six years ago "adult T cell leukemia (ATL)" was proposed as a new disease entity of T cell malignancy by K. Takatsuki's research group at the Department of Internal Medicine, Kyoto university (the 17th Annual Meeting of Japan Society of Clinical Immunology, 1976). Thereafter, increased attention has been paid to this disease in Japan because of its characteristic neoplastic cell morphology, clinical and pathologic features and the endemic distribution of patients' birthplace in southwestern Japan. At almost the same time, M. Shimoyama and Dr. K. Minato at the National Cancer Center confirmed that a majority of T cell malignancies in adult Japanese correspond to ATL (1976). Dr. M. Sasaki at the Osaka Red Cross Hospital presented the first autopsy case of ATL at the 65th Annual Meeting of the Japanese Pathological Society (1976). Later, at the Symposium entitled "Pathology of Non-Hodgkin Lymphoma" of the Japanese Pathological Society (1978), M. Hanaoka of the Institute for Virus Research, Kyoto University, Dr. M. Sakaki and others demonstrated that the pleomorphism of neoplastic cells characterized cytologic and histologic features of ATL based on their observation of 32 cases of ATL. Also at this symposium, histologic studies on ATL by Dr. T. Suchi of the Aichi Cancer Center and the Japanese Lymphoma Study Group resulted in a new category in the classification of non-Hodgkin lymphoma designated "diffuse lymphoma pleomorphic type." With the accumulation of cases of ATL and non-leukemic pleomorphic T lymphoma, both diseases were included in one category called "adult T cell leukemia-lymphoma (ATLL)" based on pathologic and clinical findings. At research centers in the ATLL-endemic area, the entire clinical picture was obtained with cytologic studies by Prof. M. Ichimaru at the Atomic Disease Institute of Nagasaki University and Prof. K. Yunoki at the Institute for Cancer Research of Kagoshima University and their colleagues; the pathologic features were clarified by Prof. E. Sato's study group at Kagoshima University and Prof. M. Kikuchi's group at the Fukuoka University. It should be noted that the progress made in these early stages was achieved through close cooperation among the above study groups.

During the period between June and August 1980, over 100 cases of ATLL were evaluated by the "Nationwide Survey on T and B Cell Malignancies" with the co-operation of 27 organizations. This survey confirmed the high incidence of T cell malignancies compared to the total lymphoid malignancies; nationwide, the incidence was 49% and in Kyushu, a southwestern area of Japan, it was 70% owing to the cluster of ATLL. These results suggested the possible involvement of microorganism in this disease. At around this time, Prof. Y. Hinuma who had come to the Institute for Virus Research, Kyoto University was asked by Hanaoka to participate in the ATLL study group in order to clarify the etiology of this disease. Initially Prof. Hinuma attempted to detect a viral antigen(s) associated with cultured ATL cells by immunofluorescence using sera of patients with ATL based on his experience with Epstein-Barr virus. Six months later in November 1980, Prof. Hinuma and Dr. K. Nagata found ATL-associated antigens in an ATL cell line (MT-1 cells) established by Dr. I. Miyoshi at the Department of Internal Medicine, Okayama University, Prof. M. Nakai at the Department of Microbiology, Osaka Medical College found virus particles in MT-1 cells under electron microscope (1981). Dr. M. Yoshida of the Cancer Institute, Tokyo, biochemically confirmed the virus was a retrovirus, and designated it ATL virus (ATLV) (1981). Their studies were epoch-making in the etiology and epidemiology of ATLL. In the survey by Prof. Hinuma, Dr. K. Tajima of the Aichi Cancer Center and others, a method was established for the ethnic study of Japanese with the detection of anti-ATLV antibody in sera of many healthy subjects in the ATLL-endemic area and persons in the non-endemic areas along the Japanese coast where patients with ATL have been found sporadically.

In the early stage of ATLL research, it was questioned whether the induction of ATLL was restricted to Japan. Thereafter, several cases of ATLL-like lymphoma with or without leukemic manifestation had been found in U.S.A. including Caucasian patients. Recently, Dr. D. Katovsky of the Royal Postgraduate Medical School, U.K. reported ATLL in West Indian patients (1982), and now the West Indies and the Caribbean Islands are considered the second ATLL-endemic area. In advance of the above reports, Dr. R. Gallo of the National Cancer Institute, U.S.A. had isolated and characterized a new type C retrovirus (human T cell lymphoma virus, HTLV) in cell lines obtained from patients, including a Caribbean, with cutaneous T cell lymphoma of peripheral T cell malignancy (1980). Now greater attention is being given to ATLL in Western countries.

The present monograph is an up-to-date summary of ATLL and its related peripheral (mature) T cell malignancies, and our present knowledge of ATL is the result of the cooperative contributions made by many investigators.

October 1982

Masao HANAOKA
Kiyoshi TAKATSUKI
Masanori SHIMOYAMA

CONTENTS

DISEASE ENTITY OF ADULT T CELL LEUKEMIA: CYTOLOGICAL ASPECTS AND GEOGRAPHIC PATHOLOGY

Masao HANAOKA

Institute for Virus Research, Kyoto University*

Adult T cell leukemia (ATL) is essentially acute lymphocytic leukemia defined both by cytology and epidemiology, that is, the proliferation of neoplastic T_2 (peripheral T) cells with highly irregular nucleus and the clustering of patients' birthplaces in southwestern Japan. For cytologic diagnosis of ATL the following criteria were proposed: nuclear polymorphism accounted for over 10% of the neoplastic T cells in the blood of adult patients which did not have a mediastinal tumor. In biopsy lymph nodes of 101 patients with ATL, diffuse lymphoma of the pleomorphic type (D-Pleo) accounted for 43% followed by 38% of the medium-sized cell type (D-Med). D-Pleo was characterized by the nuclear polymorphism of many neoplastic cells of various sizes and the appearance of giant cells. Nuclear polymorphism was also seen in many cases (71%) of D-Med and in small numbers of diffuse lymphoma, both the large cell and mixed types. Such nuclear polymorphism variant (NP) in each type and D-Pleo accounted for 74% of the entire group of biopsy lymph nodes observed histologically. Therefore both D-Pleo and NP represent the histologic feature of ATL lymph nodes. In patients with ATL, prognosis of D-Pleo and NP was poorer than that of other histologic types.

The survey of birthplaces of patients with ATL in western Japan other than Kyushu showed that almost all were distributed in underpopulated areas adjacent to the Pacific Ocean.

The development of immunological and cytochemical techniques has permitted the identification of subpopulations of human lymphoid cells. Using these tools T cell lineage has been divided into three major categories according to maturation stage: prothymocytes (T_0 cells) in the bone marrow, thymic lymphocytes (T_1 cells) in the cortex of the thymus, and peripheral T (T_2) cells circulating between the blood and lymphoid tissues except the thymus cortex. T_2 cells differentiate functionally into at least two subsets, inducer T cells and suppressor/cytotoxic T cells, which are identified by monoclonal antibodies for each surface antigen (*15*).

Neoplastic cells of T_2 cell leukemia are diverse in their sizes and shapes in contrast to homogeneous neoplastic cells with a nucleus of a fine chromatin pattern as seen in most T_0 and T_1 cell leukemia, or acute lymphoblastic leukemia in childhood and youth. T_2 cell leukemia has been classified into two major categories, monomorphic and pleo-

---

* Kawara-cho, Shogoin, Sakyo-ku, Kyoto 606, Japan (花岡正男).

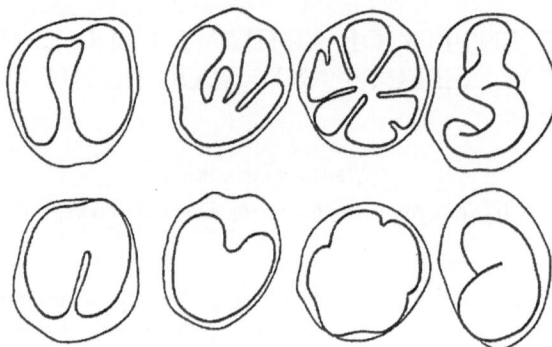

Fig. 1.   Nuclear deformation of neoplastic cells in smear preparations of the blood. Upper, various types of "nuclear polymorphism"; lower, nuclear deformation frequently also observed in lymphatic leukemia other than ATL and Sézary syndrome.

morphic groups, according to the nuclear shape of neoplastic ells in smear preparations of the blood or bone marrow (3–5).

T$_2$ cell leukemia in the monomorphic group includes diverse types found throughout the world, for example, each T cell type of chronic lymphocytic leukemia (T-CLL, small cell type), the prolymphocytic leukemia (medium-sized cell type), and the so-called leukemic reticulum cell sarcoma (large cell type). Most neoplastic cells of this group have a round nucleus with chromatin coarser than that of T$_0$ and T$_1$ neoplastic cells. The nuclear deformation of neoplastic cells in this group, if any, is slight with a single sharp clevis, a moderate convocation in one or more sides, or a notched pattern (Fig. 1).

Leukemia in the pleomorphic group is characterized by "nuclear polymorphism" in the neoplastic cells; nuclear polymorphism refers to the remarkable deformation of the nucleus, such as di- or multi-lobulation on one or all sides of the nuclear surface, and complex distortion (Fig. 1) (5). A well-known leukemia classified in this group is Sézary syndrome which is a chronic T$_2$ cell leukemia chracterized by generalized exfoliative erythrodermia. Neoplastic T$_2$ cells in Sézary syndrome have helper or helper-inducer activity for pokeweed mitogen-activated B cells resulting in differentiation toward antibody forming cells (7). The nucleus of typical Sézary cells has an irregular formation, especially in ultrastructural morphology; the nucleus is cerebriform but appears serpentine on cut section (10).

Adult T cell leukemia (ATL) is also in the pleomorphic group.

Neoplastic Cells of ATL in the Blood

Many cases of T cell leukemia in Japanese adults has been found for the past 7 years, since the first report of a case of T cell leukemia (T-CLL) in Japan by Yodoi using rabbit anti-human thymocyte sera (21). Among them a peculiar type of T cell leukemia, ATL has been noted. ATL can be characterized both morphologically and epidemiologically, that is, both by the proliferation of neoplastic T$_2$ cells with a highly convoluted nucleus, and by the clustering of patients' birthplaces in southwestern

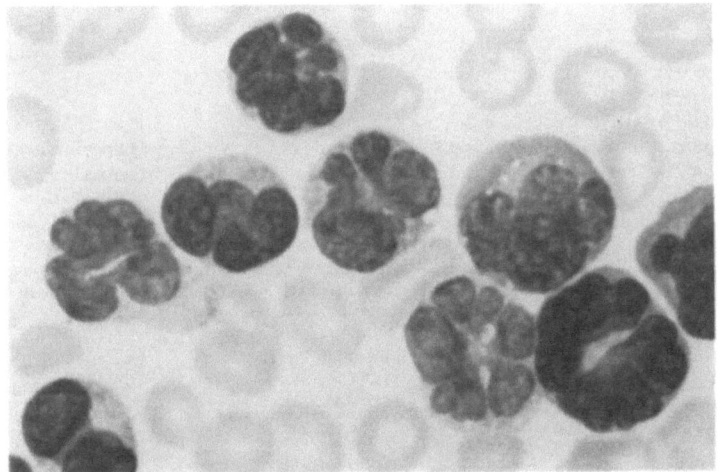

FIG. 2. Neoplastic cell in the blood of a patient with ATL. Smear, May-Giemsa staining, ×1,200.

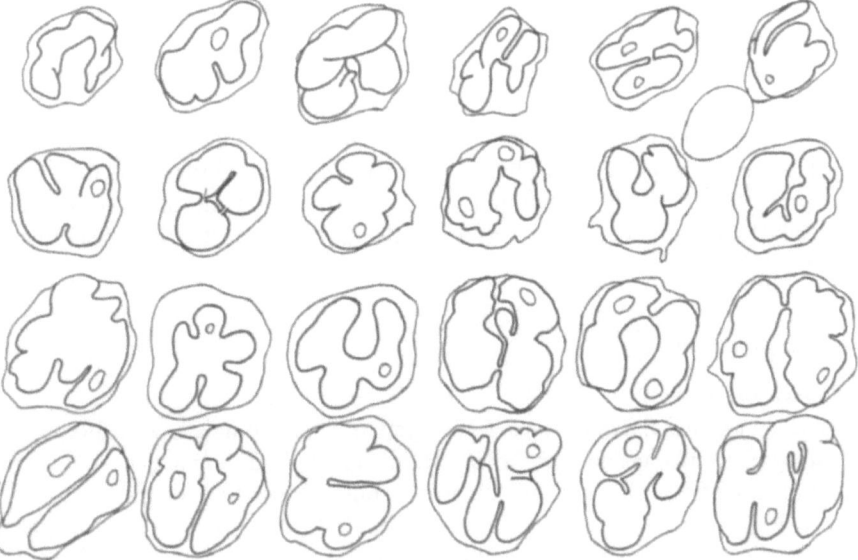

FIG. 3. Neoplastic cells on smear preparation of blood of a patient with ATL.

Japan (4, 20). Recent studies on neoplastic cells of ATL (ATL cells) using mono-clonal antibodies, immunofunctional tests and chromosomal analysis revealed a clonal growth of ATL cells originally derived from a T_2 cell subset which exhibited the suppressor-inducer activity (6, 7). This result suggests that ATL cells are derived from a different T_2 cell subset than neoplastic cells of Sézary syndrome (Sézary cells), which lack the helper activity to induce suppressor T cells (1).

In smear preparations of the blood, the nuclear polymorphism of ATL cells is

TABLE I. ATL and Sézary Syndrome

	ATL	Sézary syndrome
Neoplastic cells		
Nuclear polymorphism	⧺	⧺~ −
Immunologic function	Suppressor-inducer	Helper or helper inducer
Skin lesion	Papules, papulo-nodural eruption	Generalized exfoliative erythrodermia
Neoplastic cell infiltration	Epidermis, dermis, and subcutaneous tissues	Epidermis, dermis, and subcutaneous tissues
Main type of lymph node histology	Diffuse lymphoma, pleomorphic type and medium-sized cell type with nuclear polymorphism of neoplastic cells	Variable types with nuclear polymorphism of neoplastic cells
Duration of disease	Acute in almost all cases	Chronic
Patients' birthplaces	Clustering	Non-clustering
ATLA	Positive in almost all patients	Positive or negative

remarkable (Figs. 2, 3). The size of ATL cells are diverse and sometimes bizarre giant cells appear. Coarse heterochromatin is distributed in the nuclear periphery. May-Giemsa or PAS staining does not reveal any specific features in the cytoplasmic elements of ATL cells; in exceptional cases, azure granules or PAS positive granules are found in the cytoplasm of ATL cells.

For the cytologic diagnosis of ATL the following criteria were proposed: nuclear polymorphism accounts for over 10% of the neoplastic cells in the blood of adult patients without mediastinal tumor (5). This criteria distinguishes ATL from T_0 and T_1 cell leukemia and monomorphic T_2 cell leukemias in adults. It is difficult to distinguish ATL and Sézary syndrome from neoplastic cell morphology, but the neoplastic cell function and clinical features differ in the two diseases as summarized in Table I.

Histologic Diagnosis

1. Biopsy lymph nodes
1) Diffuse lymphoma, pleomorphic type: Japanese pathologists have been perplexed in histologically diagnosing some cases of malignant lymphoma that show a peculiar and complex feature, which is difficult to attribute to any type of the classifications of either of Rappaport, Lukes and Collins, or Kiel. This eccentric type of malignant lymphoma consists of a major figure in biopsy lymph nodes of patients with ATL. This knowledge gave us the opportunity to add a specific entity, "diffuse lymphoma, pleomorphic type (D-Pleo)," to the classification of non-Hodgkin's lymphoma established by the Lymphoma Study Group in Japan (LSG-classification) (18). In this classification, D-Pleo is defined as "a T_2 cell lymphoma showing the diffuse proliferation of multi-sized neoplastic cells with the striking polymorphism of nucleus accompanied by the apperance of giant cells" (Fig. 4). Nuclear polymorphism is the most remarkable in medium-sized neoplastic cells, and large neoplastic cells frequently have a round, clear nuclei with a prominent nucleolus resembling immunoblasts. Giant cells are defined as cells with a nucleus more than three-fold larger than that of small lymphocytes; they reveal a variety of size and shape, and most have a highly convoluted

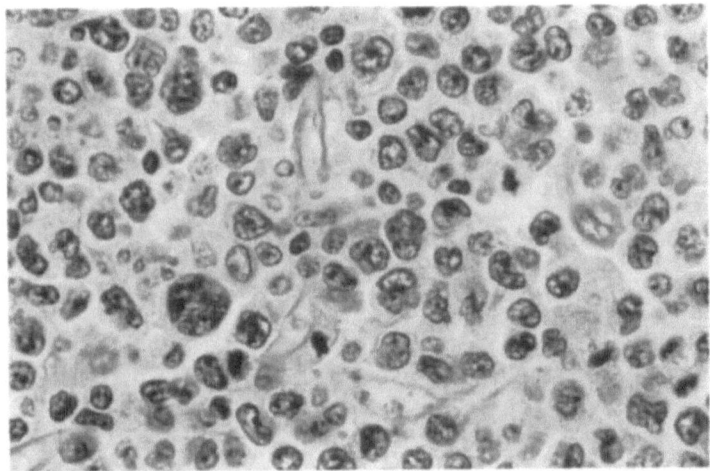

FIG. 4.   D-Pleo of biospy lymph node of a patient with ATL. Hematoxylin-eosin (H-E) staining, ×480.

TABLE II.   Biopsy Lymph Node Histology of ATL

Type	Number of cases (NP)	NP/total (%)
Diffuse lymphoma		
Small cell (D-S)	2	
Medium-sized cell (D-Med)	38 (27)	71
Mixed (D-Mix)	9 (3)	33
Large (D-L)	9 (2)	22
Pleomorphic (D-Pleo)	43	
Total	101 (75[a])	74[a]

NP, nuclear polymorphism variant.
[a] NP of each type+D-Pleo

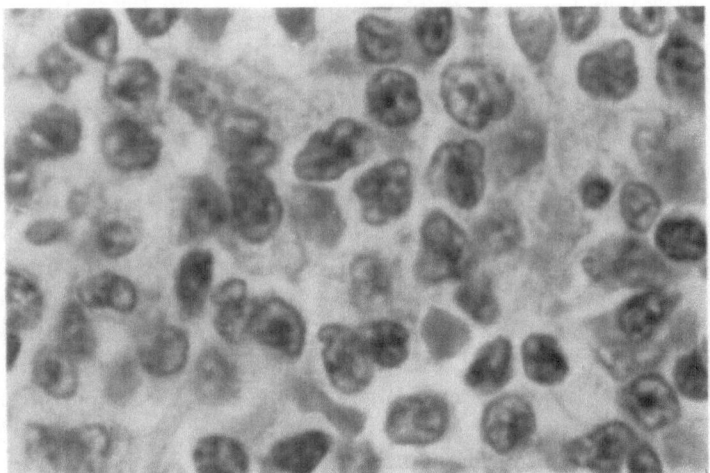

FIG. 5.   D-Pleo nuclear polymorphism variant of a biopsy lymph node of a patient with ATL. H-E staining, ×1,200.

M. HANAOKA

TABLE III.   Histologic Features of 66 Biopsy Lymph Nodes of NP in Each
Type and D-Pleo in Patients with ATL

	Number	%
Localizing of neoplastic cells in paracortical area	18	27.3
Infiltration of neoplastic cells into surrounding tissues and capsule	45	68.2
Destruction of capsule	24	36.4
Preservation of {marginal sinus	61	92.4
lymphocytes in marginal cortex	12	18.2
primary nodule	14	21.1
Formation of active germinal center	4	6.1
Infiltration of eosinophils	8	12.1
Proliferation of {macrophages	10	15.6
interdigitating cells	8	12.1
Development of postcapillary venules[a] {+	11	16.7
++	40	30.3
+++	6	9.1

[a] Grade of development of postcapillary venules: + similar to normal development; ++ better than
normal development; +++ remarkable development.

nucleus. Reed-Sternberg cells and multi-lobulated bizarre giant cells are seen in over
half the cases of ATL.

In biopsy lymph nodes obtained from 101 patients with ATL diagnosed under
the above cytologic criteria, each type of diffuse lymphoma by LSG-classification is
shown in Table II. In this classification, D-Pleo accounted for 43% followed by 38%
of D-Med type. D-Pleo in ATL lymph nodes was one of the major types, but the
rate appears to be too small to represent the general character of the histologic feature
of ATL lymph nodes (Table II).

2) *Nuclear polymorphism variant (NP) in diffuse lymphomas:* D-Pleo was characterized by both nuclear polymorphism of many neoplastic cells and the appearance of
giant cells. The former feature was seen not only in D-Pleo, but also in many cases
of D-Med (71%), and in small numbers of both types of diffuse lymphoma, mixed
and large cell types in ATL (Fig. 5). This NP in each type and D-Pleo characterized
the histologic feature of ATL lymph nodes, such lymph nodes accounted for 74% of
the entire group surveyed (Table II).

3) *Behavior or neoplastic cells in the lymph nodes and surrounding tissues:* Neoplastic
cells proliferated throughout the lymph nodes in many cases without the destruction of
the capsule and sinus. In a quarter of the ATL lymph nodes, the proliferation of neoplastic cells was restricted to the paracortical area. The infiltration of neoplastic cells
into the surrounding tissue or capsule was seen in two-thirds of the cases, but in the
majority the marginal sinus was well preserved. Frequent distribution of small or
medium-sized neoplastic cells was observed in the wall of well-developed postcapillary
venules (PCV) and in the blood and lymph, indicating the recirculation of smaller
neoplastic cells rather than the larger ones (Table III). It was not uncommon that
medium-sized neoplastic cells in the blood were of a uniform size pattern, but in lymph
nodes many large neoplastic cells proliferated.

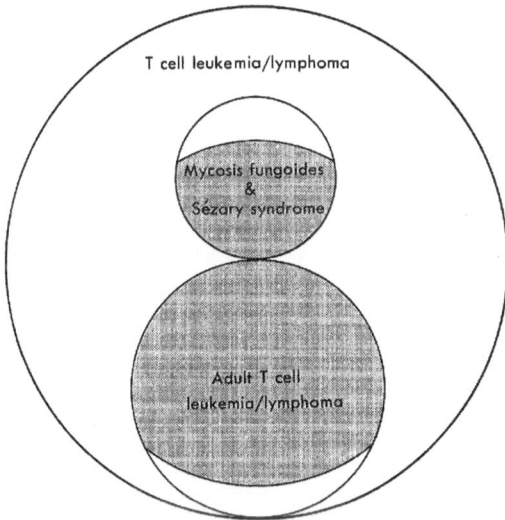

FIG. 6. Relationship of adult T cell leukemia/lymphoma, Sézary syndrome/ mycosis fungoides and D-Pleo and nuclear polymorphism variant (NP). D-Pleo+NP.

2. *ATL and T₂ lymphoma*

At present it is generally accepted that there is no essential difference between lymphatic leukemia and non-leukemic lymphoma in either subtype. Some types of lymphomas such as D-Med frequently disseminate and produce a systemic disease indistinguishable from leukemia. Non-leukemic lymphoma of the pleomorphic type in Kyushu accounted for only 20 to 30% of the total D-Pleo. The transfer from non-leukemic T_2 lymphoma to ATL was not rare.

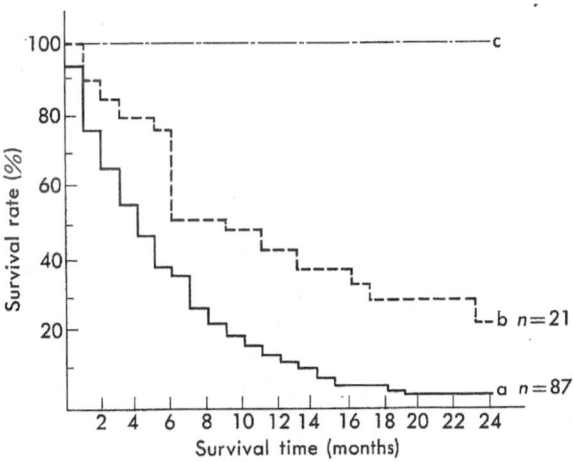

FIG. 7. Survival rates of patients with T_2 cell leukemias. a, ATL; b, T cell leukemia in adults other than ATL and Sézary syndrome; c, Sézary syndrome.

3. Neoplastic cells in autopsy lymph nodes

Cases autopsied showed that neoplastic cells had infiltrated into the interstitial tissue of almost all organs. In the lymph node, neoplastic cells lost their distinctive character such as nuclear polymorphism in many cases. Neoplastic cells of various sizes had round nuclei and floated in the mesh of pseudosinus forming compartmentalization. However, the existence of giant cells and the heterogeneous size of neoplastic cells permits a diagnosis of D-Pleo.

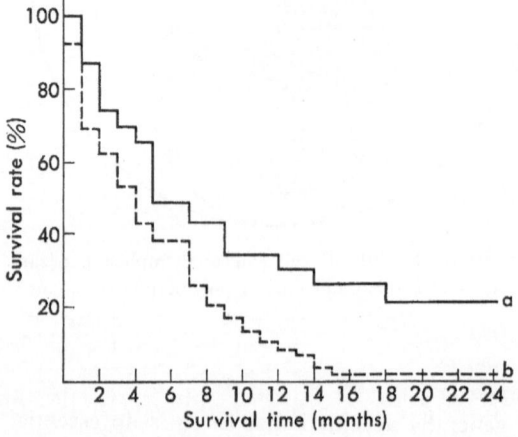

FIG. 8. Survival rates of patients with ATL. a, non-D-Pleo, non-NP ($n=23$); b, D-Pleo+NP ($n=58$). NP, nuclear polymorphism variant.

TABLE IV. Histologic Classification of Relatively Long-lived Patients with ATL

No.	Patients	Survival time (months)	Histologic type	Birthplace	Source[a]
1	H. U.	>48	D-Med, NP	Kyushu	1
2	U. S.	38	D-S	Kyushu	1
3	H. I.	>30	D-Med	Kyushu	2
4	K. N.	30	D-Mix	Kyushu	3
5	K. A.	28	D-L	Kyushu	3
6	J. T.	24	D-Pleo	Shikoku	4
7	S. K.	19	D-Med	Kyushu	3
8	S. O.	16	D-Pleo	Shikoku	4
9	A. H.	15	D-Mix	Kyushu	5
10	T. H.	15	D-Pleo	Kyushu	5
11	S. K.	14	D-Med, NP	Kyushu	3
12	Y. Y.	13	D-L	Kyushu	3
13	T. I·	13	D-Med, NP	Kyushu	3
14	T. Y.	12	D-Pleo	Shikoku	4
15	T. O.	12	D-Pleo	Shikoku	4

[a] 1, Shinko Hospital (Kobe); 2, Kansai Denryoku Hospital (Osaka); 3, Nagasaki University; 4, Uwajima City Hospital; 5, Kagoshima University.

4. Neoplastic cells in the skin and cutaneous lymphoma

ATL cells infiltrated into the subcutaneous tissues, dermis, and epidermis diffusely forming Pautlier's microabscesses. Generally nuclear polymorphism was more remarkable in ATL cells in the skin than in the lymph nodes. Giant cells with dark nuclei were also frequently found. These histologic features in the skin of ATL are similar to those of cutaneous lymphoma. The histologic pattern of lymph nodes in cutaneous lymphoma is diverse; D-Pleo is also observed in cutaneous lymphoma, *i.e.*, mycosis fungoides and Sézary syndrome. The relationship of D-Pleo in histologic entity to ATL and cutaneous lymphoma is shown in Fig. 6.

5. Histologic features and prognoses of patients with ATL

Patients with T cell malignancy other than cutaneous lymphomas had a significantly poorer prognosis than those with B cell malignancies among T_2 cell leukemias, the prognosis of patients with ATL being the worst (Fig. 7). The median survival time of 87 patients was 4.7 months while that of 21 patients with monomorphic T_2 cell leukemia was 10 months, and only 5% of the patients survived for over 2 years (5).

According to histologic features in biopsy ATL lymph nodes, the prognosis of patients with ATL was compared between 58 cases of D-Pleo and D-NP and 20 cases of non-D-NP and non-D-NP. It is clear that the prognosis of the former group was worse than that of the latter (Fig. 8). Sixty-five of the above 78 patients (83.3%) had

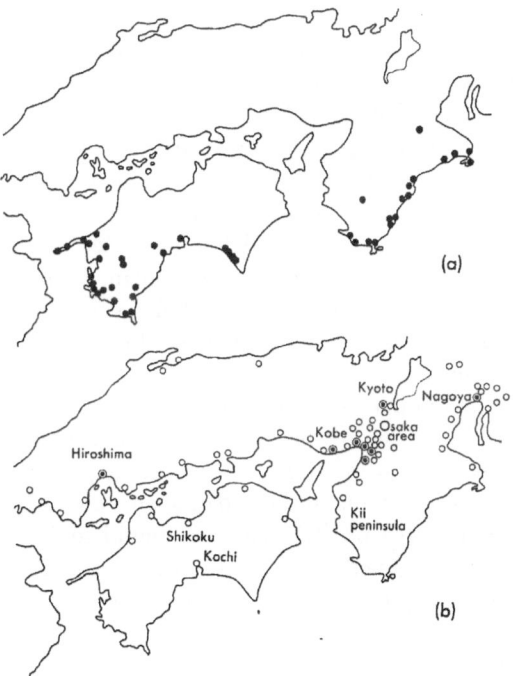

FIG. 9. Birthplaces of patients with ATL observed histologically (a) and cities of more than 100,000 population in western Japan (b), other than Kyushu (area in rectangle of the left). ○ >100,000; ⊙ >500,000.

a rapid clinical course and died within 12 months; all patients with D-Pleo died within 24 months. Histologic classification of biopsy lymph nodes in relatively long-lived patients with ATL are shown in Table IV.

Outline of Geographic Pathology of ATL

Birthplaces of patients with ATL are found in striking clusters in southwestern Japan. In a nationwide survey on T and B cell malignancies in Japan, T cell leukemia/lymphoma accounted for 45% of the total 693 cases, with 70% in the Kyushu area in contrast to 33% in Hokkaido and Honshu combined (5, 19). This high incidence of T cell leukemia/lymphoma in Kyushu was not due to the low incidence of non-T cell leukemia/lymphoma, due to the high incidence of ATL. The patients birthplaces were also found to be clustered in the southern areas of Shikoku and the Kii peninsula, especially in areas adjacent to the Pacific Ocean (Fig. 9). These "endemic areas" of ATL are warm in winter and hot in summer, and except for a few in large cities almost all the birthplaces were located in underpopulated areas (Fig. 9). There were a few patients born in well populated areas in western Japan, such as the Kyoto-Osaka-Kobe area and a zone along the Inland Sea. Some of the birthplaces were also clustered in a small area in Miyagi Prefecture, in the northern part of Japan, but there were no ATL patients born in Sendai, which is one of the largest cities in northern Japan (17).

A global scale survey is required to determine the distribution of ATL in areas other than Japan. At present a few patients with ATL diagnosed cytologically from a blood smear have been found in Taiwan (private communication from Dr. Kazuo Ohta, Aichi Cancer Center). Recently several cases resembling ATL in America have been reported. Palutke et al. investigated three cases of T cell lymphoma of the large cell type with neoplastic cells of irregular, convoluted nucleus (12). These patients had a rapid clinical course; among them, two patients were leukemic. Gaetke et al. reported a 60 year-old patient with acute T cell leukemia (2). The large neoplastic cells showing suppressor activity often had lobulated nuclei, whereas the nuclei of the smaller cells tended to be strikingly convoluted and lymph node biopsy resembled D-Pleo. Pincus et al. also presented four patients with malignant lymphomas of large multinucleated T-cell which were clinically and morphologically distinguishable from the previously described variants of T cell lymphomas (13).

Recently it was found that sera of patients with ATL reacted with cytoplasmic antigen(s), ATL-associated antigen(s) (ATLA), in MT-1 cells of the T cell line from patients with ATL established by Miyoshi et al. (8, 11). Serum anti-ATLA activity was detected in almost all patients with ATL, in most adult patients with T lymphoma, and in a quarter of the healthy adults in the endemic area of ATL (8). The anti-ATLA antibody reacted with retrovirus (ATLV) antigens found in MT-1 cells. In progress are virology studies on ATLV in which human T cell leukemia virus in cultured cells of American patients with T cell malignancy are compared (9, 14, 16). This epidemiological and virology research on ATL or ATLV is expected to contribute to the study of human oncogenesis in the near future.

Acknowledgment

These studies were supported by Grants-in-Aid #201085 and #501011 for Scientific

Research from the Ministry of Education, Science and Culture and Grant-in-Aid #54-29 for Cancer Research from the Ministry of Health and Welfare.

REFERENCES

1. Edelson, P. L. Cutaneous T cell lymphoma: Mycosis fungoides, Sézary syndrome and other variants. *J. Am. Acad. Dermatol.*, **2**, 89–106 (1980).
2. Gaeke, M. E., Verdiman, J. W., Miller, W., Madenica, M., Hopper, J. R., and Rowley, J. D. Human T-cell lymphoma with suppressor effects on the mixed lymphocyte reaction (MLR). I. Morphological and cytological analysis. *Blood*, **56**, 634–641 (1981).
3. Hanaoka, M., Shirakawa, S., Yodoi, J., Uchiyama, T., and Takatsuki, K. Adult T cell leukemia. Histological features of the lymphoid tissues. *In* "Function and Structure of the Immune System," ed. W. Müller-Ruchholts and H. K. Müller-Hermelink, pp. 613–621 (1979). Plenum Press, New York.
4. Hanaoka, M., Sasaki, M., Matsumoto, H., Tankawa, H., Yamabe, H., Tomimoto, K., Tasaka, C., Fujiwara, H., Uchiyama, T., and Takatsuki, K. Adult T cell leukemia. Histopathological classification and characteristics. *Acta Pathol. Jpn.*, **29**, 723–738 (1979).
5. Hanaoka, M. Clinical pathology of adult T cell leukemia. *Acta Haematol. Jpn.*, **44**, 1420–1430 (1981).
6. Hattori, T., Uchiyama, T., Takatsuki, K., and Uchino, H. Effect of adult T cell leukemia cells on pokeweed mitogen-induced normal B cell differentiation. *Clin. Immunol. Immunopathol.*, **17**, 287–295 (1980).
7. Hattori, T., Uchiyama, T., Toibana, T., Takatsuki, K., and Uchino, H. Surface phenotype of Japanese adult T-cell leukemia cells characterized by monoclonal antibodies. *Blood*, **58**, 645–647 (1981).
8. Hinuma, H., Nagata, K., Hanaoka, M., Nakai, M., Matsumoto, T., Kinoshita, K., Shirakawa, S., and Miyoshi, I. Antigen in an adult T-cell leukemia cell line and detection of antibodies to the antigen in human sera. *Proc. Natl. Acad. Sci. U.S.*, **78**, 6476–6480 (1981).
9. Karynarman, V. S., Sarngadharan, M. C., Poiez, B., Ruscetti, F. W., and Gallo, R. C. Immunological properties of a type C retrovirus isolated from cultured human T-lymphoma cell and comparison to other mammalian retrovirus. *J. Virol.*, **38**, 906–915 (1981).
10. Lutzner, M., Edelson, R., Schein, P., Green, I., Kirkpatrick, C., and Ahmed, A. Cutaneous T-cell lymphoma: The Sézary syndrome, mycosis fungoides and related disorders. *Ann. Intern. Med.*, **83**, 534–552 (1975).
11. Miyoshi, I., Kubonishi, I., Sumida, M., Hiraki, S., Tsubota, T., Kimura, I., Miyamoto, K., and Sato, J. A novel T-cell line derived from adult T-cell leukemia. *Gann*, **71**, 155–156 (1980).
12. Paultke, M., Tabazka, P., Weise, R. W., Axelrod, A., Palacas, C., Margolis, H., Khilanani, P., Ratnantharathorn, V., Piligian, J., Pollard, R., and Huseain, M. T-cell lymphomas of large cell type. A variety of malignant lymphomas: Histiocytic and mixed lymphocytic-histiocytic. *Cancer*, **46**, 87–101 (1980).
13. Pincus, G. S., Said, J. W., and Hargreaves, H. Malignant lymphoma, T-cell type. A district morphologic variant with large multilobulated nuclei, with a report of four cases. *Am. J. Clin. Pathol.*, **72**, 540–550 (1979).
14. Poiez, B. J., Ruscetti, F. W., Gazder, A. F., Bunn, P. A., Minna, P. A., and Gallo, E. G. Detection and isolation of type C retrovirus particles from fresh and cultured lymphocytes of patients with cutaneous T-cell lymphoma. *Proc. Natl. Acad. Sci. U.S.*, **77**, 7415–7419 (1980).

15. Reinherz, E. L. and Schlossman, S. F. The differentiation and function of human T lymphocytes. *Cell*, **19**, 821–827 (1980).
16. Reitz, M. S., Poiez, B. J., Ruscetti, F. W., and Gallo, R. C. Characterization and distribution of nucleic acid sequences of a novel type C retrovirus isolated from neoplastic human T lymphocytes. *Proc. Natl. Acad. Sci. U.S.*, **98**, 1887–1891 (1981).
17. Sato, I., Suzuki, T., Tajima, G., Arai, K., Horino, T., Takahashi, K., Sasaki, T., Endo, K., Ishida, S., Saheki, S., Mikami, M., and Yoshinaga, K. Adult T cell leukemia: Comments on the definition from clinical viewpoint. *Clin. Hematol.*, **21**, 1674 (1982) (in Japanese).
18. Suchi, T., Tajima, K., Namba, K., Wakasa, H., Mikata, A., Kikuchi, M., Mori, S., Watanabe, S., Mohori, N., Shamoto, M., Harigaya, K., Itagaki, T., Matsuda, M., Kirino, Y., Takagi, K., and Fukunaga, S. Some problem on the histological diagnosis of non-Hodgkin's malignant lymphoma. A proposal of a new type. *Acta Pathol. Jpn.*, **29**, 755–766 (1979).
19. The T- and B-cell Malignancy Study Group. Statistical analysis of immunologic, clinical and histopathologic data on lymphoid malignancies in Japan. *Jpn. J. Clin. Oncol.*, **11**, 15–38 (1981).
20. Uchiyama, T., Yodoi, J., Sagawa, K., Takatsuki, K., and Uchino, H. Adult T-cell leukemia: Clinical and hematologic features of 16 cases. *Blood*, **50**, 481–492 (1977).
21. Yodoi, J., Takatsuki, K., and Masuda, T. Two cases of T cell chronic lymphocytic leukemia in Japan. *N. Engl. J. Med.*, **290**, 572–573 (1974).

GANN Monograph on Cancer Research 28, 1982

ADULT T CELL LEUKEMIA: PROPOSAL AS A NEW DISEASE AND CYTOGENETIC, PHENOTYPIC, AND FUNCTIONAL STUDIES OF LEUKEMIC CELLS

Kiyoshi Takatsuki,[*1] Takashi Uchiyama,[*2] Yoshimi Ueshima,[*2]
Toshio Hattori,[*2] Toshio Toibana,[*2] Mitsuru Tsudo,[*2]
Yuji Wano,[*2] and Junji Yodoi[*2]

*The Second Department of Internal Medicine, Kumamoto University
Medical School[*1] and The First Division, Department of Internal
Medicine, Faculty of Medicine, Kyoto University[*2]*

Clinical observations in Japanese patients with "adult T-cell leukemia (ATL)" and cytogenetic and functional studies of the leukemic cells of this disease are reported. The pertinence of our descriptions was confirmed. This leukemia is characterized by the clustering of the patients' birthplaces; 22 of 35 patients studied in our laboratory were born in Kyushu, 11 of them in Kagoshima Prefecture. The southern part of Shikoku and the Kii Peninsula were also included in the clustering area. It is noteworthy that seaside areas and small islands appeared to have the highest incidence.

Chromosomally abnormal cells were seen in 14 of the 15 patients. These cells had a modal number of chromosomes in near diploid range in 12 patients, and in near triploid and tetraploid range in the remaining 2 patients, respectively. Eight of the 9 patients analyzed by Q-banding had clonal chromosome abnormalities. The most common abnormality was trisomy no. 7 or 7q, which was seen in 5 cases and has been primarily observed in lymphoid neoplasms. A 14q+ marker chromosome was found in 2 patients and a Dq+ in one patient; loss of a sex chromosome was found in 3 individuals.

We also studied the cell surface phenotype and the function of leukemic cells from 15 patients with ATL using OKT and Tac monoclonal antibodies, which react with differentiation antigens and define functionally distinct T-cell subsets or activated and terminally differentiated T-cells. The phenotypes of ATL cells were determined to be OKT1+, T3+, T4+, T10+, T5−, T8−, although cells from the majority of patients suppressed pokeweed mitogen (PWM)-driven Ig production and cells from all patients lacked helper activity. In addition, after cultivation with PWM, ATL cells from all patients were reactive with anti-Tac antibody.

Human neoplastic lymphoid cells have been studied for their expression of cell surface markers of T and B cells. Figure 1 shows a schematic representation of the

---

[*1] Honjo 1-1-1, Kumamoto 860, Japan (高月　清).

[*2] Kawara-cho, Shogoin, Sakuyo-ku, Kyoto 606, Japan (内山　卓, 上島嘉美, 服部俊夫, 樋端敏生, 通堂　満, 和野雅治, 淀井淳司).

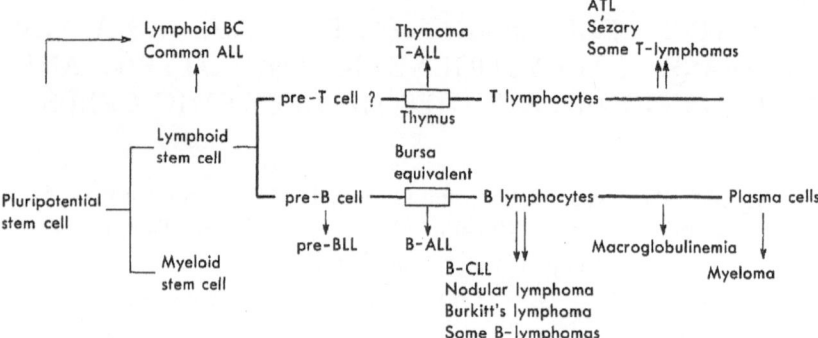

FIG. 1. Scheme of T- and B-cell differentiation and corresponding lymphoid malignancies. ALL, acute lymphocytic leukemia; CLL, chronic lymphocytic leukemia; BC, blastic crisis.

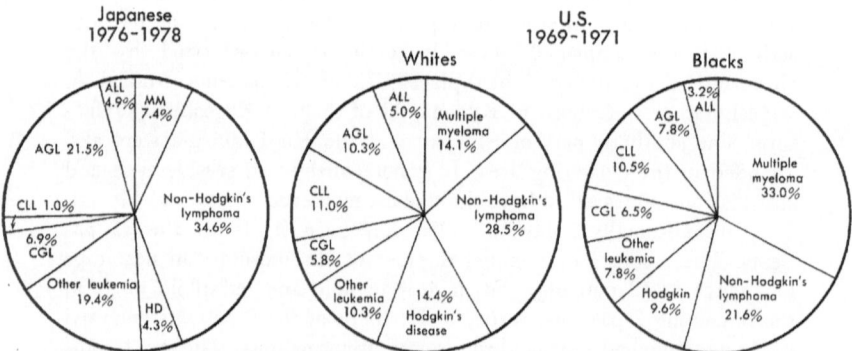

FIG. 2. Relative proportion of hematologic malignancies in the Japanese[1] and in Whites and Blacks in the United States[2]. ALL, acute lymphocytic leukemia; MM, multiple myeloma; AGL, acute granulocytic leukemia; CLL, chronic lymphocytic leukemia; CGL, chronic granulocytic leukemia; HD, Hodgkin's disease. Source: [1] Annual Report of Vital Statistics. Statistics Bureau, Ministry of Health and Welfare. [2] Blattner, W. A. Epidemiology of multiple myeloma and related plasma cell disorders. *In* M. Potter (ed.): "Progress in Myeloma," p. 6 (1980). Elsevier, Amsterdam.

correspondence of various lymphoid malignancies with the developmental stages of lymphoid cells. In adults, lymphocytic leukemias in which neoplastic cells have T-cell markers include Sézary syndrome, chronic lymphocytic leukemia of T-cell origin, and its rare variant, prolymphocytic leukemia with T-cell properties. On the other hand, it has long been noticed that there are considerable racial differences in the incidences of hematologic malignancies (Fig. 2). One of the most striking evidence is that chronic lymphocytic leukemia is an extremely rare disease in Japan. We previously reported a series of patients with "adult T-cell leukemia (ATL)" (*17, 18, 23*). The peculiar geographic distribution of the birthplaces of the patients had led us to consider this leukemia to be a new type of T-cell malignancy. It has been subsequently reported that leukemic T cells from some patients have a marked suppressive effect on pokeweed mitogen (PWM)-induecd normal B-cell differentiation (*19*). The purpose of this paper is to summarize our further clinical observations in patients with this disease and our recent studies on the leukemic cells.

Clinical Study

We studied 35 patients — 18 males and 17 females. The age at the onset of the disease ranged from 27 to 73 years, with a median of 52 years.

The predominant physical findings were peripheral lymph node enlargement (86%), hepatomegaly (77%), splenomegaly (51%), and skin lesions (49%). However, no mediastinal mass was shown in the chest X-ray and neither thymoma nor thymic involvement was demonstrated histologically in autopsied cases.

Regarding skin lesions, one of the characteristic manifestations of this leukemia, histologic examination revealed that dermal and subcutaneous infiltration was common and that epidermal infiltration like a Pautrier microabscess, not seen in the series of patients previously reported, was also found in a few patients.

The survival time ranged from one month to more than 6 years. It was previously stated that the course of this leukemia is subacute or chronic, but most of the patients studied thereafter had a rather acute course. The survival curve is shown in Fig. 3.

Hematologic findings were as already reported. Anemia was relatively mild. The white blood cell count ranged from 9,700 to 499,000. The percentage of leukemic cells in the bone marrow was relatively low compared with that in the other leukemias. Leukemic cells slightly larger than normal small lymphocytes with indented or lobulated nuclei, relatively coarsely clumped nuclear chromatin, and scant cytoplasm were predominant. Small, fairly normal-appearing, mature lymphocytes and larger atypical lymphocytes resembling Sézary cells were also occasionally found in the larger leukemic cells. In a few cases, leukemic cells were fairly uniform in size and almost all cells were the small, normal-appearing mature cells seen in classical chronic lymphocytic leukemia.

Serum immunoglobulin levels were usually within normal limits. In only one case, a small IgG spike and an antinuclear factor were transiently found. Other laboratory findings were as previously reported.

The most striking finding in our study was the clustering of the patients' birthplaces; these are shown in Fig. 4. Japan consists of four major islands — Hokkaido, Honshu, Shikoku, and Kyushu. Most of the patients studied in our laboratory lived

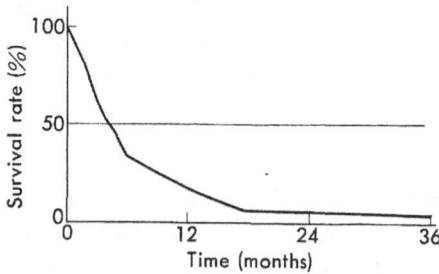

FIG. 3.   Survival rate of patients with ATL (*16*).

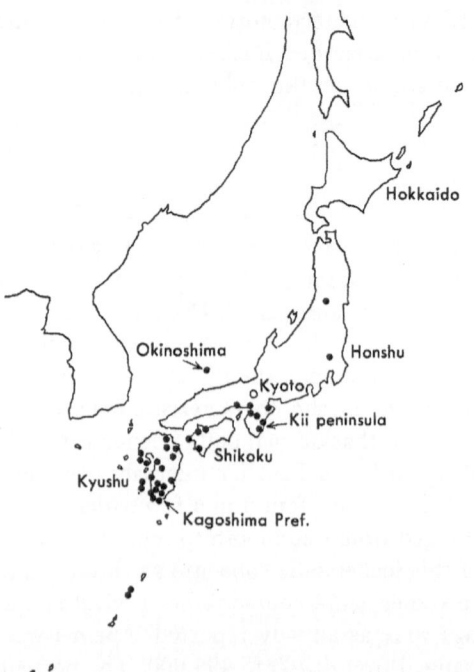

FIG. 4. Birthplaces of patients with ATL (16).

in cities near Kyoto, but, curiously, 22 of the 35 were born in Kyushu, 11 of them in Kagoshima Prefecture. Most of them had grown up in their places of birth and moved later to their present locations. It is true that many people born in Kyushu migrate to Osaka, Kyoto, Kobe, and other big cities. However, the distribution of birthplaces of the patients with ATL is unique, because this is not the case with other patients with lymphoproliferative diseases studied in our laboratory in the same period. Our findings have also been supported by recent reports from other laboratories in Japan, and the southern part of Shikoku and the Kii Peninsula are also included in the clustering area of patients with this disease. More detailed tracing of the patients' birthplaces revealed that they were frequently seaside areas or small islands. It is noteworthy that the patient found in Okinoshima who had typical clinical and hematological features of ATL had two sisters who had died of malignant lymphoma.

Clustering of the patients' birthplaces should not be overlooked in considering the etiology and pathogenesis of this disease. In the early stage of our study, we stated that attempts to elucidate leukemogenesis in this disease should be directed toward exploring the genetic background and possible viral involvement.

Cytogenetic Study

Specific chromosomal abnormalities analogous to those of the Philadelphia chromosome in chronic myeloid leukemia have not been found in any of the lymphocytic leukemias. There are few reports of cytogenetic studies on lymphocytic leukemia in which the surface markers have been studied simultaneously.

TABLE I. Cytogenetic Findings in 15 Patients with ATL (22)

Case	Source/ days in culture	Rearranged cells/total metaphases analyzed	Modal chromo- some No.	Band- ing	Modal karyotype
1	PB/1	25/25	46	Q	46, X, −Y(?), −1, 1p+, del(9)(q32), 12p+, 14q+, +2 markers
2	PB/2, 3, 4	6/11	48		48, XY, −B, +3 markers
3	PB/1	4/4	45	Q	45, XX, −1, 2q+, 14q+
	BM	0/6	46		46, XX
4	PB/1	31/31	48, 49	Q	49, XX, +7, +8, +12, 8q+, 8p+, del(10)(q23), 21q+/49, XX, +8, +12, +del(7)(p13), 8q+, 8p+, 10q−, 21q+
5	PB/1, 4	3/6	46, 47		47, XY, +marker/46, XY
6	PB/1	3/3	91		86−91
	BM	0/4	46		46, XY
7	PB/1, 4	6/6	48		48, XX, +2 markers
8	PB/1, 3	0/0			
	LN/1	7/9	48		48, XY, −B, Dq+, +3 markers
9	PB/1, 5	16/18	48	Q	48, XX, +3, −6, +7, del(10)(p13&q24), 10q+, +marker
	PHA/4	0/29	46	Q	46, XX
10	PB/1, 5	77/85	45, 46	Q	45, X, −X, −4, +t(4 ; 7)(4qter → 4p 16 : : 7q11 → 7qter)/ 46, XX/45, X, −X, −4, +t(4 ; 7)(4qter → 4p 16 : : 7q11 → 7qter), 15q+
	PHA/4	1/28	46	Q	46, XX/45, X, −X, 4p+
11	PB/1, 3	33/33	73	Q	73, XX, −Y, +1, +1, +2, +3, −6, +7, +8, +8, +11, +12, +13, +13, −16, +17, +17, +18, +19, +19, +19, +20, +22, +12p+, +9 markers
	PHA/3	0/6	46	Q	46, XY
12	PB/1, 3	51/51	47	Q	47, X, −Y, −4, +7, del(1)(q32), i(18q), 21q+, i(22q), +2 markers
	PHA/3	28/28	47	Q	47, X, −Y, −4, +7, del(1)(q32), i(18q), 21q+, i(22q), +2 markers
13	PB/1, 3	54/54	46	Q	46, XY, −10, −13, 5p+, +t(10 ; 13)(10qter → 10p 13 : : 13q32 → 13q11)21p+, +minute
	PHA/3	22/22	46	Q	46, XY, −10, −13, 5p+, +t(10 ; 13)(10qter → 10p 13 : : 13q32 → 13q11)21p+, +minute
14	PB/2, 4	0/0			
	PHA/4	17/17	48	Q	48, XX, +2 markers
15	PB/1, 3	0/0			
	PHA/3	0/40	46	Q	46, XX

PB, peripheral blood ; BM, bone marrow ; LN, lymph node ; PHA, PHA-stimulated peripheral blood.

We studied 24 patients with ATL (22). Specimens were obtained from peripheral blood, bone marrow, and lymph node. Peripheral blood mononuclear cells were separated by Ficoll-sodium metrizoate gradient centrifugation and examined after a short-term culture (24–120 hr) without phytohemagglutinin (PHA). In 10 patients, 3–4-day cultures with PHA were also prepared. Chromosome preparations were made by a slightly modified method of Moorhead et al. (7). Bone marrow was examined without prior culturing. Lymph node biopsy specimen was minced and examined after 1 day of culture. Suitable Giemsa-stained metaphases were photographed through an ordinary microscope and Q-banded metaphases through a Zeiss fluorescence microscope. In some cases (cases 1, 3, and 9), Giemsa-stained slides were restained with quinacrine mustard more than a year after the original staining. Karyotypes were arranged according to the Paris Conference (8).

Cytogenetic findings are summarized in Table I. Mitotic cells were obtained from 15 patients. 1 · of whom had chromosomally abnormal cells. The 15th patient had a normal karyotype (case 15) and was studied successfully only in a PHA culture of peripheral blood. Abnormal karyotypes were noted in cultures of unstimulated peripheral blood from 12 patients and in the lymph node of 1 patient (case 8); in 1 patient (case 14) without spontaneous mitotic cells there were abnormal mitotic cells only in PHA-stimulated peripheral blood culture. Bone marrow cells from 2 patients (cases 3 and 6) and PHA-stimulated peripheral blood culture from 3 patients (cases 9, 10, and 11) were fairly normal, whereas they had abnormal chromosomes in the unstimulated culture. Two patients (cases 12 and 13) had a similar percentage of metaphases, with abnormal chromosomes in both types of culture.

The modal chromosome number was hyperdiploid in 7 patients, pseudodiploid in 3, hyperdiploid in 2, and near triploid or tetraploid in 2.

Chromosomes from 10 patients were examined with Q-banding. One of these patients (case 15) had a normal karyotype and another (case 3) had too few mitotic cells to be analyzed. The other 8 patients had a clonal chromosome abnormality that involved most of the chromosomes. Chromosomes Nos. 11 and 20. however, were not involved in these 10 cases.

The most common single abnormality was the gain of a no. 7 chromosome, which was noted in 4 patients (cases 4, 9, 11, and 12), and a gain of 7q in one (case 10). These patients showed no other common chromosome alterations. One patient (case 9) had trisomy 3 and another (case 4) had trisomy 12 in addition to trisomy 7. The extra 7q in case 10 was translocated to the distal short arm of No. 4. This patient had the simplest karyotype in this series (45X, -X, 40+), but the other 2 cells among the 85 cells had 15q+ in addition to the original karyotype, which could be the result of karyotypic evolution.

A 14q+ marker chromosome was found in 2 patients (cases 1 and 3). Lymph node

TABLE II.   Surface Phenotype and Functional Activities of ATL Cells

Case		OKT monoclonals									la1	Tac	Function *in vitro*	
		1	3	4	5	6	8	9	10	11			Helper	Suppressor
1	32 F	+	+	+	−	−	−		+	+	−	−	−	+
2	49 M	+	+	+	−	−	−		+	+	−	+	−	−
3	31 F	+	+	+	−	−	−		+	+	−	+	−	+
4	61 M	+	+	+	−	−	−		+	−	−	+		
5	69 M	−	+	+	−	−	−		−	+	−	+		
6	70 M	+	−	+	−	−	−	+	+	+	−	+	−	−
7	55 M	+	+	+	−	−	−	−	+	+	−	+	−	−
8	65 F	+	+	+	−	−	−	+	+	+	+	+	−	+
9	55 M	+	+	+	−	−	−	−	+	+	−	−	−	+
10	46 F	+	+	+	−	−	−	−	+	+	−	+	−	+
11	41 F	+	+	+	−	− ·	−	+	+	+	+	+	−	+
12	46 M	−	−	+	−	−	−	−	+	+	−	−		
13	44 F	+	+	+	−	−	−	−	+	+	−	+		
14	60 F	+	+	+	−	−	−	−		+	+	+		
15	62 F	−	+	+	−	−	−	−		+	−	+		

cells in another patient (case 8) had a Dq+ marker, which was not examined with banding. Clinical findings of patients with trisomy 7 or 14q+ varied, yet were much the same as in patients without the abnormalities.

Our results showed a high frequency of patients with chromosomal anomalies in Japanese ATL. Although the karyotypic changes appeared to be variable, some recurring changes were noted in our series (Table II). Trisomy 7, or at least 7q, which was found in 5 of 9 banded cases, was the most frequent abnormality in our series. A 14q+ marker chromosome, perhaps the most significant marker in lymphoid malignancies (1, 5, 14, 15), was found in 2 patients (cases 1 and 3). In 2 cases of ATL including one cell line (6), a 14q+ was reported to be the result of 14q32 translocation with 12q and Yq. In our study, the fluorescent pattern of two 14q+ markers showed them to have different sizes, suggesting that they did not originate from these translocations, however, the details could not be determined because of the complex karyotypes. Thus, various chromosomes may participate in the formation of a 14q+ marker in ATL.

Leukemic T cells obtained from the patients with ATL were generally not stimulated by PHA, and sometimes only normal residual T cells were stimulated by it. However, in one patient (case 14), dividing cells with an abnormal karyotype were observed only in the PHA-stimulated culture. The dividing cells in this case may be PHA-associated leukemic T cells. Normal chromosomes in the bone marrow of 2 patients may relate to the slight infiltration of leukemic cells into the bone marrow in these patients.

Surface Marker and Functional Study

We studied the surface phenotype and the functional activities of leukemic cells from 15 patients with Japanese ATL (2). Normal peripheral blood lymphocytes (PBL) and ATL cells were separated by Ficoll-sodium metrizoate density gradient centrifugation. The viability of cells were counted by the trypan blue dye exclusion test. PBL were then separated into T and B cells by a neuraminidase-treated sheep red blood cell rosette method. One million PBL, normal T cells, B cells, or ATL cells were cultured separately in the presence or absence of PWM in RPMI 1640 medium supplemented with 10% fetal calf serum. The suppressor activity of ATL cells was examined by the addition of ATL cells (0.5, 1, 2×10^6) to 10^6 PBL. The helper activity of ATL cells was examined by the addition of ATL cells (0.1, 0.5×10^6) to 10^6 of purified normal B cells. In all experiments, cell densities were adjusted to 10^6/ml and the concentration of PWM was 10 μl/ml. Following 7 days of culture in a humid atmosphere at 37° under 5% CO_2, cells were harvested and the viabilities and cell numbers were counted. The relative proportions of cytoplasmic-immunoglobulin (CIg) positive cells among the intact cells were counted by direct immunofluorescence methods, using fluorescein (FITC) conjugated rabbit F(ab')$_2$ anti-human Ig under a Zeiss ultraviolet microscope.

In addition, ATL cells were cultured for 4 or 7 days in the presence of PWM, and these cells were used for the analysis of surface phenotype.

A panel of OK monoclonal antibodies was obtained from Drs. Patrick Kung and Gideon Goldstein. The preparation and specificity of this panel has been amply documented (3, 4, 7, 9, 10–12), OKT1 and OKT3 react with mature thymocytes and

TABLE III.   Tac and Ia Antigens on ATL Cells

Case	Tac (%)		Ia (%)	
	Fresh	After culture	Fresh	After culture
1	<1	72	3	50
2	52	54	9	<1
3	15	78	3	4
7	17	83	2	19
9	6	51		
10	32	84	3	25
11	60	95	56	75
14	30	66	59	27
15	50	78	6	72

all circulating T cells. OKT4 and OKT5/8 react with both thymocytes and with 60% and 30% of the peripheral T cells, respectively. OKT6 reacts with a majority of immature thymocytes, whereas OKT10 reacts with all immature thymocytes, some peripheral T cells, and null cells. OKIal is known to be specific for human Ia-like antigens (13). Anti-Tac monoclonal antibody reacts with activated and functionally mature T cells, including concanavalin-A-induced suppressor T cells, PWM-activated radioresistant helper T cells, PWM-activated radiosensitive suppressor T cells, and cytotoxic killer cells against allogenic cells, but no reactivity was noted with normal resting T cells, B cells, or EB-virus-transformed B cells (20, 21).

Cell surface antigens were detected by indirect immunofluorescence methods, using FITC-conjugated goat F(ab')$_2$ anti-mouse IgG (Cappel Lab., Cochranville, Pa.) as a second antibody. As a control, normal mouse IgG separated by DEAE cellulose chromatography from pooled mouse sera was used. All reagents were diluted by phosphate-buffered saline (pH 7.6, 0.15 M), supplemented with 1 mg/ml of bovine serum albumin (BSA) (Armour Pharmaceutical Co., Phoenix, Ariz.) and 0.1% sodium azide. The optimal dose of each reagent was carefully assessed, using normal peripheral blood T cells, PWM-stimulated T cells, Molt 4F, and EB-virus-transformed cell line from a normal person. Half a million ATL cells were treated with 20 liters of monoclonal antibodies (1:40 dilution for the panel of OK monoclonal antibodies; 1:5 dilution for anti-Tac monoclonal antibody containing culture supernatants) or mouse IgG (25 g/ml, E1 cm/1%=14.0 at 280 nm) for 30 min on ice. Cells were then washed twice with Hanks' balanced salt solution (Nissui, Tokyo) containing 1 mg/ml of BSA and 0.1% sodium azide. After labeling with 20 liters of a second antibody (1:20 dilution) for 30 min on ice, the percentage of reactive cells in at least 200 lymphocytes was determined under phase and fluorescent illumination as described above.

The results are summarized in Tables II and III. The phenotype of ATL cells was determined to be OKT1+, T3+, T4+, T10+, T5−, T8−, OKIal−/+, although cells from patients suppressed PWM induced normal B-cell differentiation, and cells from patients lacked helper activity in this system. In addition, after cultivation with PWM, ATL cells from all patients tested were reactive with anti-Tac monoclonal antibody. These findings suggest that ATL cells arise from peripheral mature T-cell subsets and also suggest that the transition of the surface phenotype of ATL cells to functionally mature and activated T cells occurs in culture.

Acknowledgments

We are grateful to doctors who referred patients for these immunological studies and to Dr. S. Fukuhara for instruction in the cytogenetic study.

This work was supported by a Grant-in-Aid for Cancer Research from the Ministry of Health and Welfare, and partly by grants from the Princess Takamatsu Cancer Research Fund and from the Asahi Press.

REFERENCES

1. Fukuhara, S., Shirakawa, S., and Uchino, H. Specific marker chromosome 14 in malignant lymphomas. *Nature*, **259**, 210–211 (1976).
2. Hattori, T., Uchiyama, T., Toibana, T., Takatsuki, K., and Uchino, H. Surface phenotype of Japanese adult T-cell leukemia cells characterized by monoclonal antibodies. *Blood*, **58**, 645–647 (1981).
3. Kung, P. C., Goldstein, G., Reinherz, E. L., and Scholssman, S. F. Monoclonal antibodies defining distinctive human T cell surface antigens. *Science*, **206**, 347–349 (1979).
4. Kung, P. C. and Goldstein, G. Functional developmental compartments of human T lymphocytes. *Vox. Sang.*, **39**, 121–127 (1980).
5. Manolov, G. and Manolova, Y. Marker band in one chromosome 14 from Burkitt lymphomas. *Nature*, **237**, 33–34 (1972).
6. Miyoshi, I., Sumita, M., Sano, K., Nishihara, R., Miyamoto, K., and Sato, J. Marker chromosome 14q+ in adult T-cell leukemia. *N. Engl. J. Med.*, **300**, 921 (1979).
7. Moorhead, P. S., Nowell, P. C., Mellman, W. J., Battips, D. M., and Hungerford, D. A. Chromosome preparations of leukocytes cultured from human peripheral blood. *Exp. Cell. Res.*, **20**, 613–616 (1960).
8. Paris Conference. Standardization in human chromosomes. *Birth. Defects*, **8** (1972).
9. Reinherz, E. L., Kung, P. C., Goldstein, G., and Schlossman, S. F. A monoclonal antibody with selectivity reactivity with functionally mature human thymocytes and all peripheral human T cells. *J. Immunol.*, **123**, 1312–1317 (1979).
10. Reinherz, E. L., Kung, P. C., Goldstein, G., and Schlossman, S. F. Separation of functional subsets of human T cells by a monoclonal antibody. *Proc. Natl. Acad. Sci. U. S.*, **76**, 4061–4065 (1979).
11. Reinherz, E. L., Kung, P. C., Goldstein, G., and Schlossman, S. F. A monoclonal antibody reacting with human cytotoxic/suppressor T cell subset previously defined by a heteroantiserum termed TH_2. *J. Immunol.*, **124**, 1301–1307 (1980).
12. Reinherz, E. L., Kung, P. C., Goldstein, G., Levy, R. H., and Schlossman, S. F. Discrete stages of human intrathymic differentiation: Analysis of normal thymocytes and leukemic lymphoblasts of T-cell lineage. *Proc. Natl. Acad. Sci. U. S.*, **77**, 1588–1592 (1980).
13. Reinherz, E. L., Kung, P. C., Pesando, J. M., Ritz, J., Goldstein, G., and Schlossman, S. F. Ia determinants on human T-cell subsets defined by monoclonal antibody. Activation stimuli required for expression. *J. Exp. Med.*, **150**, 1472–1482 (1979).
14. Rowley, J. D. Chromosomes in leukemia and lymphoma. *Semin. Hematol.*, **15**, 301–319 (1978).
15. Rowley, J. D. and Fukuhara, S. Chromosome studies in non-Hodgkin lymphomas. *Semin. Oncol.*, **7**, 255–266 (1980).
16. Takatsuki, K., Uchiyama, T., Ueshima, Y., and Hattori, T. Adult T-cell leukemia: Further clinical observations and cytogenetic and functional studies of leukemia cells. *Jpn. J. Clin. Oncol.*, **9** (Suppl.), 317–323 (1979).

17. Takatsuki, K., Uchiyama, T., Sagawa, K., and Yodoi, J. Adult T cell leukemia in Japan. *In* "Topics in Hematology," ed. S. Seno, F. Takaku, and S. Irino, pp. 73–77 (1977). Excerpta Medica, Amsterdam.
18. Uchiyama, T., Yodoi, J., Sagawa, K., Takatsuki, K., and Uchino, H. Adult T-cell leukemia: Clinical and hematologic features of 16 cases. *Blood*, **50**, 481–492 (1977).
19. Uchiyama, T., Sagawa, K., Takatsuki, K., and Uchino, H. Effect of adult T-cell leukemia cells on pokeweed mitogen-induced normal B-cell differentiation. *Clin. Immunol. Immunopathol.* **10**, 24–34 (1978).
20. Uchiyama, T., Broder, S., and Waldmann, T. A. A monoclonal antibody (Tac) reactive with activated and functionally mature T cells. 1. Production of anti-Tac monoclonal antibody and distribution of Tac (+) cells. *J. Immunol.*, **126**, 1393–1397 (1981).
21. Uchiyama, T., Nelson, D. L., Fleisher, T. A., and Waldmann, T. A. A monoclonal antibody (Tac) reactive with activated and functionally mature T cells. II. Expression of Tac antigen on cytotoxic killer T cells, suppressor cells and one of two types of helper T cells. *J. Immunol.*, **126**, 1398–1408 (1981).
22. Ueshima, Y., Fukuhara, S., Hattori, T., Uchiyama, T., Takatsuki, K., and Uchino, H. Chromosome studies in adult T-cell leukemia in Japan: Significance of trisomy 7. *Blood*, **58**, 420–425 (1981).
23. Yodoi, J., Takatsuki, K., and Masuda, T. Two cases of T-cell chronic lymphocytic leukemia in Japan. *N. Engl. J. Med.*, **290**, 572–573 (1974).

CELLULAR ORIGIN OF T CELL MALIGNANCIES

Masanori Shimoyama, Kensei Tobinai, Masao Hirose,
and Keisuke Minato

*Departments of Clinical Laboratory and Internal Medicine,
National Cancer Center Hospital**

Cell surface antigens of the tumor cells of 55 patients with T-cell malignancies were analyzed with 11 monoclonal antibodies, and their cellular origins were determined according to the expression of differentiation antigens.

They were divided into four major categories: 1) pre-T cell type; 2) thymic T-cell type; 3) inducer/helper T-cell type; 4) suppressor/cytotoxic T-cell type. Two cases of acute lymphoblastic leukemia (ALL) were of the pre-T cell type. Thymic T-cell type is further divided into early thymocyte type, common (cortical) thymocyte type, and mature (medullary) thymocyte type, but we did not see the mature thymocyte type in this series. Three cases of T-ALL and five of T-lymphoblastic lymphoma were of the early thymocyte type. Only one case of T-ALL was of the common thymocyte type. Of the inducer/helper T-cell type, there were 16 cases of adult T-cell leukemia (ATL) or adult T-cell leukemia-lymphoma (ATLL), eight of adult T-cell lymphoma (three of medium sized T-cell lymphoma, four of pleomorphic T-cell lymphoma, and one of large cell type T-cell lymphoma), two of T-chronic lymphocytic leukemia and two of mycosis fungoides. These results indicate that inducer/helper T-cell malignancies are still heterogeneous. On the other hand, the tumor cells of five patients with immunoblastic lymphadenopathy (IBL)-like T-cell lymphoma, one with Lennert's lymphoma and three with the mixed cell type T-cell lymphoma expressed the suppressor/cytotoxic T-cell phenotype. T-cell lymphomas of adult patients with suppressor/cytotoxic T-cell phenotype are probably the same disease. This is a new disease entity which is different from ATLL or adult T-cell lymphoma with inducer/helper T-cell phenotypeand has the following common characteristics: polyclonal hypergammaglobulinemia, no endemic distribution of patients' birthpalce, male predominance, poor prognosis, mixed cell type morphology with angioimmunoblastic and granulomatous lesions, and the same immunologic phenotype of tumor cells as suppressor/cytotoxic T-cell. The cellular origin of two cases of ATL or ATLL, five of adult T-cell lymphoma and one of mycosis fungoides could not be determined in the subset level, although they had peripheral T-cell phenotype.

The development of immunological techniques identifying human T and B lymphocytes have provided the tools to delineate the cellular origin of leukemia and lym-

---

* Tsukiji 5-1-1, Chuo-ku, Tokyo 104, Japan（下山正徳, 飛内賢正, 広瀬政雄, 湊　啓輔).

TABLE I. Reaction Specificity of Monoclonal Antibodies

Monoclonal antibodies	Immunogens[a]	Specificity	Reference	Source
OKT3	E[+] T-cell	Peripheral T-cell	Kung et al., 1979 (15)	Ortho Pharmaceutical Co. (Raritan, New Jersey)
		Mature thymocyte	Reinherz et al., 1979 (22)	
OKT4	E[+] T-cell	Inducer/helper T-cell	Reinherz et al., 1979 (19)	″
OKT6	Thymocyte	Cortical thymocyte	Bhan et al., 1980 (3)	″
OKT8	Thymocyte	Suppressor/cytotoxic T-cell	Reinherz et al., 1980 (18)	″
10.2 (anti-HuLyt-2)	E[+] T-cell	Pan T-cell	Martin et al., 1980 (16)	New England Nuclear (Boston, Massachusetts)
9.6 (anti-HuLyt-3)	PBL	E-rosette receptor	Kamoun et al., 1981 (12)	″
OKI1	E[+] T-cell	Ia-like antigen	Reinherz et al., 1979 (20)	Ortho Pharmaceutical Co.
anti-B1	Burkitt's lymphoma	B-cell specific	Stashenko et al., 1980 (27)	Sidney Farber Cancer Institute (Boston, Massachusetts)
J5	Common ALL	Common ALL specific	Ritz et al., 1980 (23)	″
OKM1	E[+] T-cell	Monocyte, granulocyte, Tγ-cell	Breard et al., 1980 (6)	Ortho Pharmaceutical Co.
anti-Mo1	Adherent PBMNC	Monocyte, granulocyte, Tγ-cell	Todd et al., 1981 (33)	Sidney Farber Cancer Institute

[a] E[+], positive rosette forming capacity with sheep erythrocytes; PBL, peripheral blood lymphocytes; PBMNC, peripheral blood mononuclear cells.

phoma (1, 4, 24). The introduction of monoclonal antibodies against normal differentiation and leukemia associated antigens in this field is likely to have made it possible to demonstrate that the lymphoid malignancies reflect the same degree of heterogeneity and maturation as is seen in normal T and B cell ontogeny (5, 7–9, 14, 17, 18, 24, 32). In this study, cell surface antigens of human T-cell malignancies were analyzed by means of 11 monoclonal antibodies whose reaction specificity we had confirmed using cultured cell lines derived from various human hemopoietic tumor cells (31). Their cellular origins were determined according to the expression of differentiation antigens. In the present study, tumor cells from 55 patients with T-cell malignancy have been analyzed with monoclonal antibodies at the National Cancer Center Hospital since December 1980. The reaction specificity and source of the 11 monoclonal antibodies used in this study are listed in Table I. The appropriate concentration of each was determined by using cultured cell lines and normal peripheral blood mononuclear cells as described previously (31, 32).

As for the morphological diagnosis, acute leukemia was diagnosed on the basis of the French-American-British co-operative Group (FAB)-classification (2) by means of May-Grünwald-Giemsa staining and peroxidase staining. Non-Hodgkin's lymphomas were diagnosed based on The Japanese Lymphoma Study Group (LSG)- classification (29). Special forms of lymphoid malignancies such as adult T-cell leukemia (ATL) (34) or adult T-cell leukemia-lymphoma (ATLL) (25), immunoblastic lymphadenopathy (IBL)-like T-cell lymphoma (26), Lennert's lymphoma (13), and mycosis fungoides

(25) were diagnosed on the basis of previously published hematological and clinical criteria.

T-cell Malignancies with Pre-T Cell or Thymic T-cell Phenotype

The reactivity of the tumor cells of six patients with T-acute lymphoblastic leukemia (T-ALL) and five with T-lymphoblastic lymphoma against monoclonal antibodies is shown in Table II. Tumor cell of two patients with ALL (Case Nos. 1, 2)

TABLE II. Reactivity of the Tumor Cells of T-ALL and T-lymphoblastic Lymphoma with Monoclonal Antibodies

| | Differentiation stage | | | | | | | | | | |
| | Pre-T (T_0) (C/T hybrid) | | Early thymocyte (T_1) | | | | | | | | Common thymocyte (T_1) |
Case No.	1 S. K.	2 A. T.	3 T. H.	4 H. N.	5 O. Y.	6 T. A.	7 K. H.	8 H. H.	9 B. O.	10 O. S.	11 O. M.
Age	15	5	36	79	19	7	35	30	31	33	39
Sex[a]	M	M	F	F	M	F	F	M	M	M	M
Diagnosis	C/T-ALL		T-ALL			T-lymphoblastic lymphoma					T-ALL
Specimen[b]	BM	PB	BM	BM	PB	BM	LN	LN	LN	LN	BM
Lymphoid cells (%)	96	78	98	80	90	82	82	92	90	94	80
Tumor cells (%)	90	52	95	75	88	80	76	90	90	84	70
OKT3 (%)	1	38	2	3	3	1	11	12	14	15	12
OKT4 (%)	0	18	3	0	1	0	6	17	10	9	77[e]
OKT6 (%)	0	0	0	0	0	0	0	4	8	0	69
OKT8 (%)	2	14	0	1	2	1	4	9	6	11	71
10.2 (%)	2	67	68	77	29	82	19	28	16	20	76
9.6 (%)	96	39	0	4	90	3	80	22	26	13	72
ERFC (%)	68	26	2	4	54	0	26	31	32	9	54
OKI1 (%)	69	16	22	3	0	1	—[f]	22	9	5	8
α-B1 (%)	0	7	0	0	0			6	4	12	4
J5 (%)	50	42	0	0	0		0	0	0	0	0
OKM1 (%)	0	3	0	4	2	0		7	4	0	3
α-Mo1	0	0		6	0			0		0	
S-Ig[c] (%) γ	2	11	1	8	8	0	1	12	7	9	18
α	0	7	0	1	0	0	0	5	5	3	2
μ	0	2	0	0	0	0	1	3	3	4	1
δ	0	1	4	0	0	0	0	9	6	9	2
κ	2	5	0	0					9		10
λ	0	8	4	2					6		5
C-Ig[d] (μ)	—	—	—	—	—	—	—	—	—	—	—

[a] M, male; F, female.
[b] BM, bone marrow; PB, peripheral blood; LN, lymph node.
[c] S-Ig, surface immunoglobulins.
[d] C-Ig, cytoplasmic immunoglobulins.
[e] Italic figures indicate cells judged to have positive reactivity.
[f] — indicates negative result by heteroantisera against Ia-like antigen.

not only reacted with J5, but also expressed a definitive T-cell nature, either pan-T cell antigen (10.2-reactive) or rosette-forming capacity with sheep erythrocytes (ERFC). Therefore, these two cases are judged to belong to the C/T hybrid type, which was defined in the study for cultured cell lines (31). The tumor cells of one of the two patients with ALL also reacted with OKI1 (reactive with Ia-like antigen).

The tumor cells of three patients with ALL and five with lymphoblastic lymphoma (Case Nos. 3–10) expressed a definitive T-cell nature (10.2, 9.6 and/or ERFC), but reacted with neither J5 (reactive with cALL antigen) nor OKT-series monoclonal antibodies. According to the differentiation schemas of T-cells proposed by Reinherz et al. (18) and Tobinai et al. (31), these eight cases are judged to belong to the early thymocyte type.

The tumor cells of one patient with ALL (Case No. 11) reacted with OKT4, OKT6, and OKT8, in addition to showing positive reactivity with 10.2, 9.6, and ERFC. This surface phenotype is the same as that of normal common (cortical) thy-

TABLE III. Reactivity of the Tumor Cells of

Differentiation stage								19		20	21	
Case No.	12	13	14	15	16	17	18	19 M. M.		20 K. H.	21 Y. Y.	
	N. H.	T. T.	Y. K.	A. I.	I. I.	T. C.	A. K.					
Age	48	55	38	54	58	62	73	56		46	42	
Sex	F	F	M	M	M	F	M	M		F	M	
Diagnosis Histology[a]								Med			Med	
Specimen[b]	PB	PB	PB	PB	PB	PB	PB	PB	LN	PB	PB	LN
Lymphoid cells (%)	90	77	60	85	90	85	90	94	92	94	90	96
Tumor cells (%)	62	60	30	66	34	68	90	92	88	90	88	82
OKT3 (%)	53	56	11	46	20	0	53	81	78	92	63	58
OKT4 (%)	62	44	30	64	13	15	91	91	88	16	40	46
OKT6 (%)	0	0	0	0	0	0	0	0	0	0	0	0
OKT8 (%)	9	9	2	10	14	1	4	15	18	6	16	20
10.2 (%)							89	93	91	90	83	54
9.6 (%)							90	90	90	66		67
ERFC (%)	57	58	33	32	48	42	71	87	78	88	71	56
OKI1 (%)	—	—	—	—	—	—	3	9	8	11	9	24
α-B1 (%)							1	0	9	0	8	21
J5 (%)							0	0	0	0		0
OKM1 (%)								0	0	0		0
α-Mo1 (%)								11	2			
S-Ig (%) γ	5	1	10	32	6	28	6	9	6	10	18	19
α	1	2	2	5	3	1		0	16	1		4
μ	0	2	1	18	5	1		6	2	0		14
δ	2	4	1	4	5	1		2	10	2		9
κ								18	12	2		21
λ								8	6	1		9
C-Ig (μ)	—	—	—	—	—	—	—	—	—	—	—	—

[a] Med, medium-sized cell type; Mix, mixed type; Pleo, pleomorphic type.
[b] LN, lymph node at onset; PB, peripheral blood at relapse; LN, lymph node at relapse.

mocytes, as reported by Reinherz *et al.* (*18*). Therefore, this case is judged to belong to the common thymocyte type.

T-cell Malignancies with Inducer/Helper T-cell Phenotype

The reactivity of the tumor cells of 18 patients with ATL or ATLL, 13 with adult T-cell lymphoma (four with medium-sized T-cell lymphoma, six with pleomorphic T-cell lymphoma, three with large cell type T-cell lymphoma), two with T-chronic lymphocytic leukemia (T-CLL), and three with mycosis fungoides is shown in Tables III and IV. Tumor cells from 16 out of the 18 ATL patients had ERFC, but those from two ATL patients (Case Nos. 27, 29) did not have ERFC, and one of them (Case No. 29) did not react with 10.2 and 9.6. All other ATL patients who were examined for reactivity with 10.2 and 9.6 reacted with these antibodies. No tumor cells from any of the 18 patients with ATL reacted with OKT6 and OKT8. Tumor cells from most

ATL or ATLL with Monoclonal Antibodies

Inducer/helper T-cell

22	23		24	25		26			27	28		29	
K. S.	T. M.		O. S.	T. U.		S. A.			A. S.	T. A.		S. K.	
62	53		65	43		34			33	31			
M	F		F	F		M			F	F		M	
ATL or ATLL													
		Mix	Pleo		Med	Pleo		Pleo			Pleo		Pleo
PB	PB	LN	LN	PB	LN	LN	PB	LN	PB	PB	LN	PB	LN
98	96	89	88	98	96	94	96	94	88	98	96	96	98
96	95	80	80	80	80	90	94	90	72	81	90	96	78
88	29	42	21	78	68	72	86	71	52	78	84	28	13
54	91	86	78	80	56	26	82	66	38	82	92	4	4
0	0	0	8	0	0	0	0	0		0	0	0	0
0	4	9	11	15	28	8	3	6	8	14	13	3	9
90	82	85	76	66	76	88	83	88	56	81	85	8	10
94	89	79	81	76	74	86	91	56		13	91	10	13
84	58	45	22	44	43	73	61	17	9	65	79	9	12
62	85	57	47	46	53	52	32	85	14	0	8	44	62
0	0	4	26	16	33	0	0	7		0	0	0	0
0	0	0	7	0	3	2	3	0		0	0	0	0
	0	2	17	4	8	0	9	0			0	0	0
3	4	12	20	14	21	3	7	11	7	8	6	4	2
0	3	2	5	2	6	5	2	5		1	0	0	3
0	1	3	16	1	16	4	1	5		0	0	0	0
4	4	6	12	1	19	9	1	3		0	0	3	0
1	5	13	12	3	22	6	5.	10		5	2	1	5
2	2	5	13	0	12	7	0	4		0	0	2	0
—	—	—	—	—	—	—	—	—		—	—	—	—

Other abbreviations are the same as in Table II.

M. SHIMOYAMA ET AL.

Table IV. Reactivity of the Tumor Cells of Adult T-cell Lymphoma,

Differentiation stage							
Case No.	30 T. S.	31 Y. K.	32 O. T.	33 A. A.	34 H. K.	35 S. Y.	36 T. K.
Age	34	50	78		51	77	35
Sex	M	F	F	M	M	F	M
Diagnosis							Adult T-cell
Histology	Med	Med	Med	Med	Pleo	Pleo	Pleo
Specimen	LN	LN	LN	PB	LN	LN	LN
Lymphoid cells (%)	70	95	94	98	92	90	91
Tumor cells (%)	66	86	64	94	48	51	42
OKT3 (%)	65	92	59	63	56	80	43
OKT4 (%)	50	88	62	7	16	47	45
OKT6 (%)	0	0	0	0	0	0	0
OKT8 (%)	11	5	5	4	13	32	29
10.2 (%)	62	95	78	74	62	72	71
9.6 (%)	55	92	71	17	46	80	72
ERFC (%)	31	83	71	5	22	78	19
OKI1 (%)	+	20	29	6	23	28	63
α-B1 (%)		0	6	0	16	5	26
J5 (%)		86	0	3	0	0	0
OKM1 (%)		0	6	0	0	2	13
α-Mo1 (%)		0			0	0	
S-Ig (%) γ		3	9	8	16	5	28
α		2	2	6	2	1	3
μ		0	2	5	14	1	26
δ		2	3	8	12	2	31
κ		1	7	7	13	2	8
λ		0	3	3	9	3	10
C-Ig (μ)	—	—	—		—	—	—

[a] L, large cell type. [b] A, ascites. Other abbreviations are the same as in previous tables.

(15) of them reacted with both OKT3 and OKT4, those from one ATL patient (Case No. 17) reacted with only OKT4, and those from two ATL patients (Case Nos. 16, 29) reacted with OKT3, but not with OKT4. OKT3 has been reported to react with most peripheral T-cells and mature (medullary) thymocytes (*18*), and OKT4 has been reported to react specifically with inducer/helper T-cell (*19*). Therefore, the OKT4 reactive 16 ATL cases are judged to express inducer/helper T-cell phenotype. The two OKT4 negative but OKT3 positive ATL cases are judged to have peripheral T-cell phenotype, but their subset origin cannot be defined. The tumor cells of the 18 patients with ATL expressed Ia-like antigen which can be detected by OKI1. Anti-B1, OKM1, anti-Mo1, and J5 did not react at all with tumor cells from these ATL patients.

The reactivity of the tumor cells of 12 patients with adult T-cell lymphoma (four with medium-sized T-cell lymphoma, six with pleomorphic T-cell lymphoma, two with large cell type T-cell lymphoma), two with T-CLL and three with mycosis fun-

T-CLL, and Mycosis Fungoides with Monoclonal Antibodies

Inducer/helper T-cell

37 U.A.	38 I.N.	39 S.I.	40 Y.M.	41 O.E.	42 M.T.	43 K.S.	44 M.T.	45 O.S.	46 T.Y.
70	58	68	75	49	74	44	71	54	66
M	M	M	F	F	F	M	M	F	F
lymphoma					T-CLL		Mycosis fungoides		
L or Pleo	Mix or Pleo	L or Pleo	L^a	L			Med	Med	Med
LN	LN	LN	LN	A^b	PB	PB	LN	Skin	Skin
91	88	90	94	86	98	99	88	96	89
80	70	84	85	80	98	99	80	90	46
5	46	20	8	12	99	91	82	74	71
89	62	82	89	0	79	92	78	83	26
0	0	0	0	0	0	0	5	0	0
1	8	6	1	0	0	2	12	1	39
	74	84	33	1	98	96	83	86	
	68	79	74	84	96	98	85	91	
82	71	80	91	27	98	43	55	95	70
	9	9	8	32	0	74	64	63	
	3	8	1	0	0	0	5	0	
	0	0	0	0	0	0	0	0	
	0	4	5	0	0	0	3	0	
	0	2		0		0	1		
5	3	2	5	0	0	4	17	2	
0	2	2	0	0	0	0	5	0	
0	0	5	0	0	3	2	14	0	4
0	2	10	0	0	0	2	6	0	
	1	14	4	0	0	4	6	0	
	0	3	4	0	0	0	9	1	
—	—	—	—	—	—	—	—	—	—

goides is shown in Table IV. Tumor cells of all 17 patients with these T-cell malignancies had at least one of the ERFC, E-R antigens detected by monoclonal antibody 9.6 or pan-T cell antigen detected by monoclonal antibody 10.2, but had no reactivity with either OKT6 or OKT8. Tumor cells from most (12) patients with these T-cell malignancies were OKT4 positive and OKT8 negative, indicating that these tumor cells had the same inducer/helper T-cell phenotype as ATL. The tumor cells of the five patients (Case No. 33, medium sized T-cell lymphoma; Case Nos. 34 and 35, pleomorphic T-cell lymphoma; Case No. 41, large cell type T-cell lymphoma; Case No. 46, mycosis fungoides) were OKT3 positive, but both OKT4 and OKT8 were negative, indicating that they had peripheral T-cell phenotype with specific subset undetermined. Ia-like antigen was positive in about half of the cases. Anti-B1, OKM1, and anti-Mo1 was not reactive, but J5 were exceptionally reactive with tumor cells of a certain case (Case No. 31).

T-cell Malignancies with Suppressor/Cytotoxic T-cell Phenotype

The reactivity of the tumor cells of five patients with IBL-like T-cell lymphoma, one with Lennert's lymphoma and three with mixed cell type T-cell lymphoma is shown in Table V. Tumor cells from all these patients not only had ERFC, E-R antigen detected by monoclonal antibody 9.6 and pan-T cell antigen detected by monoclonal antibody 10.2 in the cases examined for reactivity of these monoclonal antibodies, but also reacted with both OKT3 and OKT8. However, they did not react with OKT4 and OKT6, indicating that the tumor cells had suppressor/cytotoxic T-cell phenotype, because both OKT3 and OKT8 positive and OKT4 negative T-cell have been reported

TABLE V. Reactivity of Tumor Cells of IBL-like T-cell Lymphoma, Lennert's Lymphoma, and Mixed Cell Type T-cell Lymphoma with Monoclonal Antibodies

Differentiation stage	Suppressor/cytotoxic T-cell													
Case No.	47	48			49	50			51		52	53	54	55
	S.R.	H.K.			Y.I.	S.R.			S.M.		K.T.	H.S.	K.T.	I.S.
Age	50	80			36	71					60	66	67	43
Sex	M	M			M	M			M		M	M	M	M
Diagnosis or Histology	IBL-like T-cell lymphoma										Lennert[c]	Mix	Mix	Mix
Specimen	LN	LN[a]	PB[b]	LN[b]	LN	LN[a]	PB[b]	LN[b]	LN[a]	LN[b]	LN	LN	LN	LN
Lymphoid cells (%)	86	84	94	80	70	96	98	91	76	52	76	84	84	99
Tumor cells (%)	60	46	90	76	34	41	90	70	15	38	48	76	42	39
OKT3 (%)	39	65	92	48	39	88	93	63	67	21	72	82	52	66
OKT4 (%)	0	42	2	1	9	23	18	8	43	7	26	0	21	10
OKT6 (%)	2	0	0	0	1	0	0	0	0	0	0	0	0	0
OKT8 (%)	47	42	88	72	24	52	76	67	11	20	45	75	41	44
10.2 (%)					40	83	94	63	70	55	49	48	61	64
9.6 (%)					40	92	95	76	73	51	71	78	54	74
ERFC (%)	55	56	79		67	67	78	73	72	54	70	74	58	34
OKI1 (%)	+	+	+		20	65	83	59	17	49	+	20	81	58
α-B1 (%)					5	5	3	5	11	27		0	31	24
J5 (%)					0	0	0	0	0	0		0	0	0
OKM1 (%)					3	4	4	1	3	10		0	0	0
α-Mo1 (%)					3	7	0		0			0		
S-Ig (%) γ	24	33	5		20	14	9	7	22		8	12	5	9
α	6	2	0		3	8	3	6	14		0	0	7	2
μ	1	30	0		30	5	2	9	28		2	0	2	18
δ	0	0	0		15	8	0	6	6		0	0	6	6
κ	9	11			7	6	5		10				9	6
λ	17	10			6	3	13		9				6	13
C-Ig (μ) (%)	0	40			3	2	—		—		2	0	—	—

[a] LN, lymph node at onset; PB, peripheral blood at onset.
[b] LN, lymph node at relapse; PB, peripheral blood at leukemic phase.
[c] Lennert, Lennert's lymphoma.
Other abbreviations are the same as in previous tables.

to be suppressor/cytotoxic T-cells (18). Tumor cells of the seven patients expressed Ia-like antigen. Anti-B1, J5, OKM1, and anti-Mo1 did not react with the tumor cells of any of the six cases examined. In case No. 48, the lymph node at onset was found to contain as many OKT4-positive cells as OKT8-positive cells, because many normal lymphocytes were mixed with tumor cells. However, after leukemic transformation almost all the cells, both in peripheral blood and lymph nodes, were judged to be tumor cells morphologically, and found to react specifically with OKT8. In most cases of this type of lymphoma, morphologically detectable tumor cells in the initially biopsied lymph nodes are usually seen in less than 50% of the cells. Therefore, frequent repeated examinations were done in these cases. In Case No. 51, as the lymph node at onset was found to contain many normal lymphocytes and some granulocytes, it is difficult to judge the reactivity of the tumor cells. At relapse, however, about 70% of the lymphoid cells in the biopsied lymph node were found to be tumor cells which reacted with OKT3 and OKT8, although about half of the cells in the lymph node were granulocytes and histiocytes.

Estimation of Cellular Origin of T-cell Malignancies

The reactivity of the tumor cells of 55 patients with T-cell malignancies whose differentiation and subset could be determined is summarized in Table VI. These malignancies could be divided into four major categories according to their differentiation antigens: 1) Pre-T cell malignancy; 2) thymic T-cell malignancy; 3) inducer/helper T-cell malignancy; and 4) suppressor/cytotoxic T-cell malignancy. Pre-T cell malignancy can be identified as the C/T hybrid type. Two cases of childhood ALL belonged to the pre-T cell malignancy (T_0). Thymic T-cell malignancy (T_1) is further divided into early thymocyte type, common (cortical) thymocyte type and mature (medullary) thymocyte type. Three cases of T-ALL and five cases of T-lymphoblastic lymphoma belonged to the early thymocyte type. Only one case of T-ALL belonged to the common thymocyte type. However, we did not see the mature thymocyte type in this series. Peripheral T-cell malignancy is divided into the inducer/helper T-cell malignancy, and suppressor/cytotoxic T-cell malignancy. Tumor cells of 16 patients with ATL or ATLL, three with medium-sized adult T-cell lymphoma, four with pleomorphic adult T-cell lymphoma, and one with large cell type adult T-cell lymphoma, two with T-CLL and two with mycosis fungoides expressed the inducer/helper T-cell phenotype. Tumor cells of two patients with ATL, one with medium-sized adult T-cell lymphoma, two with pleomorphic adult T-cell lymphoma and two with large cell type adult T-cell lymphoma, and one with mycosis fungoides expressed the peripheral T-cell phenotype, but their specific subset phenotype could not be determined. On the other hand, tumor cells of five patients with IBL-like T-cell lymphoma, one with Lennert's lymphoma and two with the mixed cell type T-cell lymphoma expressed the suppressor/cytotoxic T-cell phenotype.

These results indicate that the inducer/helper T-cell malignancies are still heterogeneous. Mycosis fungoides, ATL or ATLL and some T-CLL have been reported to be different diseases (16), although the immunological phenotype of the tumor cells was found to be the same. ATL and some adult T-cell lymphomas have been considered to be the same disease, even though their morphologic diagnosis is different (11, 25).

TABLE VI. Cellular Origin of T-cell Malignancies

Differentiation	J5	10.2 (pan-T)	9.6 (ERFC)	OKT3	OKT4	OKT6	OKT8	OKI1	Tumor	No. of cases
Pre-T (T$_0$) C/T hybrid	+	+	−∼+	−	−	−	−	+∼−	C/T-ALL	2
Thymic-T (T$_1$)									T-ALL	3
Early thymocyte	−	+	−∼+	−	−	−	−	−	NHL, Lb[d]	5
Common thymocyte	−	+	+	−	+	+	+	−	T-ALL	1
Mature thymocyte	−	+	+	+	−/+	−	−/+	−		
Peripheral-T (T$_{2-3}$)									ATL, ATLL	16 (+2)[a]
Inducer/helper T-cell	−	+	+	+	+	−	−	−/+	NHL[b], Pleo	4 (+2)
									NHL, medium	3 (+2)
									NHL, large	1 (+1)
									T-CLL	2
									MF[c]	2 (+1)
Suppressor/ cytotoxic T-cell	−	+	+	+	−	−	+	−/+	IBL-like	5
									Lennert	1
									NHL, Mixed	3

Abbreviations are the same as in previous tables.
[a] Number of cases in parenthesis indicates number of cases with specific subset undetermined.
[b] NHL, non-Hodgkin's lymphoma.
[c] MF, mycosis fungoides.
[d] Lb, lymphoblastic.

Recent advances in immunology show that inducer/helper T-cells characterized by the presence of T4-antigen may be divided into at least two subsets: one with helper function for pokeweed mitogen-stimulated immunoglobulin production of B-cells and the other with immunoregulatory (suppressor) function for the same system (21, 28). More recently Thomas et al. (30) analyzed T- and B-cell interactions with monoclonal antibodies, and reported the existence of functional heterogeneity within the T4-antigen positive subset. In order to establish a more precise cellular origin of each heterogeneous inducer/helper T-cell tumor, it is further necessary to conduct subset analyses of these T4-antigen-positive tumors.

It has been reported that the antibody against ATL-associated antigen (ATLA) can be detected in the sera of almost all patients with ATL (10). Anti-ATLA antibody in the patient's serum or ATLA itself in the tumor cell might become a useful marker to distinguish ATL from other inducer/helper T-cell malignancies.

We have proposed a new disease entity called IBL-like T-cell lymphoma (26) which is T-cell lymphoma in adult but different from ATL or ATLL, and is characterized by polyclonal hypergammaglobulinemia, poor prognosis, male predominance, no endemic distribution of patients' birthplace, and mixed cell type morphology with angioimmunoblastic and granulomatous lesions. All IBL-like T-cell lymphoma were found to have the suppressor/cytotoxic T-cell phenotype. In addition to this, Lennert's lymphoma and the mixed cell type T-cell lymphoma which were associated with granulomatous lesions and polyclonal hypergammaglobulinemia were also found to have the suppressor/cytotoxic T-cell phenotype. Clinical manifestations as well as immunologic phenotype of these lymphomas were almost the same, although the morphological diagnoses were different. Therefore, T-cell lymphomas in adult with suppressor/cytotoxic T-cell phenotype, characterized by polyclonal hypergammaglobulinemia, male predominance, poor prognosis, no endemic distribution of patients' birthplace and mixed cell type morphology with angioimmunoblastic and granulomatous lesions is probably the same disease and a new disease entity which is completely different from ATL or ATLL. However, it is necessary to determine in the future why lymphoma of the suppressor/cytotoxic T-cell phenotype is frequently associated with granulomatous lesions and polyclonal hypergammaglobulinemia.

In the case of T-cell malignancies whose subsets cannot be determined in one examination, repeated examination of tumor cells at the appropriate phase is indicated, because contaminated normal T-cells sometimes interfere with accurate judgment of the tumor cell reaction.

REFERENCES

1. Aisenberg, A. C. and Bloch, K. J. Immunoglobulins on the surface of neoplastic lymphocytes. *N. Engl. J. Med.*, **287**, 272–276 (1972).
2. Benett, J. M., Catovsky, D., Daniel, M. T., Flandrin, G., Galton, D.A.G., Gralnick, H. R., and Sultan, C. (FAB Co-operative Group). Proposals for the classification of the acute leukemias. *Br. J. Hematol.*, **33**, 451–458 (1976).
3. Bhan, A. K., Reinherz, E. L., Poppema, S., McClusky, R. T., and Schlossman, S. F. Location of T-cell and major histocompatibility complex antigens in the human thymus. *J. Exp. Med.*, **152**, 771–782 (1980).
4. Borella, L. and Sen, L. T-cell surface markers on lymphoblasts from acute lymphocytic leukemia. *J. Immunol.*, **111**, 1257–1261 (1973).
5. Boumsell, L. I., Bernard, A., Reinherz, E. L., Nadler, L. M., Ritz, J., Coppin, H., Richard, Y., Dubertret, L., Degos, L., Lemerle, J., Flandrin, G., Dausset, J., and Schlossman, S. F. Surface antigens on malignant Sézary and T-CLL cells correspond to those of mature T-cells. *Blood*, **57**, 526–530 (1981).
6. Breard, J., Reinherz, E. L., Kung, P. C., Goldstein, G., and Schlossman, S. F. A monoclonal antibody reactive with human peripheral blood monocytes. *J. Immunol.*, **124**, 1943–1948 (1980).
7. Greaves, M. F., Rao, J., Hariri, G., Verbi, W., Catovsky, D., Kung, P. C., and Goldstein, G. Phenotypic heterogeneity and cellular origins of T-cell malignancies. *Leukemia Res.*, **5**, 281–299 (1981).
8. Hattori, T., Uchiyama, T., Toibana, T., Takatsuki, K., and Uchino, H. Surface phenotype of Japanese adult T-cell leukemia cells characterized by monoclonal antibodies. *Blood*, **58**, 645–647 (1981).
9. Haynes, B. F., Metzgar, R. S., Minna, J. D., and Bunn, P. A. Phenotypic characterization of cutaneous T-cell lymphoma: Use of monoclonal antibodies to compare with other malignant T-cells. *N. Engl. J. Med.*, **304**, 1319–1323 (1981).
10. Hinuma, Y., Nagata, K., Hanaoka, M., Nakai, M., Matsumoto, T., Kinoshita, K., Shirakawa, S., and Miyoshi, I. Adult T-cell leukemia: Antigen in an ATL cell line and detection of antibodies to the antigen in human sera. *Proc. Natl. Acad. Sci. U.S.*, **78**, 6476–6480 (1981).
11. Ichimaru, M., Kinoshita, K., Kamihira, S., Ikeda, S., Yamada, Y., and Amagasaki, T.

T-cell malignant lymphoma in Nagasaki district and its problems. *Jpn. J. Clin. Oncol.*, **9** (Suppl.), 337–346 (1979).

12. Kamoun, M., Martin, P. J., Hansen, J. A., Brown, M. A., Siadek, A. W., and Nowinski, R. C. Identification of a human T lymphocyte surface protein associated with the E-rosette receptor. *J. Exp. Med.*, **153**, 207–212 (1981).

13. Kim, H., Jacobs, C., Warnke, R. A., and Dorfman, R. F. Malignant lymphoma with a high content of epitheloid histiocytes: Distinct clinicopathologic entity and a form of so-called "Lennert's lymphoma." *Cancer*, **41**, 620–635 (1978).

14. Kung, P. C., Berger, C. L., and Goldstein, G. Cutaneous T cell lymphoma: Characterization by monoclonal antibodies. *Blood*, **57**, 261–266 (1981).

15. Kung, P. C., Goldstein, G., Reinherz, E. L., and Schlossman, S. F. Monoclonal antibodies defining distinctive human T cell surface antigens. *Science*, **206**, 347–349 (1979).

16. Martin, P. J., Hansen, K. A., Nowinski, R. C., and Brown, M. A. A new human T cell differentiation antigen: Unexpected expression on chronic lymphocytic leukemia cells. *Immunogenetics*, **11**, 429–439 (1980).

17. Nadler, L. M., Ritz, J., Hardy, R., Pesando, J. M., Schlossman, S. F., and Stashenko, P. A unique cell surface antigen identifying lymphoid malignancies of B cell origin. *J. Clin. Invest.*, **67**, 134–140 (1981).

18. Reinherz, E. L., Kung, P. C., Goldstein, G., Levey, R. H., and Schlossman, S. F. Discrete stages of human intrathymic differentiation: Analysis of normal thymocytes and leukemic lymphoblasts of T-cell lineage. *Proc. Natl. Acad. Sci. U.S.*, **77**, 1588–1592 (1980).

19. Reinherz, E. L., Kung, P. C., Goldstein, G., and Schlossman, S. F. Further characterization of the human inducer T-cell subset defined by monoclonal antibody. *J. Immunol.*, **123**, 2894–2896 (1979).

20. Reinherz, E. L., Kung, P. C., Pesando, J. M., Ritz, J., Goldstein, G., and Schlossman, S. F. Ia determinants on human T-cell subsets defined by monoclonal antibody. *J. Exp. Med.*, **150**, 1472–1482 (1979).

21. Reinherz, E. L., Strelkauskas, A. F., O'Brien, C., and Schlossman, S. F. Phenotypic and functional distinction between the TH_2^+ and JRA^+ T cell subsets in man. *J. Immunol.*, **123**, 83–86 (1979).

22. Reinherz, E. L., Kung, P. C., Goldstein, G., and Schlossman, S. F. A monoclonal antibody with selective reactivity with functionally mature human thymocytes and all peripheral human T cells. *J. Immunol.*, **123**, 1312–1317 (1979).

23. Ritz, J., Pesando, J. M., Notis-McConarty, J., Lazarus, H., and Schlossman, S. F. A monoclonal antibody to human acute lymphoblastic leukaemia antigen. *Nature*, **283**, 583–585 (1980).

24. Shimoyama, M. Cellular origin, differentiation and classification of leukemia and lymphoma cells as based on surface marker analysis. *Acta Haematol. Jpn.*, **42**, 897–917 (1979).

25. Shimoyama, M., Minato, K., Saito, H., Kitahara, T., Konda, C., Nakazawa, M., Ishihara, K., Watanabe, S., Inada, N., Nagatani, T., Deura, K., and Mikata, A. Comparisons of clinical, morphologic and immunologic characteristics of adult T-cell leukemia-lymphoma and cutaneous T-cell lymphoma. *Jpn. J. Clin. Oncol.*, **9** (Suppl.), 357–372 (1979).

26. Shimoyama, M., Minato, K., Saito, H., Takenaka, T., Watanabe, S., Nagatani, T., and Naruto, M. Immunoblastic lymphadenopathy (IBL)-like T-cell lymphoma. *Jpn. J. Clin. Oncol.*, **9** (Suppl.), 347–356 (1979).

27. Stashenko, P., Nadler, L. M., Hardy, R., and Schlossman, S. F. Characterization of a human B lymphocyte specific antigen. *J. Immunol.*, **125**, 1678–1685 (1980).

28. Strelkauskas, A. V., Schauf, V., Wilson, B. S., Chess, L., and Schlossman, S. F. Isolation and characterization of naturally occurring subclasses of human peripheral blood T cells with regulatory functions. *J. Immunol.*, **120**, 1278–1282 (1978).

29. Suchi, T., Tajima, K., Nanba, K., Wakasa, H., Mikata, S., Kikuchi, M., Mori, S., Watanabe, S., Mohri, N., Shamoto, M., Harigaya, K., Itagaki, T., Matsuda, M., Kirino, Y., Takagi, K., and Fukunaga, S. Some problems on the histopathological diagnosis of non-Hodgkin's malignant lymphoma: A proposal of a new type. *Acta Pathol. Jpn.*, **29**, 755–776, 1979.

30. Thomas, Y., Rogozinski, L., Irigoyen, O. H., Friedman, S. M., Kung, P. C., Goldstein, G., and Chess, L. Functional analysis of human T cell subsets defined by monoclonal antibodies. IV. Induction of suppressor cells within the OKT4+ population. *J. Exp. Med.*, **154**, 459–467 (1981).

31. Tobinai, K., Hirose, M., Minato, K., and Shimoyama, M. The reaction specificity of various monoclonal antibodies and cellular origin and differentiation of cultured cell lines derived from human leukemias and lymphomas. *Jpn. J. Clin. Oncol.*, **11**, 469–480 (1981).

32. Tobinai, K., Hirose, M., Yamada, H., Minato, K., and Shimoyama, M. Cellular origin of human lymphoid malignancies as based on immunologic analysis of membrane differentiation antigens. *Jpn. J. Clin. Oncol.*, **12**, 73–90 (1982).

33. Todd, R. F. III, Nadler, L. M., and Schlossman, S. F. Antigens on human monocytes identified by monoclonal antibodies. *J. Immunol.*, **126**, 1435–1442 (1981).

34. Uchiyama, T., Yodoi, J., Sagawa, K., Takatsuki, K., and Uchino, H. Adult T-cell leukemia: Clinical and hematologic features of 16 cases. *Blood*, **50**, 481–492 (1977).

GANN Monograph on Cancer Research 28, 1982

BIOPSY OF ADULT T CELL LEUKEMIA

Masahiro Kikuchi, Tetsuji Mitsui, Tadaaki Eimoto,
Reiko Toyooka, and Masayoshi Nishiuchi
*First Department of Pathology, School of Medicine, Fukuoka University**

Twenty-eight cases of adult T-cell leukemia (ATL) were examined histologically on lymph nodes.

Histologically the cases showed common features, *i.e.*, a diffuse proliferation of atypical lymphoid cells varying in size and nuclear configuration, presence of giant nuclear cells of cerebriform and/or Reed-Sternberg type, mild proliferation of epithelioid venules with features of atypical lymphoid cells passing through the wall, and preserved peripheral sinuses. The same histologic features, except lower incidences of atypical cells through the wall of epithelioid venules, were also found in 13 cases of non-leukemic counterpart. Clinically ATL showed frequent skin rash (57.1%) and had a rapid fatal course with a 50% actuarial survival rate of 4 months, but its histological counterpart revealed occasional skin rash (18.2%) and a longer course of 10 months. Both the patients with ATL and those with its non-leukemic counterpart revealed a positive reaction with ATL-associated antigen, and the tumor cells in both groups showed a similarly positive dot-like reaction for acid α-naphthyl acetate esterase and acid esterase positive reactivities and had a positive reaction with OKT4. These results indicated that ATL and its non-leukemic counterpart might be categorized in one special histological group of peripheral T-cell lymphoma of inducer/helper cells but had rather different clinical behavior.

Recently a kind of leukemia which presents some characteristic clinicohematological features has been recognized as adult T-cell leukemia (ATL) by Takatsuki and his group (*16*). The leukemia is characterized by an appearance of abnormal leukemic cells with lobulated or cloverleaf-like nuclei and by frequent occurrence in natives of southwestern Japan. The patients show mild lymphadenopathy and frequent skin rash with a rapid clinical course despite strong chemotherapy. Furthermore, the patients have antibodies for ATL-associated virus antigen (ATLA) (*3, 4*). In this paper we describe biopsy findings of lymph nodes in these patients.

During the period from 1979 to early 1982, 115 cases of malignant lymphoma which had been examined for surface markers were filed in the Department of Pathology, Fukuoka University which is situated on Kyushu Island, the endemic area of ATL. Of these 115 cases there were 83 cases of T-cell malignancy, including 28 cases of ATL with an appearance of typical lobulated abnormal tumor cells in peripheral blood which we confirmed (Photo 1).

---

* Nanakuma 34, Nishi-ku, Fukuoka 814-01, Japan (菊池昌弘, 三井徹次, 栄本忠昭, 豊岡玲子, 西内正好).

M. KIKUCHI ET AL.

Clinical Findings

The age range of the patients at the time of biopsy was 33–78 years, with a median age of 52 years. The ratio of males to females was 2.1: 1. The usual observable symptoms were mild lymphadenopathy (100%), fatigue (100%), and skin rash (57.1%). Leukocytosis over 10,000 per cmm (maximum 53,700 per cmm) was observed in 15 patients (53.6%). Atypical lymphocytes appeared in numbers of from 432 to 28,950 per cmm with a median of 9,464. Important clinical features and hematological findings are summarized in Table I. Eighty percent of the patients had died within 1 year with a 50% survival rate of 4 months. The actuarial survival rate of ATL is shown in Fig. 1.

TABLE I. Summary of Clinicohematological Data of ATL

	ATL	Non-leukemic counterpart	Total
No. of cases	28	11	39
Age (year old)	33–78	34–80	33–80
(median)	(52)	(62)	(52)
Sex (M/F)	2.1	1.8	2.0
Actuarial 50% survival rate (months)	4	10	5
Fatigue (%)	100	100	100
Lymphadenopathy (%)	100	100	100
Skin rash (%)	57.1	18.2	46.2
Leukocytosis over 10,000 (%)	53.6	9.2	41.0
Atypical cell/cmm	432–28,950	0	432–28,950
(median)	(9,464)		(9,464)

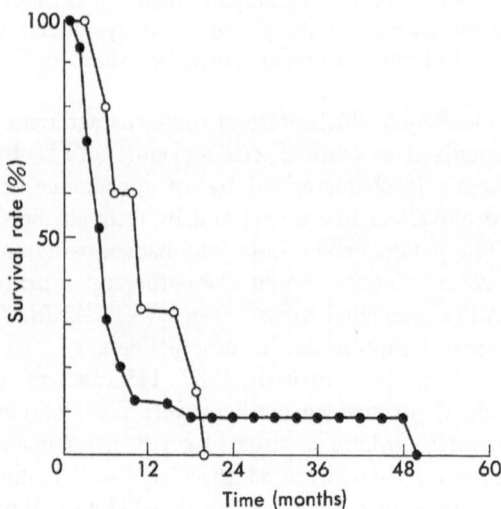

FIG. 1. Actuarial survival rate of ATL and its non-leukemic counterpart. ● ATL (28 cases); ○ non-leukemic counterpart (11 cases).

Pathological Features

All cases documented lymph nodal involvement of the lymphoma cells. Histologically the infiltrate assumed a diffuse growth pattern, with architectural obliteration and focal extension of the infiltrate beyond the capsule. In 5 cases incomplete involvement was demonstrated with preservation of follicles which were surrounded by neoplastic cells. Histologically ATL was classified by its cellular structures and sizes into three groups, *i.e.*, medium-sized, large cell, and pleomorphic types, by the Japanese Lymphoma Study Group (LSG)-classification (*15*).

1. Medium-sized type (12 cases)

The lymphoma cells in non-cohesive monotonous proliferation were 6–8 μm, 1.5 times the diameter of small lymphocytes in the same sections. Frequently the nuclei assumed mulberry, maple leaf or walnut seed shapes. The chromatin was delicate and finely dispersed. Nucleoli were indistinct or small and ranged from one to three per nuclei. Scant quantities of amphophilic cytoplasm were observed. Cell borders were well defined. Mitoses (average 12/10 high power fields) were frequent (Photo 2). Only a few giant cells with cerebriform, Reed-Sternberg type or bizarre nuclei were intermingled. Histiocytes were occasionally seen in 9 cases, but eosinophils and plasma cells were rare. Vascularity was not prominent. In 12 cases features of atypical lymphoid cells passing through the epithelioid venules were conspicuous. Arrangements of atypical lymphoid cells around the small vessels in a concentric configuration were seen in one case (Photo 3). This histology represented the irregular nuclear subtype of the medium-sized cell type (*7, 11*).

2. Large cell type (4 cases)

Histologically lymphoma cells were composed predominantly of lymphoid cells with large nuclei of 10 μm or more in diameter, irregular in shape with one to three distinct nucleoli and thick nuclear membrane. They always occupied over 50% of the tumor cells. The cytoplasm was usually abundant with amphophilic or pale staining characters (Photo 4). Mitoses were frequent (average 16/10 high power fields). A few giant cells of cerebriform or Reed-Sternberg type or multiple nuclei were detected in 2 cases. Epithelioid venules were slightly increased with swollen endothelial cells. Features of a few small atypical lymphoid cells through the wall were observed in 2 cases. This histology was consistent with that of the common subtype which has been reported in another paper (*11*).

3. Pleomorphic type (12 cases)

This type was characterized by a diffuse non-cohesive proliferation of lymphoma cells, irregular in size and with nuclear configuration of maple leaf-like, walnut seed or convoluted figures (Photo 5). The proportion of cells in the different sizes varied, but medium-sized cells were generally dominant. The cytoplasm of the tumor cells was usually obvious, but narrow. Occasionally cells with abundant amphophilic cytoplasm were intermingled. Mitoses were frequent (average 13/10 high power fields). Among these lymphoma cells there were considerable numbers of giant cells (Photo 6) which had cerebriform (Photo 7) or Reed-Sternberg type (Photo 8) or bizarre nuclei; these were easily recognized with low power magnification. Occasionally epithelioid venules were well developed with straight elongation and with atypical small lymphoid cells in the wall (Photo 9). Reactive histiocytes were increased in 7 cases. Plasma cells and eosinophils were rarely encountered. Peripheral sinuses were well preserved and contained atypical lymphoid cells in all cases (Photo 10). T-zone distribution of the lymphoma cells was apparent with preserved lymphoid follicles in 2 cases.

Other Peripheral T-Cell Lymphomas

Histological findings the same as ATL were found in 11 non-leukemic cases: 2 medium-sized, 6 large cells, and 3 pleomorphic types. The patients in this group showed similar clinical features with a longer clinical course and lesser occurrence of skin rash, as shown in Table I.

Besides these cases, 9 of the medium-sized type categorized in a monomorphic subtype presented a monotonous proliferation of cells with less irregular nuclei with no giant cells; 14 of the large cell type showed a prominent proliferation of clear or immunoblastic cells (clear cell or immunoblastic subtype). The detail of the histology of such cases has been reported in another paper (11).

T-chronic lymphocytic leukemia (CLL), mycosis fungoides Sézary syndrome, Lennert's lymphoma and other specific histological groups were also found in peripheral T-cell malignancy, but these cases were few in number and detailed clinicopathological findings cannot yet be summarized.

Histochemistry

Neoplastic cells showed little or no cytoplasmic pyroninophilia and minimal cytoplasmic basophilia with Giemsa stain. Acid α-naphthyl acetate esterase (ANAE) activity revealed a distinct pattern of cytoplasmic positivity (Photo 11), generally defined by a single strongly positive dot. This staining pattern contrasted sharply with strong diffuse cytoplasmic positivity observed in histiocytes. Acid phosphatase (AcP) determination demonstrated strong punctate cytoplasmic staining with tartrate-sensitive reaction in all cases (Photo 12).

Naphthol AS-D chloroacetate esterase activity was absent. Net-like membranous reaction for ATPase activity was positive, as was true of B lymphocytes in all examined cases (Photo 13). The non-leukemic counterpart of ATL demonstrated the same reaction on these enzymes.

Electron Microscopy

Twenty cases of ATL were observed electron microscopically. The characteristic fine structures of these cases were tumor cells showing slight to marked nuclear irregularity with convoluted-shape predominance, a speckled chromatin pattern of the large cells, prominent lysosomes, and glycogen accumulation in addition to the difference in cellular distribution. Medium-sized and small lymphoid cells showed finely dispersed chromatin with prominent marginal heterochromatin, frequent multivesicular bodies and lipid droplets. Segments of endoplasmic reticulum were seen but those of smooth endoplasmic reticulum associated with cytoplasmic vesicles were predominant (Photos 14, 15). Details have been reported in another paper (*1*).

Immunologic Studies by Monoclonal Antibodies for T Cells

To define the nature of the malignant T-cell population in ATL, characterization was performed by monoclonal antibodies on OKT 3, 4, 6, 8, M, and Ia (Ortho). All 7 examined nodes had a positive reactivity with anti OKT4, known to define helper/inducer cells. The non-leukemic counterpart of ATL also showed the same reactivity. The patients had no activity with anti OKT8, a marker for suppressor/cytotoxic cells. Results are tabulated in Table II.

TABLE II. Monoclonal Antibodies (%) for T Cells in ATL

ATL Case No.	Histology	Material[a]	OKT3	OKT4	OKT6	OKT8	M	Ia	E-rosette
ML 75	Medium	LN	29	60	3	8	9	36	92
ML 78	Medium	PB	96	87	7	15	10	20	89
ML 167	Medium	LN	71	51	11	27	18	32	65
ML 179	Medium	LN	52	85	0	3	1	47	70
ML 187	Large	PB	95	93	7	10	13	10	48
ML 161	Pleo	LN	73	62	2	3	2	58	59
ML 183	Pleo	PB	21	58	3	10	9	21	83
Non-leukemic counterpart									
ML 21	Large	LN	24	34	8	11	17	35	—
ML 189	Large	LN	30	83	6	11	7	15	68
ML 76	Pleo	LN	70	73	11	12	25	28	97

[a] LN, lymph node; PB, peripheral blood; Pleo, pleomorphic type.

Detection of Anti ATLA Antibodies

Sera from 5 patients of ATL were tested for presence of antibodies to ATLA. All gave positive results in the anti-ATLA test. Three cases of non-leukemic counterpart of ATL which had been tested also gave positive reactivity.

DISCUSSION

ATL proposed by Takatsuki *et al.* (*16*) appears to be a new disease entity not only by its frequent endemic occurrence in natives in southwestern Japan and characteristic clinical features but also by the presence of antibodies for ATLA in sera of the patients (*3*).

Hanaoka *et al.* (*2*) summarized the histology of this disease: 1) Diffuse proliferation of the neoplastic cells; 2) pleomorphism of the neoplastic cells with markedly deformed nuclei; 3) heterogenous histological features of lymph nodes admixed with a cluster of normal lymphocytes, proliferation of macrophages and well developed high endothelium venules; and 4) high incidence of skin lesions due to the infiltration of neoplastic cells. Kikuchi *et al.* (*7*) had insisted the importance of pleomorphism of neoplastic cells

TABLE III. Histology of Lymph Nodes in ATL

	ATL	Non-leukemic counterpart	Total
No. of cases	28	11	39
Medium-sized cell type	12	2	14
Large cell type	4	6	10
Pleomorphic type	12	3	15
Tumor cell features	Variable in size and shape, mixed small to large		
Nuclei	Maple leaf, mulberry, walnut seed, convoluted		
Nucleoli	Small, usually one to three		
Chromatin	Relatively homogenous distribution		
Mitoses	Usually 10-20 per 10 high power fields		
Giant cells	Cerebriform, Reed-Sternber, or Hodgkin's cell type, or other bizarre type		
Epithelioid venules	Slightly increased with a straight line		
Atypical cells through wall of epithelioid venules	24 (85.7%)	3 (27.2%)	27 (69.2%)
Preserved peripheral sinus	23 (82.1%)	6 (53.5%)	29 (74.4%)
Residual lymph follicles	5 (17.9%)	1 (9.2%)	6 (15.4%)
Compartmentalization	12 (42.9%)	3 (27.3%)	15 (38.4%)
Eosinophils	3 (10.7%)	0 (0.0%)	3 (7.7%)
Plasma cells	1 (3.6%)	1 (0.9%)	2 (5.1%)
Histiocytes	20 (71.4%)	4 (36.3%)	24 (61.5%)
Reticulum cells	13 (46.4%)	7 (63.4%)	20 (51.3%)

and the presence of giant cells with a highly deformed nuclear configuration. Suchi *et al.* (*14*) had proposed a new histological type for a special kind of lymphoma in Japan and considered that the type gave the core histology of ATL. Watanabe *et al.* (*20*) confirmed these results. After accumulations of histological materials of ATL, Kikuchi *et al.* (*7*) reported that ATL consisted not only of the pleomorphic type, but of medium-sized and large cell types by LSG-classification. Ichimaru *et al.* (*5*) reported similar results. In our series ATL showed 3 histological types of LSG: Medium-sized, large cell, and pleomorphic types. Common histological findings of these cases were presence of highly deformed nuclear cells with variation in size, giant cells being more than 4 times the small lymphocytes in nuclear diameter, mild proliferation of epithelioid venules with features of atypical lymphoid cells through the wall, and preserved peripheral sinuses. The main histological findings are tabulated in Table III. In addition to the pleomorphic type they categorized an irregular nuclear subtype in the medium-sized type and a common subtype in the large cell type. No cases showed a monomorphic subtype in the medium-sized, or an immunoblastic or clear cell subtype in the large cell type. These features were observable not only in ATL but also in the non-leukemic counterpart of ATL.

Cytochemical features of dot-like accumulation of ANAE and AcP were useful to speculate the immunological subsets of peripheral T-cell markers as previously reported (*7*). ATP was not characteristic for B-cells as reported by Mikata *et al.* (*10*) because the enzyme also reacted positively on the membrane of ATL. No differences were present between ATL and its non-leukemic counterpart for these enzymatic reactions.

We have already reported on the ultrastructural features of ATL (*1*). The characteristic fine structures of the tumor cells included nuclear irregularity with superconvolution, a speckled chromatin pattern, predominant lysozome and glycogen accumulation. Kaiserling *et al.* (*6*) and Said *et al.* (*12*) have also reported similar features in cases of T-zone lymphoma and T-immunoblastic sarcoma, respectively. Most of these features we reported seemed to be common figures of peripheral T-cell lymphoma (*13*).

Monoclonal antibodies on the surface of ATL cells were detected by several anti-T cell subset antibodies as shown in Table II. Positivity of OKT3 indicated that ATL might be a neoplasia of helper/inducer type of peripheral T cell. These functional characters were similar to those of the mycosis fungoides-Sézary syndrome group but in ATL a suppressor effect on pokeweed mitogen (PWM)-induced B-cell differentiation (*18*) and phytohemagglutinin (PHA) response of normal lymphocytes (*17*) in culture by the tumor cells was reported. This discrepancy between the surface markers and function of tumor cells *in vitro* suggests that the observed suppression might be due to some nonspecific cytostatic effect of these tumor cells on surrounding cells with no immunological relevance (*17*). It has been reported that nearly 100% of the patients with ATL show a positive reaction to ATLA (*3*). All 10 cases of ATL and its non-leukemic counterpart examined in our series revealed positive reactivities. In Fukuoka, the district in which we performed this research, about 17% of the sera of people over 40 years of age with no hematological disorders showed a positive reaction to ATLA (*4*). So the data we obtained strongly suggested the relationship between ATL and its counterpart concerning pathogenesis.

Finally, we conclude that ATL and its non-leukemic counterpart seem to be categorized from both an immunological and a histological point of view as a single pleomorphic group, which includes not only pleomorphic type but an irregular subtype of medium-sized and common pleomorphic variants of large cell type in LSG-classification. However, to separate the ATL into three variants seems to be clinically useful, because the prevalence of smaller cells (medium-sized and small cells) in histology might indicate a more rapid course and more frequent leukemic changes than the predominantly larger cell cases shown in Table IV. Furthermore, ATL showed a more frequent skin rash (57.1%) and rapid clinical course (with a 50% survival rate of 4 months) than those of its non-leukemic counterpart (skin rash 18.2% and 50% survival rate of 10 months). So, leukemic manifestation appeared to be the important sign to predict prognosis of the patients. Relationship of this disease entity to T-zone lymphoma or the mixed "blastic/cytic" lymphoma of T type of Lennert (*8*, *14*), T-immunoblastic sarcoma of Lukes (*9*), and peripheral T-cell lymphoma of Waldron *et al.* (18) remains undefined. All these diseases show similar nuclear irregularity in size and shape, T-

TABLE IV. Relation of Histology to Survival and Skin Rash in ATL and Its Non-leukemic Counterpart

Histology by LSG-classification	No. of cases	Actuarial 50% survival rate (months)	Skin rash (%)	ATL (%)
Medium-sized cell type	14	3	42.9	85.7
Large cell type	10	10	30.0	40.0
Pleomorphic type	15	5	60.0	80.0
Total	39	5	46.2	71.8

zone distribution and reactive epithelioid venules, but skin involvements and leukemic changes are not as frequent as the pleomorphic type of LSG-classification. We examined only the endemic region of ATL, so a detailed analysis of differences of ATL to these diseases should be performed to clarify the pathogenesis and cause of local occurrence of ATL.

Acknowledgments

This work was supported by a Grant-in-Aid for Cancer Research from the Japanese Ministry of Health and Welfare. We are deeply grateful to Prof. Y. Hinuma, Kyoto University, and Dr. H. Sato, Kyushu University, for kind examination of antibodies to ATLA in sera of the patients. We also are indebted to Miss K. Kawasaki for secretarial assistance and to Mr. T. Nishimura for photography.

REFERENCES

1. Eimoto, T., Mitsui, T., and Kikuchi, M. Ultrastructure of adult T-cell leukemia/lymphoma. *Virchow Arch., Cell Pathol.*, **38**, 189–208 (1981).
2. Hanaoka, M., Sasaki, M., Matsumoto, H., Tankawa, M., Yamabe, H., Tomimoto K., Tasaka, C., Fujiwara, H., Uchiyama, T., and Takatsuki, K. Adult T cell leukemia. Histological classification and characteristics. *Acta Pathol. Jpn.*, **29**, 723–738 (1979).
3. Hinuma, Y., Nagata, K., Hanaoka, M., Nakai, M., Matsumoto, T., Kinoshita, K., Shirakawa, S., and Miyoshi, I. Adult T-cell leukemia: Antigen in an ATL cell line and detection of antibodies to the antigen in human sera. *Proc. Natl. Acad. Sci. U.S.*, **78**, 6476–6480 (1981).
4. Hinuma, Y., Komoda, H., Chosa, T., Kondo, T., Kobakura, M., Takenaka, T., Kikuchi, M., Ichimaru, M., Yonoki, K., Sato, I., Matsuo, R., and Hanaoka, M. Antibodies to adult T-cell leukemia virus associated-antigen (ATLA) in sera from patients with ATL and controls in Japan: A nationwide seroepidermiologic study. *Int. J. Cancer* **29**, 631–635 (1982).
5. Ichimaru, M., Kamihira, S., and Kinoshita, K. Chemotherapy and immunological deficiency of malignant lymphoma in view of surface marker—Characteristics of malignant lymphoma in Nagasaki district—. *Gan to Kagakuryoho (Cancer and Chemotherapy)*, **8**, 995–1006 (1981) (in Japanese).
6. Kaiserling, E. Ultrastructure of non-Hodgkin's lymphomas. *In* "Malignant Lymphomas Other Than Hodgkin's Disease," ed. K. Lennert, pp. 471–528 (1978). Springer-Verlag, Berlin-Heidelberg-New York.
7. Kikuchi, M., Mitsui, T., Matsui, N., Sato, E., Tokunaga, M., Hasui, K., Ichimaru, M., Kinoshita, K., and Kamihira, S. T-cell malignancies in adults: Histopathological studies of lymph nodes in 110 patients. *Jpn. J. Clin. Oncol.* **9** (Suppl.), 407–422 (1979).
8. Lennert, K. Lymphocytic lymphoma of T-zone type (T-zone lymphoma). *In* "Histophathology of Non-Hodgkin's Lymphomas," pp. 41–44 (1981). Springer-Verlag, Berlin-Heidelberg-New York.
9. Lukes, R. J., Parker, J. W., Taylor, C. R., Tindle, B. H., Cramer, A. D., and Lincoln, T. L. Immunologic approach to non-Hodgkin lymphomas and related leukemias. Analysis of the results of multiparameter studies of 425 cases. *Semin. Hematol.*, **15**, 322–351 (1978).
10. Mikata, A., Harigaya, K., Suzuki, H., Ohishi, T., Tutsumi, Y., Suzuki, S., Watanabe, S., and Kageyama, K. Enzyme histochemistry of non-Hodgkin's lymphomas. *Acta Pathol. Jpn.*, **29**, 739–758 (1979).

11. Mitsui, T., Kikuchi, M., Eimoto, T., Nishiuchi, M., and Toyooka, R. Non-Hodgkin's lymphoma in northwestern Kyushu Island of Japan: Clinicopathological studies based on the Japanese classification of malignant lymphoma. *Acta Pathol. Jpn.*, unpublished.

12. Said, J. W. and Pinkus, G. S. Immunoblastic sarcoma of the T cell type. An ultrastructural study of five cases. *Am. J. Pathol.*, **101**, 515–525 (1981).

13. Shamoto, M., Murakami, S., and Zenke, T. Adult T-cell leukemia in Japan. An ultrastructural study. *Cancer*, **47**, 1804–1811 (1981).

14. Stein, H., Tolksdorf, G., and Lennert, K. T-cell lymphomas. A cell origin-related classification on the basis of cytologic, immunologic, and enzyme cytochemical criteria. *Path. Res. Pract.*, **171**, 197–215 (1981).

15. Suchi, T., Tajima, K., Nanba, K., Wakasa, H., Mikata, A., Kikuchi, M., Mori, S., Watanabe, S., Mohri, N., Shamoto, M., Harigaya, K., Itagaki, T., Matsuda, M., Kirino, Y., Takagi, K., and Fukunaga, S. Some problems on the histopathological diagnosis of non-Hodgkin's malignant lymphoma.—A proposal for a new type—. *Acta Pathol. Jpn.*, **29**, 755–776 (1979).

16. Takatsuki, K., Uchiyama, T., Sagawa, K., and Yodoi, J. Adult T cell leukemia in Japan. *In* "Topics in Hematology," ed. S. Seno, F. Takaku, and S. Irino, pp. 73–77 (1977). Excerpta Medica, Amsterdam.

17. Tatsumi, E., Takiuchi, Y., Domae, N., Shirakawa, S., Uchino, H., Baba, M., Yasuhira, K., and Morikawa, S. Suppressive activity of some leukemic T cells from adult patients in Japan. *Clin. Immunopathol.*, **15**, 190–199 (1980).

18. Uchiyama, T., Sagawa, K., Takatsuki, K., and Uchino, H. Effect of adult T cell leukemia cells on pokeweed mitogen-induced normal B cell differentiation. *Clin. Immunol. Immunopathol.*, **10**, 24–34 (1978).

19. Waldron, J. A., Leech, J. H., Glick, A. L., Flexner, J. M., and Collins, R. D. Malignant lymphoma of peripheral T-lymphocyte origin. *Cancer*, **40**, 1604–1617 (1977).

20. Watanabe, S., Shimosato, Y., and Shimoyama, M. Lymphoma and leukemia of T-lymphocytes. *In* "Pathology Annual, Part 2," ed. S. C. Sommers and P. P. Rosen, pp. 155–203 (1981). Appleton-Century-Crofts, New York.

EXPLANATION OF PHOTOS

PHOTO 1. Characteristic leukemic cell with lobated nucleus. Giemsa staining, ×1,950.

PHOTO 2. Medium-sized cell type. Diffuse proliefration of tumor cells with maple leaf-like nuclei. Hematoxylin-eosin (H-E) staining, ×780.

PHOTO 3. Medium-sized cell type. Concentric arrangement of tumor cells around small blood vessels. H-E staining, ×780.

PHOTO 4. Large cell type. Proliferating large lymphoid cells and some neoplastic giant cells with many reactive histiocytes. H-E staining, ×780.

PHOTO 5. Pleomorphic type. Diffuse proliferation of small, medium-sized and large lymphoid cells accompanied by neoplastic giant cells. H-E staining, ×390.

PHOTO 6. Pleomorphic type. Details of tumor cells with maple leaf-like nuclei and giant cells. H-E staining, ×780.

PHOTO 7. Pleomorphic type. Giant cell with cerebriform nucleus. H-E staining, ×1,950.

PHOTO 8. Pleomorphic type. Giant cell of Reed-Sternberg type. H-E staining, ×1,950.

PHOTO 9. Pleomorphic type. Atypical lymphoid cells passing through well developed epithelioid venules. H-E staining, ×780.

PHOTO 10. Pleomorphic type. Preserved peripheral sinuses containing tumor cells. PAS staining, ×195.

PHOTO 11. Acid α-naphthyl acetate esterase (ANAE). Dot or pointed reaction. ×780.

PHOTO 12. Acid phosphatase (AcP). Dot or perinuclear capping reaction. ×780.

PHOTO 13. ATPase. Apparent membranous reaction. ×780.

Photo 14.   Electron micrograph of ATL showing an infiltration of large and some medium-sized cells. Note the markedly irregular nuclei. The large cell nuclei show scattered heterochromatin ("speckled" pattern) as well as prominent nucleoli. × 3,250.

Photo 15.   Higher power view showing the cytoplasmic details as well as nuclear irregularity of tumor cells. Note abundant polysomes, prominent vesicles in many cells, and poorly developed rough endoplasmic reticulum (ER). × 8,250.

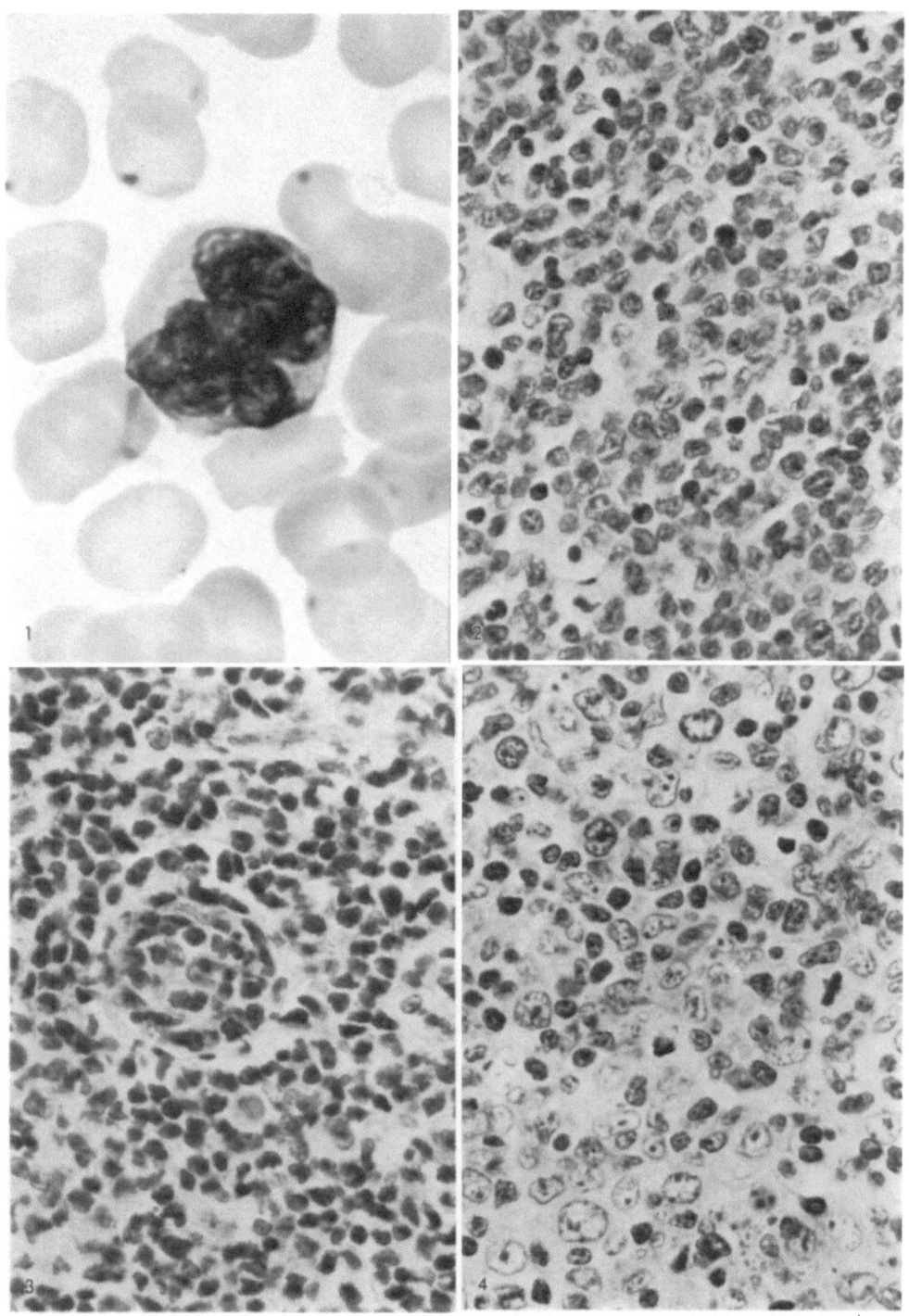

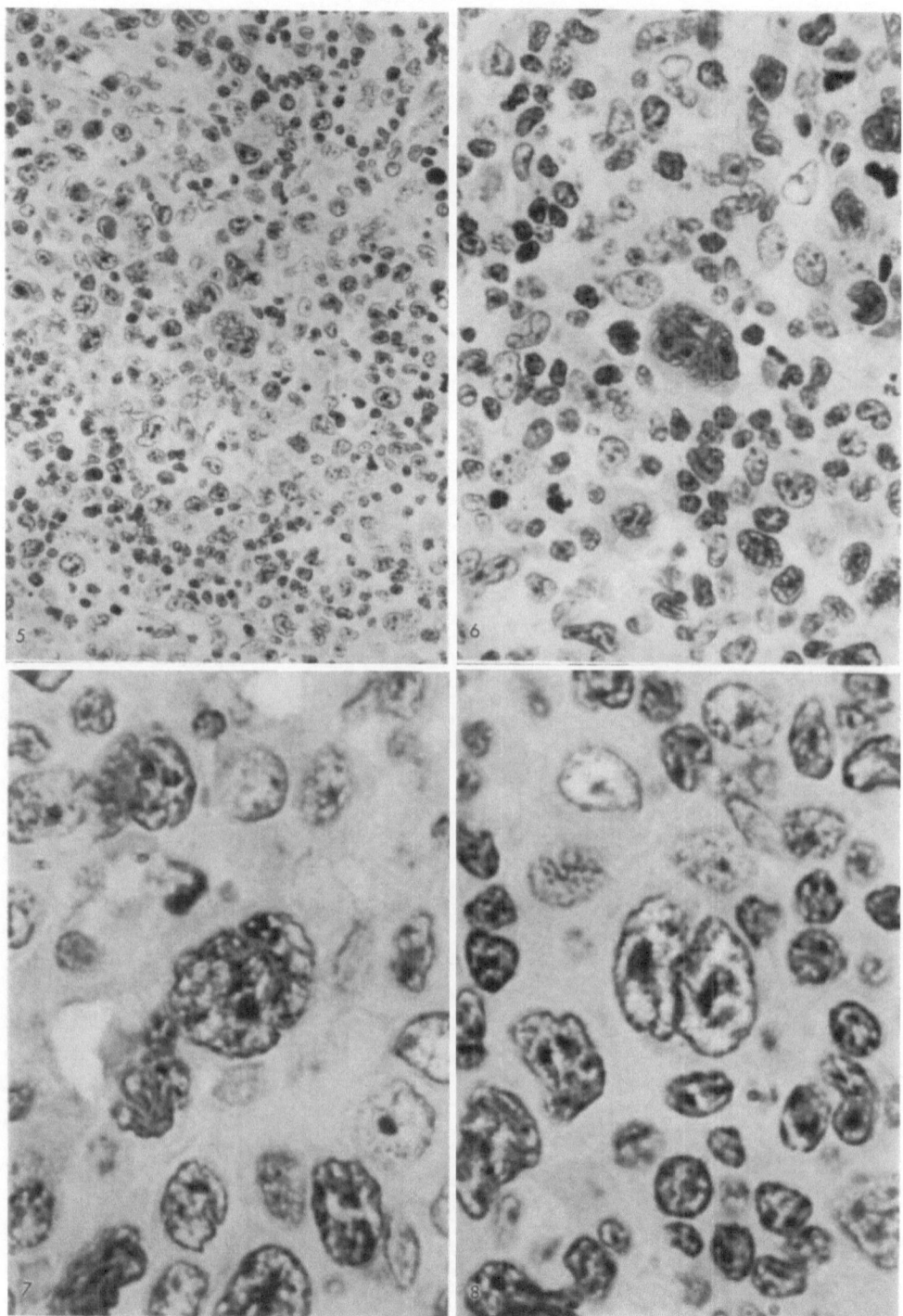

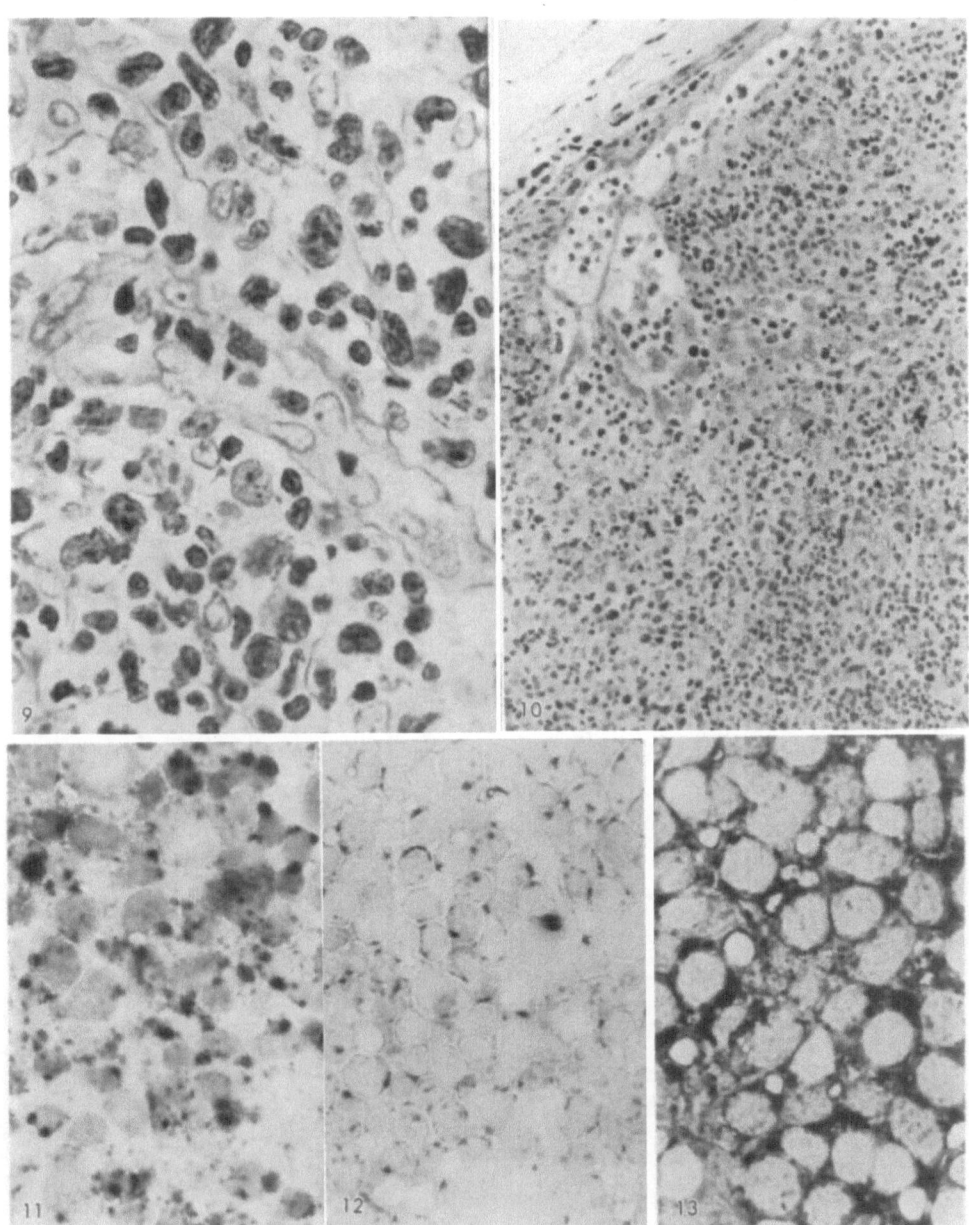

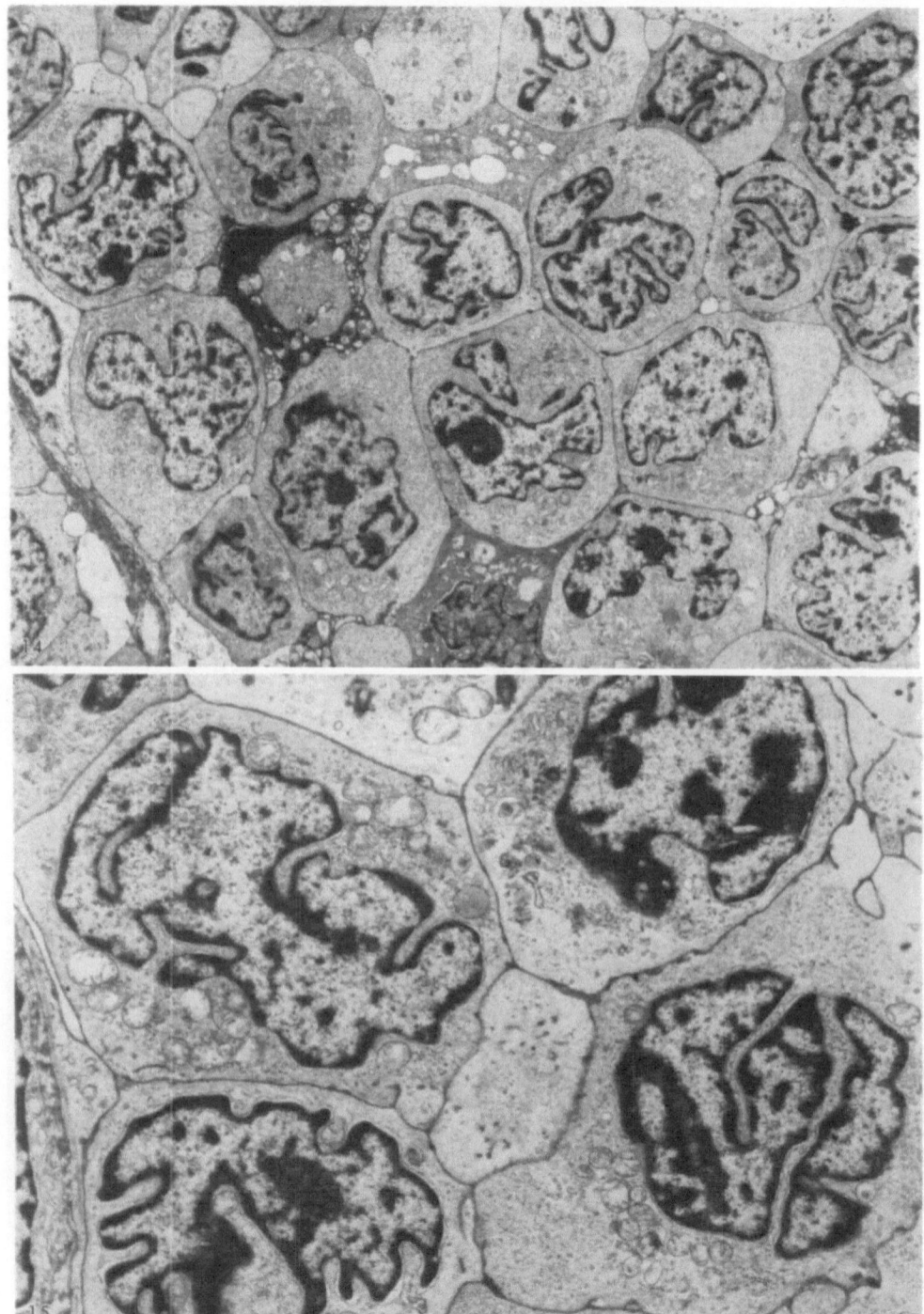

AUTOPSY FINDINGS OF ADULT T CELL LYMPHOMA-LEUKEMIA

Eiichi Sato, Kazuhisa Hasui, and Masayoshi Tokunaga

*Department of Pathology, Faculty of Medicine, Kagoshima University**

Based on a histological evaluation of 48 autopsy cases in which 75 biopsy specimens were compared, this report indicates that adult T cell lymphoma-leukemia appears to originate from the peripheral lymphatic tissues. The tumor cells reveal a more conspicuous pleomorphism at autopsy than in biopsy. Among the three groups of adult T cell leukemia, peripheral T cell lymphoma, and cutaneous T cell lymphoma, classified by the clinical course, some subtle differences are discerned in biological behavior, the spread of tumor cells and the response to therapy. Most of the patients died rapidly of severe lung complications, mainly because of opportunistic infections of *Pneumocystis carinii*, cytomegalovirus, herpes virus, *Aspergillus*, *Candida* or *Cryptococcus*. These resulted from an immunodeficiency which is detectable morphologically as a severe depletion of the normally functioning lymphocytes, even from uninvolved lymphatic organs such as the spleen and the tonsil.

Despite the fairly good descriptions of the histological and ultrastructural appearances of tumor cells in adult T cell lymphoma-leukemia (ATLL) based on the observation of biopsy specimens (*2, 4, 5, 7, 14, 19, 20, 25*), documentation of autopsy findings seems rare. This is despite the fact that some 6 years have elapsed since the identification of adult T cell leukemia (ATL) by Takatsuki *et al.* as a disease entity (*15, 22*).

Our previous reports (*10, 21*) and some others (*2, 17*) on the autopsy findings of ATLL indicate that most of the patients with ATLL died of severe complications of the lung, caused by immunodeficiency after chemotherapy.

In this report we present further results of observations on 48 necropsy subjects with a clinical diagnosis of ATLL by the analysis of tumor cell markers which were autopsied in our department during the 6 years from 1976 to 1981. The clinical records and histological material of these patients were reviewed. Seventy-five biopsy specimens of the lymph nodes or the skin from 37 patients were also available for the study, and these histological findings were compared with those of the autopsy material.

The autopsy cases were divided into three groups, ATL, peripheral T cell lymphoma (PTML), and cutaneous T cell lymphoma (CTCL), according to the clinical course (*1, 3, 9, 11*).

Twenty-five cases which revealed a leukemic manifestation at the time of the first hospitalization were grouped as ATL. PTML was experienced by 17 patients who showed a swelling of lymph nodes or tonsils and were not leukemic at the early stage

* Usuki-cho 1208-1, Kagoshima 890, Japan (佐藤栄一, 蓮井和久, 徳永正義).

of the disease. Six patients were classified as CTCL whose skin tumors preceded the development of universal symptoms and no signs of leukemia or lymphoma were initially seen. Cases with typical findings of mycosis fungoides were excluded from this study.

Clinical Data

Age: The age of the 48 patients at autopsy ranged from 22–76 years (Table I). Their average age was 57.4 years for males and 50.4 years for females.

Sex: There were 30 males and 18 females.

Clinical course: The average duration of the disease from onset of symptoms to death was 4.9 ± 2.8 months for ATL, 10.4 ± 8.3 for PTML, and 39.5 ± 16.0 for CTCL. The

TABLE I. Clinical Data: Age and Sex by Disease Type

Age	ATL		PTML		CTCL		TTL
	Male	Female	Male	Female	Male	Female	
20–		1		1			2
30–				1			1
40–	3	2	3	2			10
50–	7	5	3	1	2	1	19
60–	4	3	4	1	3		15
70–			1				1
Total	14	11	11	6	5	1	48

TABLE II. Major Initial Signs and Symptoms in ATL by Disease Type

	ATL	PTML	CTCL
Skin eruption and tumor	5 (20%)	4 (23.5%)	6 (100%)
Lymph node swelling	7 (28%)	11 (64.7%)	0
Tonsilar swelling	1 (4%)	2 (11.8%)	0
Leukemia	9 (36%)	0	0
Fever	2 (8%)	2 (11.8%)	0
General fatigue	12 (48%)	0	0
Loss of appetite	2 (8%)	0	0
Headache	2 (8%)	0	0
Nausea and vomiting	2 (8%)	0	0
Abdominal pain and discomfort	6 (24%)	4 (23.5%)	0
Diarrhea	1 (4%)	1 (5.9%)	0
Lumbago	2 (8%)	2 (11.8%)	0
Joint pain	1 (4%)	2 (11.8%)	0
Pneumonia	1 (4%)	1 (5.9%)	0
Cough	2 (8%)	2 (11.8%)	0
Dyspnea	1 (4%)	0	0
Sputum	2 (8%)	1 (5.9%)	0
Hepatomegaly	2 (8%)	0	0
Splenomegaly	2 (8%)	0	0
Osteolytic lesion	1 (4%)	1 (5.9%)	0
No. of cases	25	17	6

average period of time from clinical diagnosis to death was 4.0 ± 3.1 months for ATL, 5.5 ± 3.3 for PTML, and 39.5 ± 16.0 for CTCL. The major initial signs and symptoms are listed in Table II.

Therapy: Most of the patients had received combined chemotherapy such as VEPA, VEMP, MEPA, or ACOPP (*6, 9*).

Histopathology

1. Lymph node

In the biopsy material from the lymph nodes, the histology of ATLL in Kagoshima has mostly been characterized by its polymorphous features and termed the "pleomorphic type" according to the classification proposed by the Japanese Lymphoma Study Group (LSG-classification) (*13*). However, in detailed observations of more than 130 cases, we have noted that the histological features are extremely variegated, showing a relatively monomorphous pattern to a highly polymorphous appearance, modified not only by the shape of the tumor cells themselves but also by the amount of intermingling of other non-neoplastic components such as histiocytes and plasma cells.

The histology of lymph nodes from autopsy materials reveals a much more advanced variety than in biopsy, influenced partly by many kinds of therapy, infections, and partly by the mode of proliferation or spread of the tumor cells. Generally speaking, the tumor cells at autopsy showed a highly conspicuous pleomorphism with the frequent appearance of giant cells containing Reed-Sternberg's cell-like nuclei and other bizarre features, although there were rare exceptions in which the tumor cells disclosed less pleomorphism at autopsy than in biopsy (Photos 1, 2). It was not infrequently observed that different findings were obtained from the lymph nodes at different sites in the same subject (Photos 3, 4). Among the lymph nodes involved, the retroperitoneal nodes revealed the most prominent feature of tumor cell proliferation and cellular variety, including most notably several kinds of giant cells. The axillary, cervical and/or inguinal lymph nodes sometimes showed loosely dispersed or sporadic infiltration of tumor cells, despite the fact that massive growth was seen in the retroperitoneal nodes. The prevalence of involvement by sites of the lymph nodes is given in Table III.

Comparing the size of lymph nodes of ATL with that of PTML, the former gave an impression of smaller swelling than the latter in rough estimation. In evaluating the histology of autopsy materials, a relatively loose or sparse proliferation was present in 8 cases of ATL, whereas such proliferation was seen in only 3 at biopsy. On the other hand, the loosened proliferation was evaluated only in one case of PTML at autopsy

TABLE III. Lymph Node Involvement in ATLL

Location of lymph node	Positive/No. examined	Percent
Cervical	35/47	74.5
Axillary	20/38	52.6
Mediastinal	28/47	59.6
Bronchial	36/48	75.0
Abdominal	31/48	64.6
Retroperitoneal	31/48	64.6
Inguinal	22/48	45.8

and a highly massive or packed growth pattern was common in PTML, although cohesiveness was usually lost in the autopsy materials as a postmortem phenomenon. Probably related to the effect of the drugs, an extremely decreased parenchyma in lymph nodes was occasionally demonstrated, especially in the cases of CTCL. In such cases only the skeletal framework composed of sinus lining cells, lymph and blood vessels, some fibrocytes, abundant histiocytes, and a few lymphocytes remained (Photos 5, 6). Other findings in relation to the effect of the treatment were extensive necrosis of tumor tissue surrounded by histiocytes and fibroblasts, focal fibrosis and pyknosis of tumor cell nuclei. In some cases activated histiocytes were proliferating in the sinuses and medullary cords, phagocytizing many degenerative materials and erythrocytes (Photos 7, 8). The starry sky appearance was rare in ATLL.

2. Tonsil

Among the cases with initial involvement of the tonsils two were autopsied, terminating in systemic invasion of the tumor cells. The secondary involvement of the tonsils was histologically confirmed in 22 cases (59.5%). In many cases, the parenchyma of the tonsil and lymphatic apparatus of the Waldeyer's ring tended to be atrophic.

3. Thymus

None of the autopsy cases showed enlargement of the thymus in gross observation. Microscopically a few atypical cells were very occasionally seen in this organ which was generally very small (Table IV). Thus, neither the origin nor the obvious involvement of ATLL was recognized in the thymus.

4. Spleen

The spleen was the organ most frequently involved in ATLL (81.3%). Usually a diffuse or reticular-like infiltration of tumor cells was observed in the red pulp, in the sinuses, around the trabeculae and/or around and in the lymphoid follicles; in the latter

TABLE IV.   Visceral Involvement in ATLL

	Positive/No. examined	Percent
Spleen	39/48	81.3
Liver	29/48	60.4
Tonsil	22/37	59.5
Bone marrow	28/42	58.3
Lung	26/48	54.2
Adrenal	24/48	50.0
Kidney	20/48	41.7
Pancreas	15/48	31.3
Stomach	14/48	29.2
Urogenital	14/48	29.2
Intestine	12/48	25.0
Central nervous system	7/28	25.0
Esophagus	10/48	20.8
Heart	8/48	16.7
Thyroid	8/48	16.7
Thymus	3/45	6.3

case a vague nodular pattern was shown. There was also the combined feature of nodular and diffuse infiltration in some cases when the amount of tumor cells was plentiful (Photos 9, 10). A distinct nodular lesion composed of an admixture of mononuclear cells and bizarre multinucleated giant cells was found in one female case of ATL with an 11 year history of skin rash (Photo 4).

In the majority of cases, lymphocytes around the small arteries, T zone lymphocytes, were decreased in degrees from mild to complete depletion (Photo 11).

5. Liver

Although hepatosplenomegaly has sometimes been pointed out clinically (9), the involvement of the liver was generally not as severe as the spleen. The tumor cells were diffusely scattered or sporadically infiltrating in the sinusoid or aggregated in Glisson's sheaths, when present.

6. Bone marrow

Bone marrow was involved in more than half of the cases, although it was occasionally inconspicuous, probably due to the effect of therapy. There was a case where the first symptom appeared as a bone tumor and swelling of lymph nodes was not apparent. An amputation of the left leg was performed after the pathological diagnosis of T cell lymphoma. Four months later, autopsy disclosed a mild infiltration of tumor cells mainly in the paratracheal and inguinal lymph nodes. The patient died of a generalized infection of cytomegalovirus and *Cryptococcus* after strong chemotherapy (Photo 12).

7. Lung

The lung was involved quite frequently in ATLL, although the degree and the involvement sites varied. Sometimes it was difficult to distinguish neoplastic cells from the lymphoid infiltrates when they were of the small cell type.

Besides the involvement, severe complications were very conspicuous in many cases of ATLL. Several kinds of opportunistic infections were observed, among them *Pneumocystis carinii*, cytomegalovirus, herpes virus, *Aspergillus*, *Candida*, *Cryptococcus*, and *Klebsiella* were most common agents (Table V; Photos 13–15). There were sometimes mixed infections, causing a severe interstitial pneumonia and associated with the exudation of protein-rich fluid, edema, hyaline membrane formation and hemorrhage, occasionally without a cellular reaction. Formation of abscess and cavity, diffuse fibrosis and granulomatous lesions were also not infrequently noticed. A fresh deposition of calcium along the alveolar septa due to hypercalcemia was seen in 11 patients (Photo 16).

TABLE V. Prevalence of Opportunistic Infection in 48 Autopsy Subjects with ATL

Agents	No. case	Percent
Cytomegalovirus	24	50.0
Pneumocystis carinii	17	35.4
Herpes virus	6	12.5
Aspergillus	5	10.4
Cryptococcus	3	6.25

8. Other organs

The adrenals were frequently involved, predominantly in the deep cortex. More than one-third had ATLL in the kidney, pancreas, and gastro-intestinal tract. The heart and the thyroid had the least involvement. In the central nervous system, there were mild but suspicious infiltrations in the leptomeniges. Some cases showed an increased number of macrophages in the arachnoid where tumor cells were not obviously found. In one case of CTCL, neoplastic bizarre giant cells invaded destructively into the perivascular area of the white matter of the cerebrum (Photos 17–20).

COMMENTS

These studies seem to confirm that ATLL originates from the peripheral lymphatic system including the tonsils and possibly the bone marrow. It exhibits an extremely variable histopathological appearance, not only in its own neoplastic cells but also by a coexistence of "reactive" cells. The results of these studies also suggest that the mode of tumor cell growth, the biological behavior and response to therapy appear to be somewhat different among the 3 groups of ATL, PTML, and CTCL, even though they all represent T cell malignancies of peripheral origin and manifest leukemic features sooner or later.

Total effacement of the normal structure of the lymph nodes by ATLL was a usual finding in the autopsy materials, in contrast to occasional partial retention of normal structure in biopsy (2). Generally, the basal stromal architecture was discernible in autopsy cases, especially in ATL and CTCL, with mild swelling of the lymph nodes in which cellular proliferation was strongly suppressed by combined chemotherapy, resulting in severe depletion of normal lymphocytes not only from the lymph nodes but also from other lymphatic organs including the spleen. These processes of reduction of normal lymphocytes may so alter the peripheral blood that the decreased population of T cells which bear receptors for IgG and of K cells are detectable (26). In such a condition of T cell deficiency, combined with the possible influences of the suppressor function of tumor cells (23), several opportunistic infections may develop rapidly. Most patients with ATLL died of severe lung complications, many of which are shown as interstitial pneumonia. However, it is of note that an interstitial fibrosis can be caused by the side-effects of cyclophosphamide in patients with malignant lymphoma (12).

From the histological appearances seen in biopsy materials, it has been repeatedly emphasized that ATLL has a resemblance to Hodgkin's disease, mycosis fungoides (MF) and to histiocytic medullary reticulosis. As a matter of fact, some cases of ATLL have been confused with Hodgkin's disease (16, 24). For the differential diagnosis, attention should be focused on atypism of small lymphocytes intermingling in the background (8). The relationship of ATLL to MF has not yet been elucidated. In our series, some cases of CTCL strongly resembled MF, even though the dermatological findings differed (3). The autopsy examination disclosed a different mode of spreading: MF has been said to invade preferentially the T zone of the spleen (18), whereas CTCL did not. However, CTCL in this series might be in an intermediate position to MF and the usual ATLL, as a relatively prolonged clinical course of the disease has been noted in CTCL (11).

REFERENCES

1. Broader, S. and Bunn, P. A. Cutaneous T-cell lymphomas. *Semin. Oncol.*, **7**, 310–331 (1980).
2. Hanaoka, M., Sasaki, M., Matsumoto, H., Tankawa, H., Yamabe, H., Tomimoto, K., Tasaka, C., Fujiwara, H., Uchiyama, T., and Takatsuki, K. Adult T cell leukemia histological classification and characteristics. *Acta Phathol. Jpn.*, **29** (5), 723–738 (1979).
3. Kaneko, K. Clinical and histopathological studies on cutaneous lymphoma with special reference to prognostic factors. *Jpn. J. Dermatol.*, **91**, 1817–1830 (1981).
4. Katsuda, K. Clinicopathological study of malignant lymphoma involving Waldeyer's ring. *Otologia*, **25** (Suppl. 5), 664–676 (1979).
5. Kikuchi, M., Mitsui, T., Matsui, N., Sato, E., Tokunaga, M., Hasui, K., Ichimaru, M., Kinoshita, K., and Kamihira, S. T-cell malignancies in adults: Histopathological studies of lymph nodes in 110 patients. *Jpn. J. Clin. Oncol.*, **9** (Suppl.), 407–422 (1979).
6. Lymphoma Study Group. Combination chemotherapy with vincristine, cyclophosphamide (Endoxan), prednisolone and adriamycin (VEPA) in advanced adult non-Hodgkin's lymphoid malignancies: Relation between T-cell or non-T-cell phenotype and response. *Jpn. J. Clin. Oncol.*, **9** (Suppl.), 397–406 (1979).
7. Matsumoto, T., Matsumoto, M., Yunoki, K., Hanada, S., Nomura, K., and Hashimoto, S. *In vitro* generation of multinucleated giant cells from pleomorphic T-cell leukemia-lymphoma lymphocytes. *Jpn. J. Clin. Oncol.*, **9** (Suppl.), 451–458 (1979).
8. Mikata, A. Hodgkin's disease. *In* "Atlas of Malignant Lymphoma According to New Classification," ed. M. Kojima, S. Iijima, M. Hanaoka, and T. Suchi, pp. 79–84 (1981). Bunko-do, Tokyo (in Japanese).
9. Nomura, K. and Matsumoto, M. Clinical features of adult T-cell leukemia in Kagoshima, the southernmost district in Japan—Comparison with T-cell lymphoma—. *Acta Haematol. Jpn.*, **44**, 1444–1457 (1981).
10. Sato, E., Tokunaga, M., and Hasui, K. Pathology of non-Hodgkin's lymphoma in Kagoshima prefecture, with special reference to adult T cell lymphoma. *Jpn. J. Clin. Hematol.*, **20**, 1070–1082 (1979).
11. Shimoyama, M., Minato, K., Saito, H., Kitahara, T., Konda, C., Nakazawa, M., Watanabe, S., Inada, N., Nagatani, T., Deura, K., and Mikata, A. Comparisons of clinical, morphologic and immunologic characteristics of adult T-cell leukemia-lymphoma and cutaneous T-cell lymphoma. *Jpn. J. Clin. Oncol.*, **9** (Suppl.), 357–372 (1979).
12. Snider, G. L. and Mark, E. J. Diffuse pulmonary infiltrates in a patient with lymphoma —Case records of the Massachusetts General Hospital. *N. Engl. J. Med.*, **306**, 469–476 (1982).
13. Suchi, T., Tajima, D., Nanba, K., Wakasa, H., Mikata, A., Kikuchi, M., Mori, S., Watanabe, S., Mohri, N., Shamoto, M., Harigaya, K., Itagaki, T., Matsuda, M., Kirino, Y., Takagi, K., and Fukunaga, S. Some problems on the histopathological diagnosis of non-Hodgkin's malignant lymphoma—A proposal of a new type—. *Acta Pathol. Jpn.*, **29** (5), 755–776 (1979).
14. Suchi, T. and Tajima, K. Peripheral T-cell malignancy as a problem in lymphoma classification. *Jpn. J. Clin. Oncol.*, **9** (Suppl.), 443–450 (1979).
15. Takatsuki, K. Clinical features of T and B lymphocytic tumors—with special reference to T cell leukemia as a new disease entity. *J. Jpn. Med. Assoc.*, **75**, 379–387 (1976).
16. Teshima, S. and Watanabe, S. Hodgkin's disease in Japan—An examination on 110 cases in National Cancer Hospital—. *J. Jpn. Soc. RES*, **19**, 347–355 (1979) (in Japanese).
17. Terashi, S., Yoshii, H., Otsuji, A., Kaneko, Y., Koike, M., Nagi, Y., and Isaka, H.

Histopathological studies on autopsy cases of adult T-cell leukemia. *Proc. Jpn. Cancer Assoc.*, **37**, 278 (1978) (in Japanese).

18. Thomas, L. B. and Rappaport, H. Mycosis fungoides and its relationship to other malignant lymphomas. *In* "The Reticuloendothelial System," ed. J. W. Rebuck, C. W. Berard, and M. R. Abell, pp. 243–261 (1975). The Williams & Wilkins Co., Baltimore.
19. Tokunaga, M. and Sato, E. Non-Hodgkin's lymphomas in a southern prefecture in Japan: An analysis of 715 cases. *Cancer*, **46**, 1231–1239 (1980).
20. Tokunaga, M., Sato, E., Tanaka, S., and Sakai, M. Malignant lymphoma occurring in Kagoshima prefecture, Japan: Pathological and descriptive epidemiological survey based on 849 biopsy materials. *Gann*, **69**, 673–678 (1978).
21. Tokunaga, M., Hasui, K., Sato, E., and Terashi, S. An autopsy study of non-Hodgkin's lymphoma in Kagoshima prefecture. *Proc. Jpn. Cancer Assoc.*, **39**, 271 (1980) (in Japanese).
22. Uchiyama, T., Yodoi, J., Sagawa, K., Takatsuki, K., and Uchino, H. Adult T-cell leukemia: Clinical and hematologic features of 16 cases. *Blood*, **50**, 481–492 (1977).
23. Uchiyama, T., Sagawa, K., Takatsuki, K., and Uchino, H. Effect of adult T cell leukemia cells on pokeweed mitogen-induced normal B cell differentiation. *Clin. Immunol. Immunopathol.*, **10**, 24–34 (1978).
24. Wakasa, H. Hodgkin's disease in Asia, particularly in Japan. *Natl. Cancer Inst. Monogr.*, **36**, 15–22 (1973).
25. Waldron, J. A., Leech, J. H., Glick, A. D., Flexner, J. M., and Collins, R. D. Malignant lymphoma of peripheral T-lymphocyte origin. *Cancer*, **40**, 1604–1617 (1977).
26. Yagi, Y., Hasui, K., and Sato, E. Population of killer cells and T-cells bearing receptors for IgG in lymphoproliferative disorders, with special reference to adult T-cell malignant lymphoma-leukemia. *Jpn. J. Clin. Oncol.*, **11** (2), 299–306 (1981).

EXPLANATION OF PHOTOS

PHOTO 1.   Biopsy of cervical lymph nodes, revealing monotonous proliferation of large lymphoma cells. Hematoxylin-eosin (H-E) staining, ×132.

PHOTO 2.   Autopsy: same case as in Photo 1. More advanced pleomorphism than in Photo. 1. ×132.

PHOTO 3.   Biopsy: pleomorphic type containing relatively conspicuous non-neoplastic histiocytic cells with pale staining. H-E staining, ×132.

PHOTO 4.   Same case as in Photo 3. A nodular lesion in the spleen composed of highly atypical tumor cells. ×132.

PHOTO 5.   Autopsy, cervical lymph node, showing pronounced depletion of lymphocytes perdominantly from the paracortex. H-E staining, ×10.

PHOTO 6.   Axillary lymph node, showing a well preserved framework of the stroma, due to depletion of lymphocytes. H-E staining, ×10.

PHOTO 7.   Autopsy: marked proliferation of histiocytes and sporadic infiltration of atypical lymphoid cells. The feature has a resemblance to histiocytic medullary reticulosis. H-E staining ×13.2.

PHOTO 8.   High power view of Photo 7. A pattern similar to hemophagocytic reticulosis. H-E staining, ×132.

PHOTO 9.   Spleen: vague nodular proliferation of lymphoma cells in and around the area of white pulp. H-E staining, ×10.

PHOTO 10.   Spleen: high power view of Photo 8. Periarterial zone composed of variable cells. H-E staining, ×100.

PHOTO 11.   Spleen: severe depletion of lymphocytes in the periarterial zone. H-E staining, ×132.

PHOTO 12.   Peripancreatic lymph node with infection of *Cryptococcus* (pale staining), showing marked histolytic figure. ×132.

PHOTO 13.   Lung: showing interstitial pneumonia with many cytomegalic inclusion bodies, protein-rich exudate filling the alveolar lumen. H-E staining, ×50.

PHOTO 14.   Lung: methenamine silver stain, demonstrating *Pneumocystis carinii.* Atypical lymphocytes in alveolar septa and cytomegalic inclusions are also found. Methenamine-Silver impregnation. ×100.

PHOTO 15.   Lung: deposition of calcium along the alveolar septa due to hypercalcemia. H-E staining, ×25.

PHOTO 16.   Tongue: herpetic infection causing an ulcer. H-E staining, ×25.

PHOTO 17.   Photos 17–20 are taken from the same subject. The skin biopsied 4 years before death, showing a proliferation of hyperconvoluted relatively small cells. ×66.

PHOTO 18.   Lymph node biopsied 3 months before death. Note massive proliferation of large cells with distinct nucleoli. ×132.

PHOTO 19.   Skin at autopsy. Conspicuous proliferation of bizarre giant cells in contrast to the figure in Photo 17. ×132.

PHOTO 20.   Cerebrum: note perivascular infiltration of highly atypical tumor cells. H-E staining, ×66.

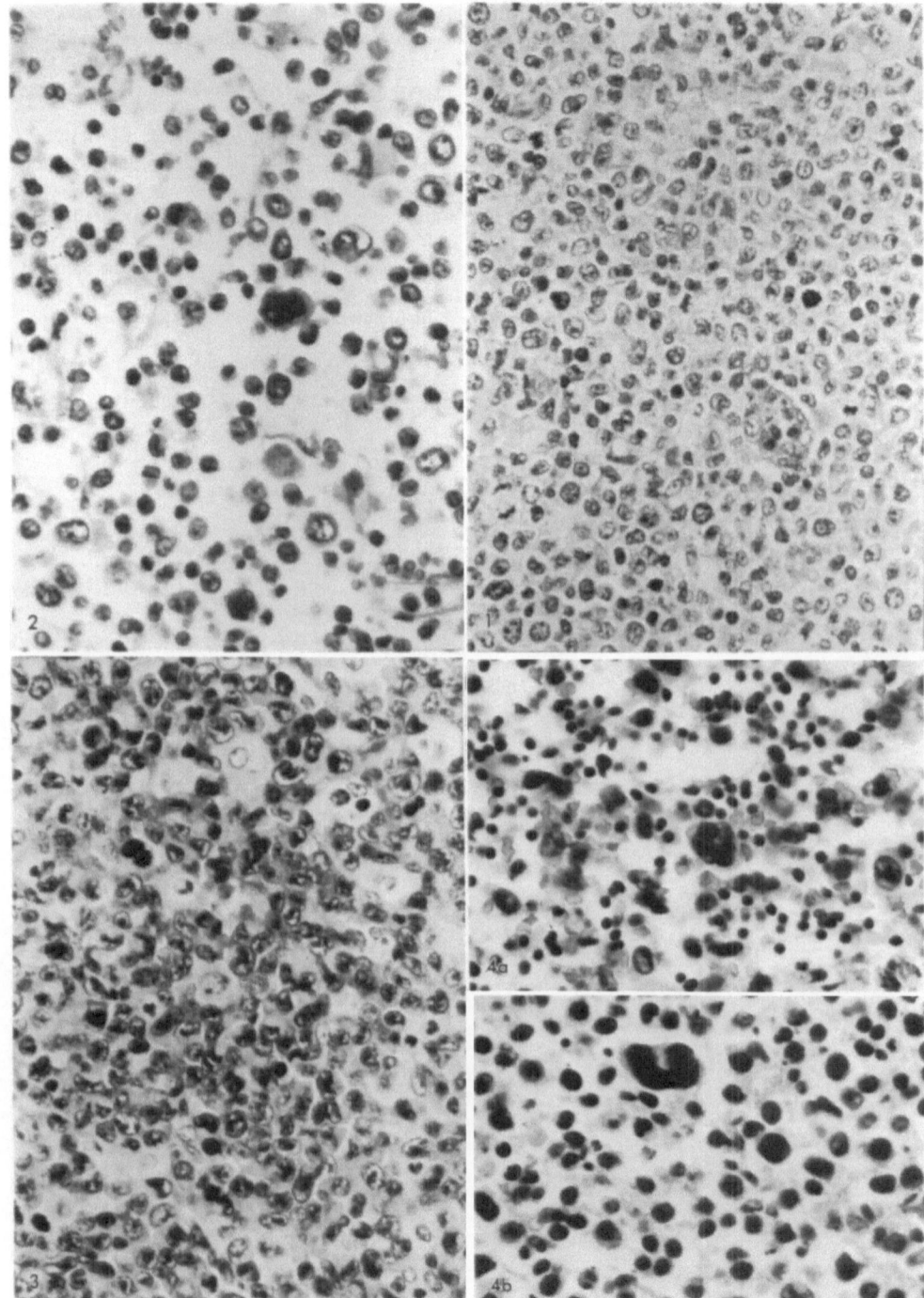

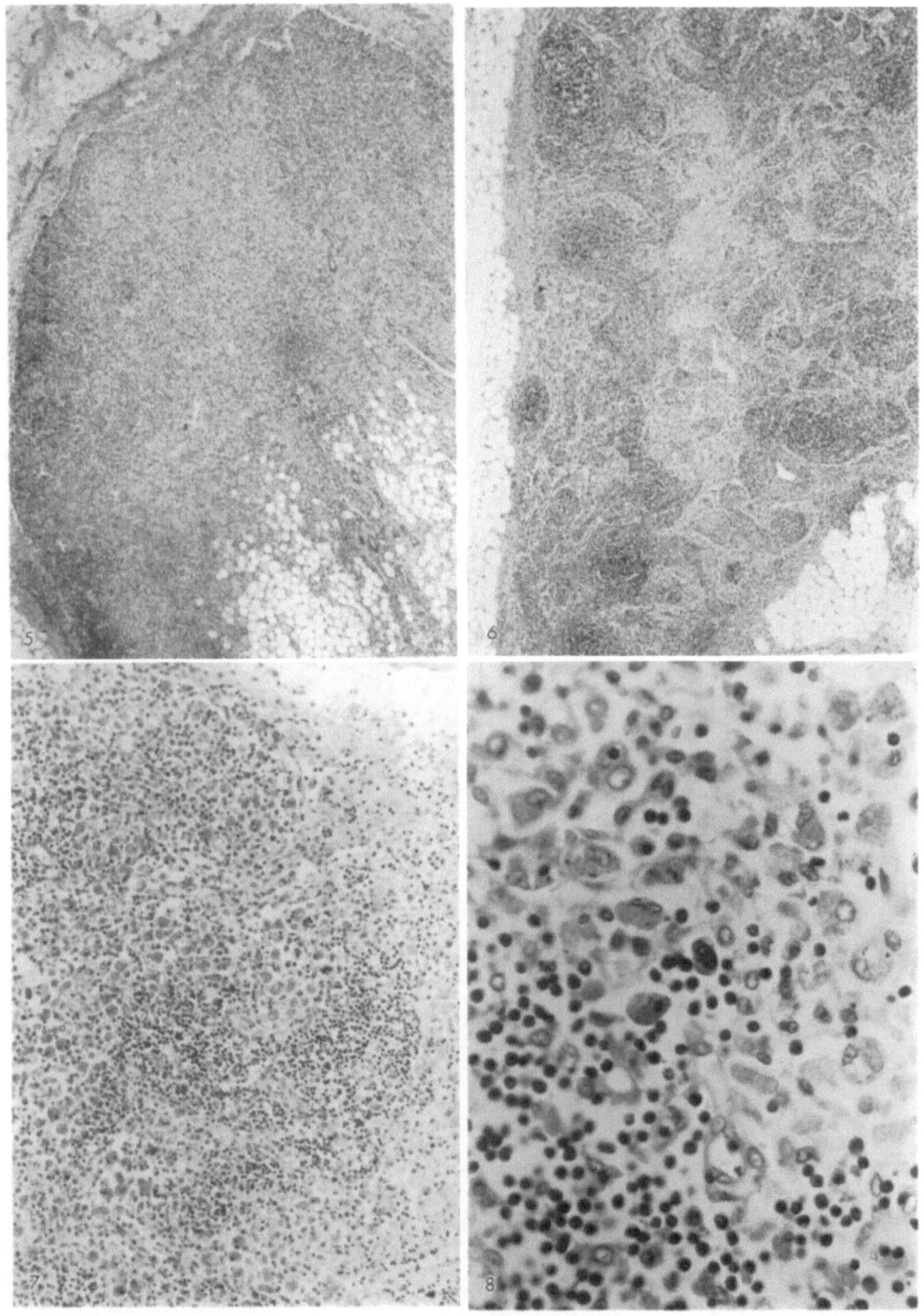

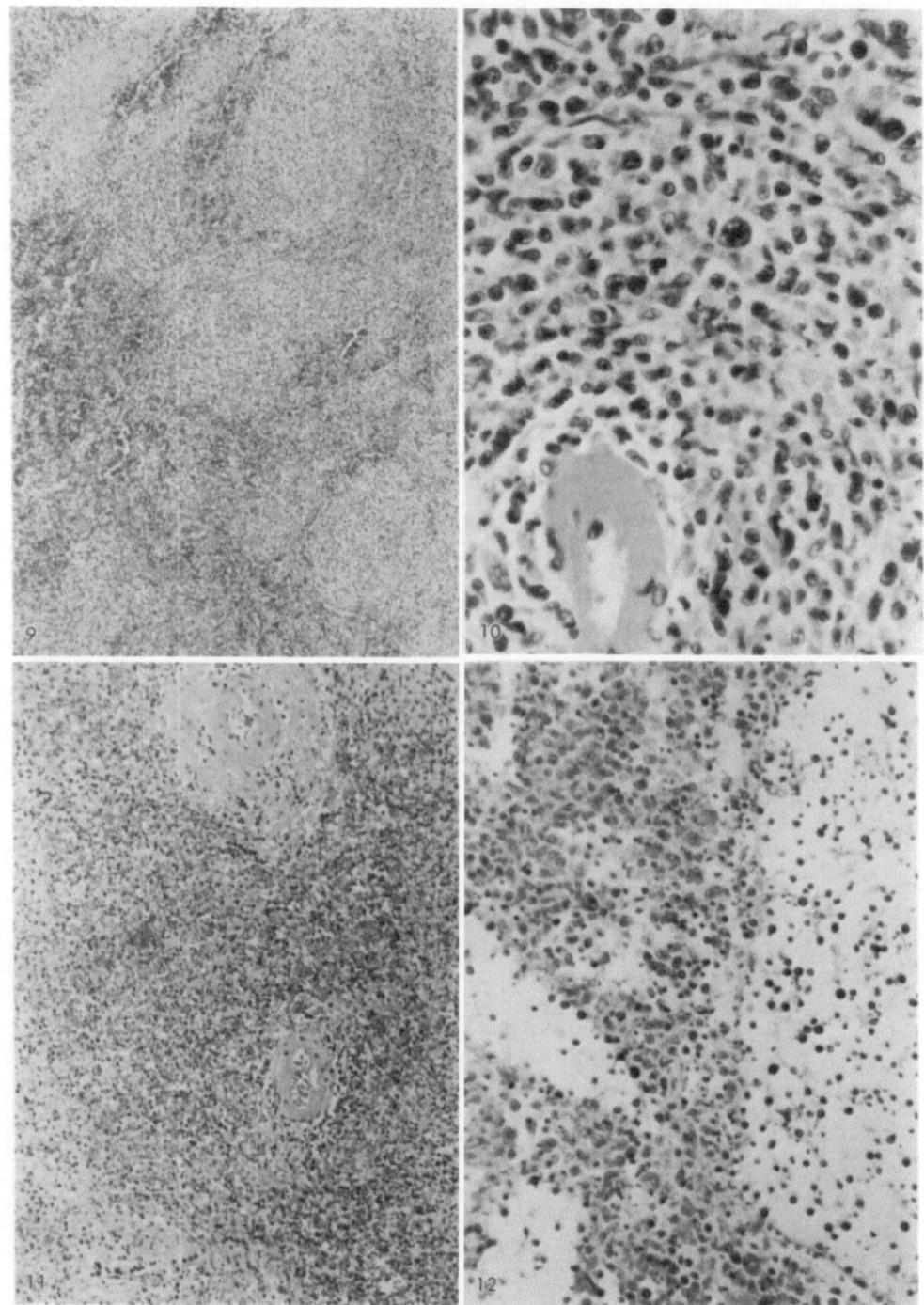

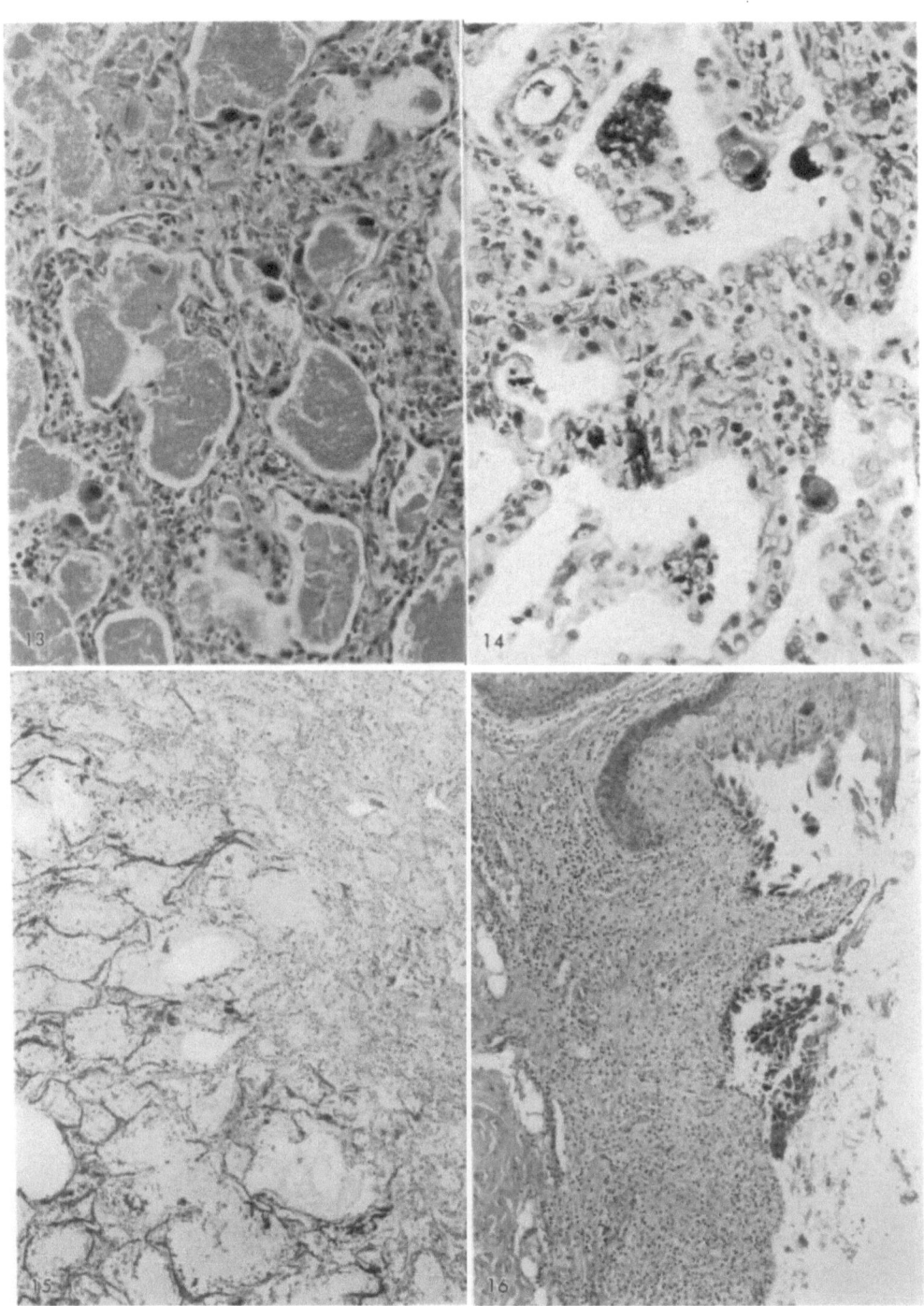

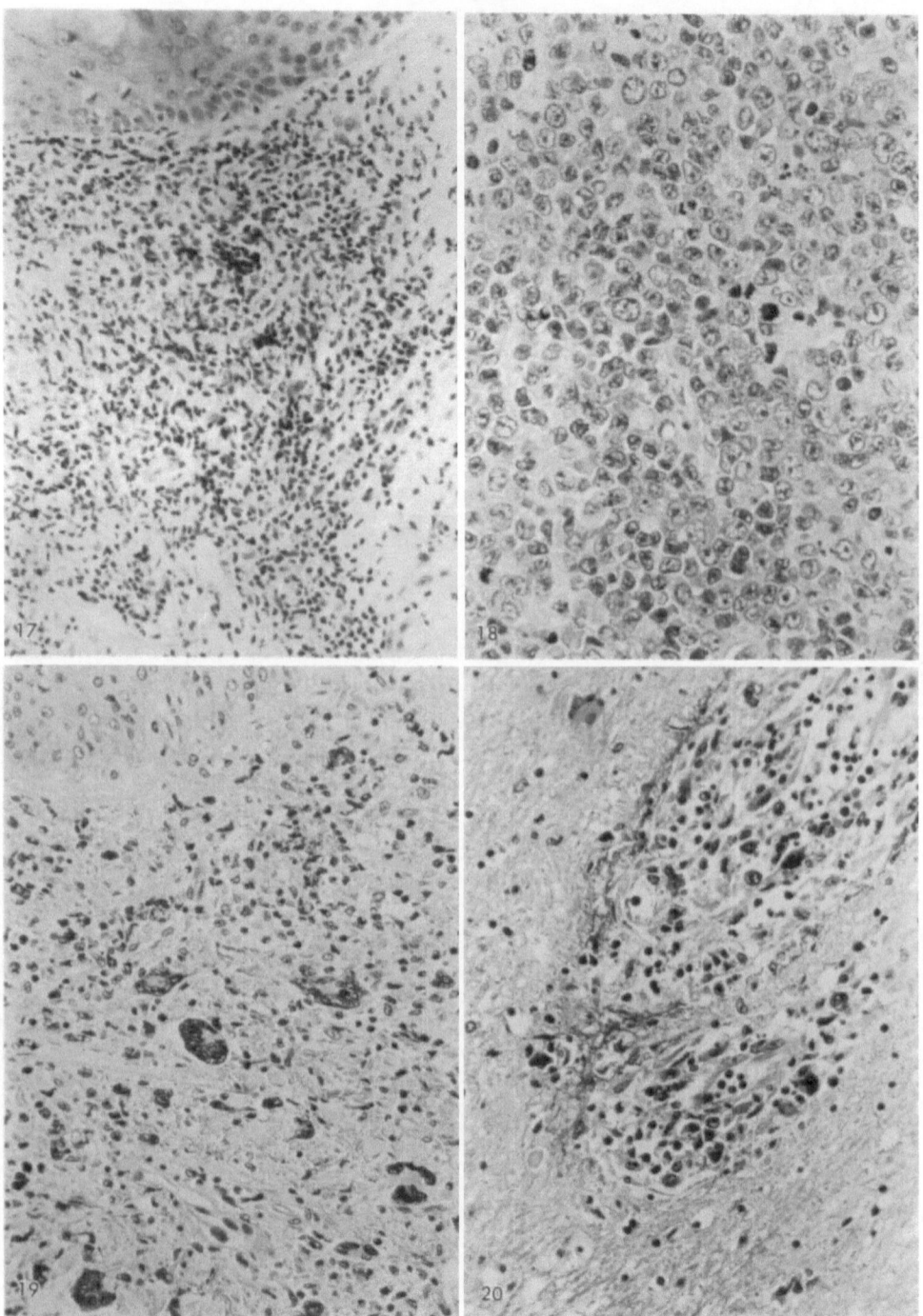

GANN Monograph on Cancer Research 28, 1982

ULTRASTRUCTURE AND DNA CYTOPHOTOMETRY OF ADULT T CELL LEUKEMIA-LYMPHOMA

Masayoshi Tokunaga, Kazuhisa Hasui, and Eiichi Sato

*2nd Department of Pathology, Faculty of Medicine, Kagoshima University**

The cellular characteristics of 34 cases of adult T-cell leukemia-lymphoma (ATLL) were analyzed by electron microscopy. The most prominent feature of ATLL was nuclear pleomorphism, primarily characterized by nuclear convolution, multilobulation, and fragmentation; the pleomorphic type particularly showed marked variation in nuclear size and shape. There were large cells which resembled Reed-Sternberg (R-S) cells in the pleomorphic type, but these differed from the true R-S cells of Hodgkin's disease because the nucleoli were not as prominent and the cytoplasm was poorly differentiated and contained abundant polysomes. Numerous Gall body-like lipid droplets, clustered dense bodies, and glycogen were observed in the cytoplasm. The DNA cytophotometry of the leukemic cases showed a histogram pattern of cellular proliferation in the diploid range with an increased S phase, and the pleomorphic type showed great variation in nuclear diameter and DNA content.

Malignant lymphomas of the T-cell type consist of a heterogeneous group derived from various stages of T-cells. They comprise a broad morphologic and clinical spectrum including lymphoblastic, "Lennert" type, mycosis fungoides, Sézary syndrome, node-based T-cell lymphoma, and adult T-cell leukemia-lymphoma (ATLL) (*1*). A special type of T-cell derived neoplasia named "adult T-cell leukemia (ATL)" appears to occur endemically in Japan (*3, 5, 8 9*). This ATL is a malignant lymphoma which occurs primarily in the lymph node, Waldyer's ring and bone marrow. This tumor is characterized morphologically by nuclear pleomorphism of the neoplastic cells with markedly deformed nuclei, and histological heterogeneous features frequently including an admixture with clusters of normal lymphocytes, proliferation of histiocytes and dendritic cells, and well developed venules (*3*). An ultrastructural study of 18 cases of ATLL showed a characteristic fine structure of slight to marked nuclear irregularity with convoluted-shape predominance, a speckled chromatin pattern of the large cells, prominent lysosomes, and glycogen accumulation in addition to the difference in cellular distribution (*2*). Similar findings (*6, 8*) of ultrastructural study of ATLL were previously reported. This report will include the ultrastructural features citing 34 patients of ATLL. Among 34 cases examined, 13 developed leukemia, and all of these leukemic patients died within 17 months with a median survival of 2.75 months. Among 21 non-leukemic cases, 15 patients died within a year and the median survival was 7 months. All of the patients examined were adults with a mean age of 57 years. The

---

* Usuki-cho 1208-1, Kagoshima 890, Japan (徳永正義, 蓮井和久, 佐藤栄一).

TABLE I. Histological Types of ATL Examined

	Number of cases	
	Leukemic group	Non-leukemic group
Diffuse lymphoma		
Small cell type	0	0
Medium-sized cell type	4	9
Mixed type	5	5
Large cell type	1	4
Pleomorphic type	3	3
Total	13	21

incidence in males was higher than in females, 2:1 in the leukemic cases and 3:1 in the non-leukemic cases.

Examination with the light microscope revealed a diffuse type growth pattern in all of the cases. Histological types of the cases studied using the classification of the Japanese Lymphoma Study Group (LSG) (7) are shown in Table I.

Electron Microscopic Findings under Low Power Magnification

All of the cases were characterized, as shown by light microscopy, by the preservation of the sinus structure and small venules, particularly in the leukemic cases. As shown in Photo 1, tumor cells of varied size and shape were observed in the tissue and dilatated sinuses. The tumor cells in the tissue had a tendency to become attached to each other (Photo 2) and also to the normal lymphocytes and histiocytes. Photo 3 shows the tumor cells in the skin attached to a histiocyte by long villi.

Nuclear Findings

The most distinctive feature of the ATLL was its nuclear appearance, even though the nuclear size differed in various histological types. The most characteristic type of ATLL "pleomorphic type" varied in size from that of a small lymphocyte to large histiocyte-like cells (Photo 1). Sometimes there were large multinucleated giant cells with nuclei resembling mirror images similar to Reed-Sternberg (R-S) cells in pleomorphic type. However, the nucleoli in these cells were not as prominent and the cytoplasm contained abundant polysomes instead of the prominent nucleoli and well developed cytoplasmic organelles characteristic of the true R-S cell. The nuclear shape ranged from ovoid in configuration with simple indentation to irregular with deep indentation and cleavage planes. Multilobulated nuclear shape observed in Sézary syndrome is also a prominent feature of ATLL (Photo 4). The nuclear chromatin profiles also varied, ranging from finely granular and dispersed to a clump of heterochromatin. The nucleoli were generally small and discrete but in some cases they were prominent and tended to be centrally located.

Cytoplasmic Findings

The cytoplasm varied from sparse to plentiful and showed undifferentiated organelles as well as ribosomes and rough endoplasmic reticulum. The pleomorphic type showed variable amounts of cytoplasm and contained abundant ribosomes with a few mitochondria. The cells with abundant cytoplasm showed increased numbers of mitochondria, endoplasmic reticulum and polysomes (Photo 4). There was a tendency toward an increase in nuclear irregularity with the decreasing number of mitochondria, endoplasmic reticulum, and polysomes. Then the cells of the medium-sized and mixed cell types showed relatively well developed organelles. In a few cases, poorly differentiated laminated rough endoplasmic reticulum was observed. The electron-lucent cytoplasm contained scattered polysomal aggregates and an inconspicuous Golgi apparatus. These findings were characteristic features of large T-immunoblasts (Photo 6). These features of the nuclear size and shape are thought to be the most representative characteristics of the pleomorphic type of ATLL. The medium-sized cell and mixed types with medium-sized and large cell were relatively uniform in size but numerous non-neoplastic elements such as lymphocytes, plasma cells, and histiocytes were observed (Photo 5). The large cell type also characterized by relatively uniform large cells measured more than 12 μm in diameter. These nuclei contained a fine chromatin pattern with peripheral clumping, as in immunoblasts.

Lysosomes, occasional lipid droplets and myelinated bodies were observed. More than 85% of the leukemic patient group and 71% of the non-leukemic patient group had groups of Gall-bodies (Photos 2, 6). Clustered dense bodies were also seen in 38% of the former and 24% of the latter group. Forty-six percent of the leukemic group and 24% of the non-leukemic group contained intracytoplasmic glycogen granules and sometimes glycogen pools, as shown in Photo 7.

Nuclear DNA Cytophotometry of ATLL

Twenty cases of ATLL were studied by nuclear DNA cytophotometry. The nuclear DNA content of cells in Feulgen stained imprint preparations of lymph nodes was measured with an Olympus BHQ cytophotometric microscope. The two parameters of nuclear size and nuclear DNA value were used in the analysis for the purpose of understanding the cell kinetics of the neoplastic lymphocytes of both leukemic and non-leukemic ATLL (4).

Representative cases of leukemic and non-leukemic ATLL are given in Fig. 1 a, b. A leukemic case of the medium-sized type showed a mode at 13 μm in the nuclear size histogram and a bimodal pattern with a mode value of 8 arbitrary units (A.U.) in the DNA histogram (Fig. 1a). In the density scattergram, a high density area was seen in the central zone and low density areas were spreading into the larger and smaller values in DNA content as well as in nuclear size. The nuclear size histogram in the case of the non-leukemic pleomorphic type showed a wider distribution than that of the leukemic case and the DNA histogram showed a multimodal distribution (Fig. 1b). In the density scattergram of this case, a high density area was not obvious but the cells were almost evenly distributed from the left lower zone to the right upper zone. The results of these scattergrams indicated that a considerable number of cells in leukemic cases were in the

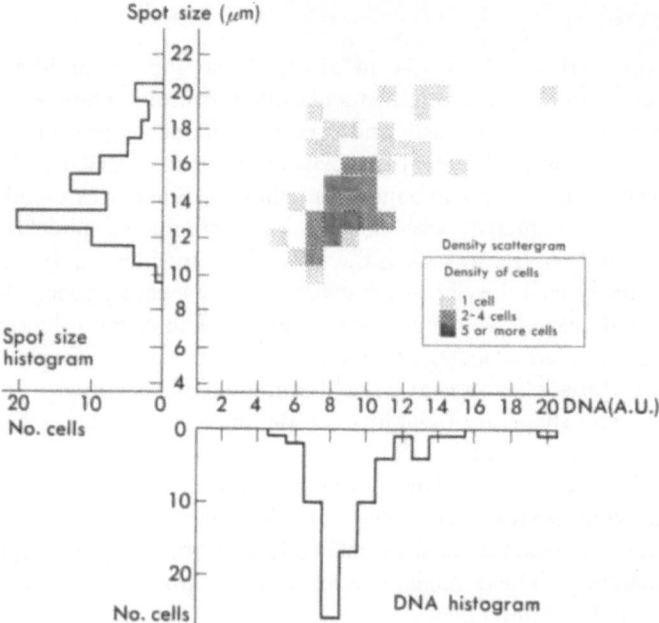

Fig. 1a.   DNA and nuclear size histogram of medium-sized type.

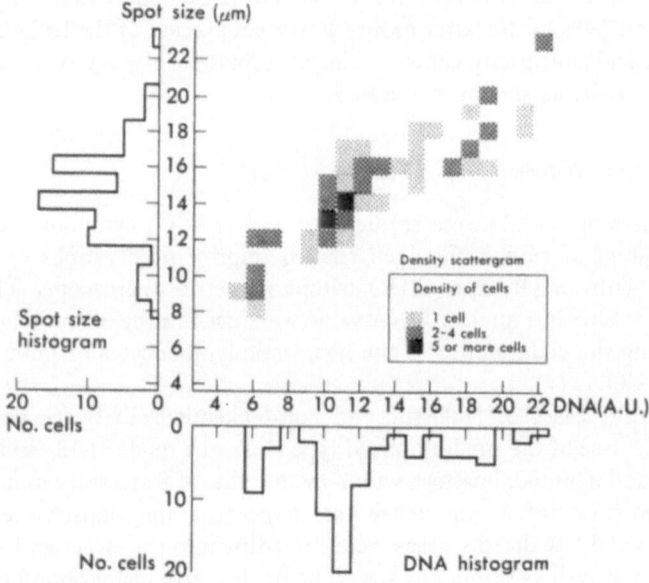

Fig. 1b.   DNA and nuclear size histogram of pleomorphic type.

S phase and some were in the pre-M phase with a mode in the diploid region. In the case of non-leukemic pleomorphic type, many tumor cells appeared to be in the S or pre-M phase randomly, showing proliferation with high heteroploidy.

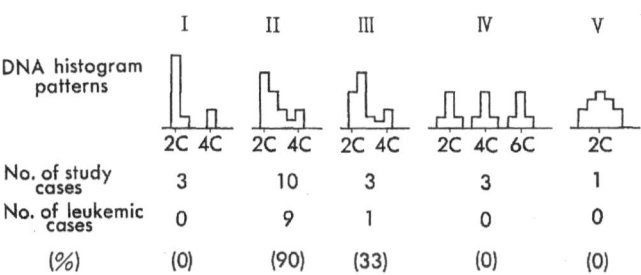

FIG. 2. Standardized DNA histogram patterns and number of cases.

In order to understand the leukemic tendency of ATLL from the viewpoint of cell kinetics, standardized histograms calculated from the mean DNA value of the mode sized nuclei were prepared. The following five standardized histogram patterns were obtained (Fig. 2). I) Diploid range proliferation: S phase fraction was low. II) Diploid range proliferation: S phase fraction was high but the mode was in 2C. III) Diploid range proliferation: S phase fraction was high and the mode was above 2C. IV) Diploid and tetraploid range proliferation. V) Monopeak with ploidy reduction pattern.

Most of the leukemic cases showed the pattern of type II or III (Fig. 2). Accordingly, it was concluded that the tumor cells of leukemic cases were proliferating predominantly in the diploid range with a high fraction in the S phase and that the cells showed a less variable nuclear feature than in the non-leukemic ATLL.

REFERENCES

1. Collins, R. D., Waldron, J. A., and Glick, A. D. Results of multi-parameter studies of T-cell lymphoid neoplasms. *Am. J. Clin. Pathol.*, **74** (Suppl. 4), 699–707 (1979).
2. Eimoto, T., Mitsui, T., and Kikuchi, M. Ultrastructure of adult T-cell leukemia-lymphoma. *Virchows Arch., Cell Pathol.*, **38**, 189–208 (1981).
3. Hanaoka, M., Sasaki, M., and Matsumoto, H. Adult T-cell leukemia: Histopathological classification and characteristics. *Acta Pathol. Jpn.*, **29**, 723–738 (1979).
4. Hasui, K. Cell kinetic analysis of adult T-cell leukemia-lymphoma. *J. Jpn. Soc. Res.*, **20**, 189–201 (1980) (in Japanese).
5. Kikuchi, M., Mitsui, T., and Matsui, N. T-cell malignancies in adults. Histopathological studies of lymph nodes in 110 patients. *Jpn. J. Clin. Oncol.*, **9** (Suppl.), 407–422 (1979).
6. Shamoto, M., Murakami, S., and Zenke, T. An ultrastructural study of adult T-cell leukemia. *Cancer*, **47**, 1804–1811 (1981).
7. Suchi, T., Tajima, K., and Nanba, K. Some problems on the histopathological diagnosis of non-Hodgkin's malignant lymphoma—a proposal of a new type. *Acta Pathol. Jpn.*, **29**, 755–776 (1979).
8. Tokunaga, M., Hasui, K., Wakimoto, J., and Sato, E. Elecrton microscopical study of adult T-cell lymphoma. *Proc. Jpn. Cancer Assoc., The 38th Annual Meeting*, 253 (1979) (in Japanese).
9. Uchiyama, T., Yodoi, J., Sagawa, K., Takatsuki, K., and Uchino, H. Adult T-cell leukemia: Clinical and hematologic features of 16 cases. *Blood*, **50**, 481–492 (1977).

EXPLANATION OF PHOTOS

PHOTO 1. Electron micrograph of the pleomorphic type demonstrates tumor cells of varied size and shape in the tissue and sinuses. ×2,000.

PHOTO 2. Note the tumor cells in the lymph node attached to each other with smooth cellular margins. ×6,600.

PHOTO 3. Tumor cells infiltrating in the dermis interdigitated with histiocyte processes. ×8,200.

PHOTO 4. Note the nuclear lobulation and poorly developed cytoplasmic organelles. ×6,000.

PHOTO 5. Note the cellular variety infiltrating in the tissue. × 3,400.

PHOTO 6. Note an atypical mitotic cell retaining some Gall-body-like dense bodies, and an immunoblastic type cell with abundant polysomes. ×5,300.

PHOTO 7. Note intracytoplasmic glycogen pool and nuclear pleomorphism. ×8,500.

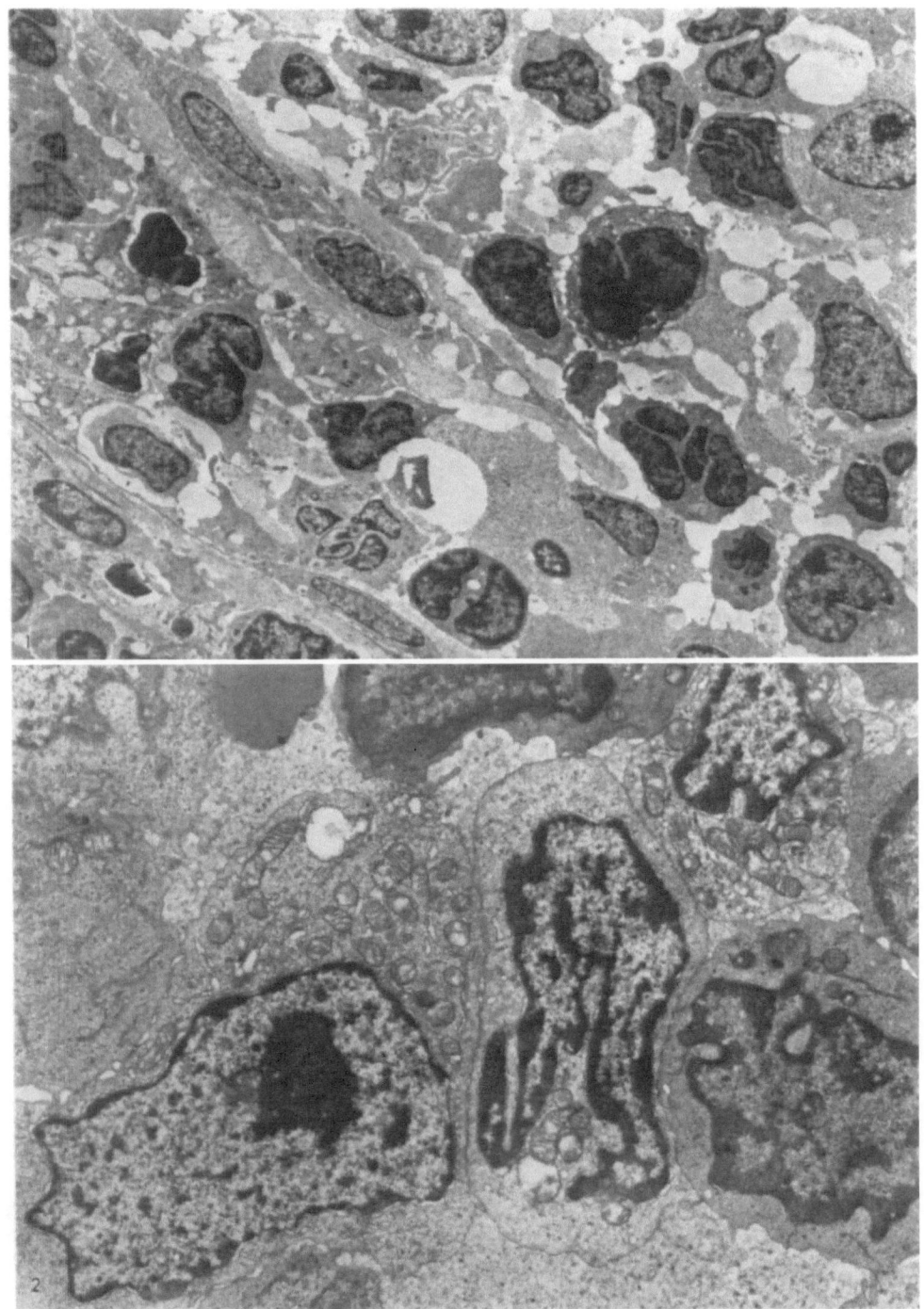

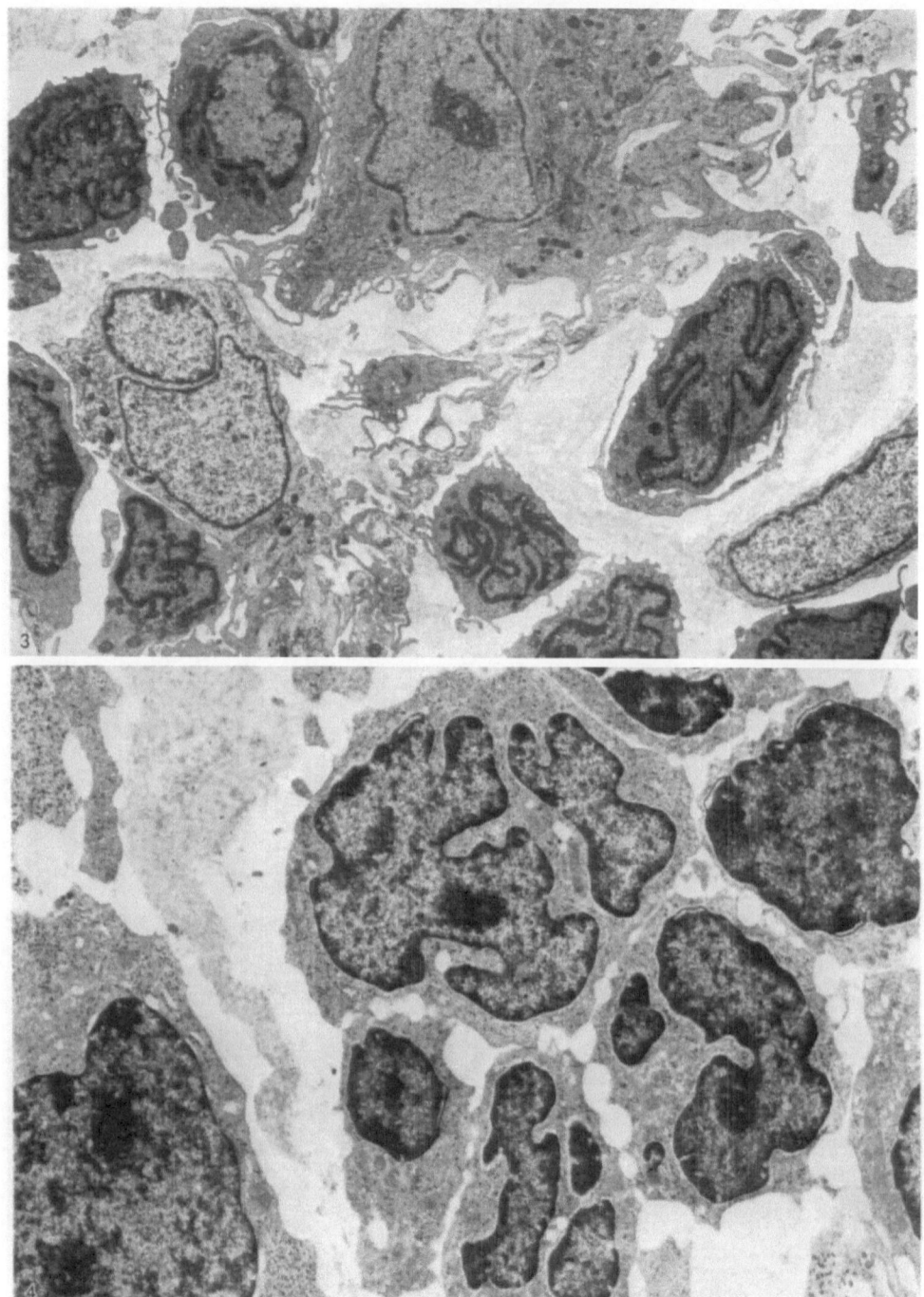

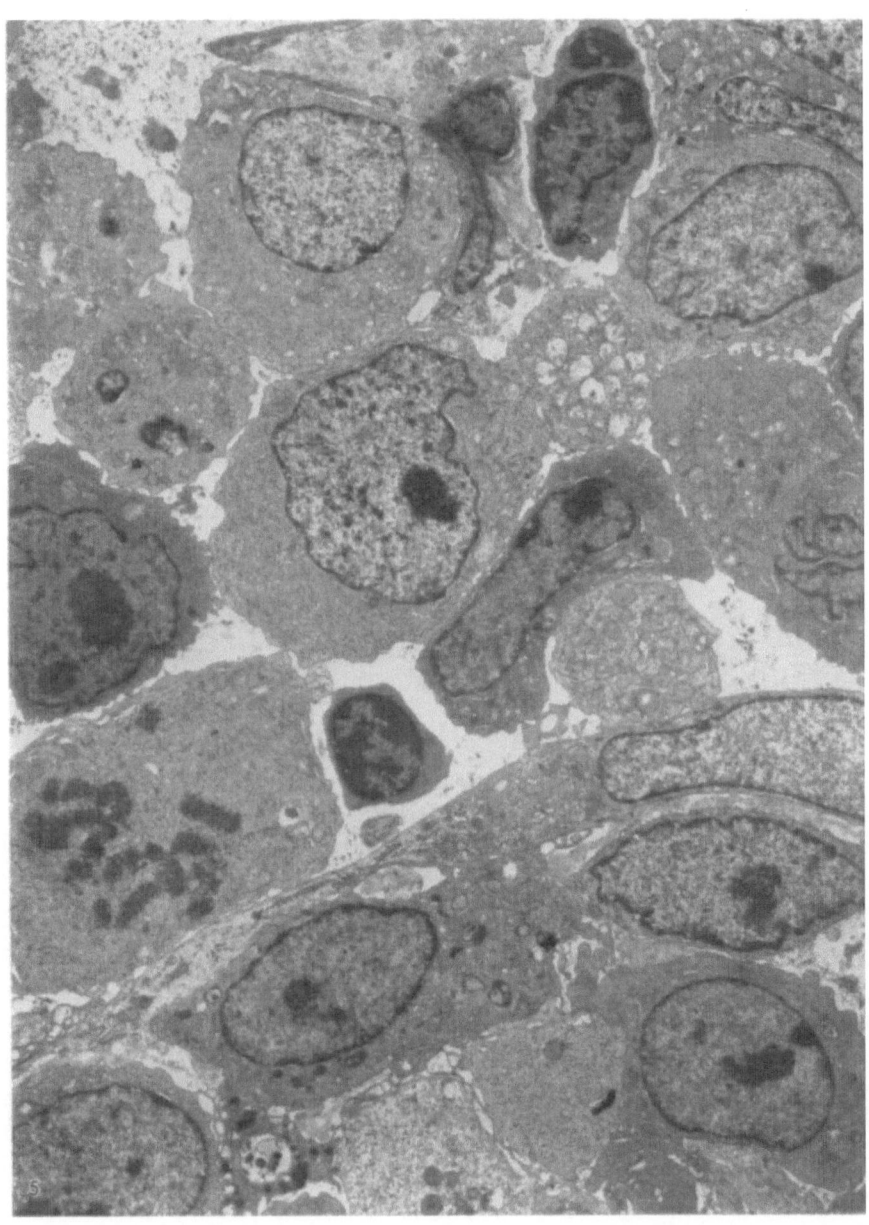

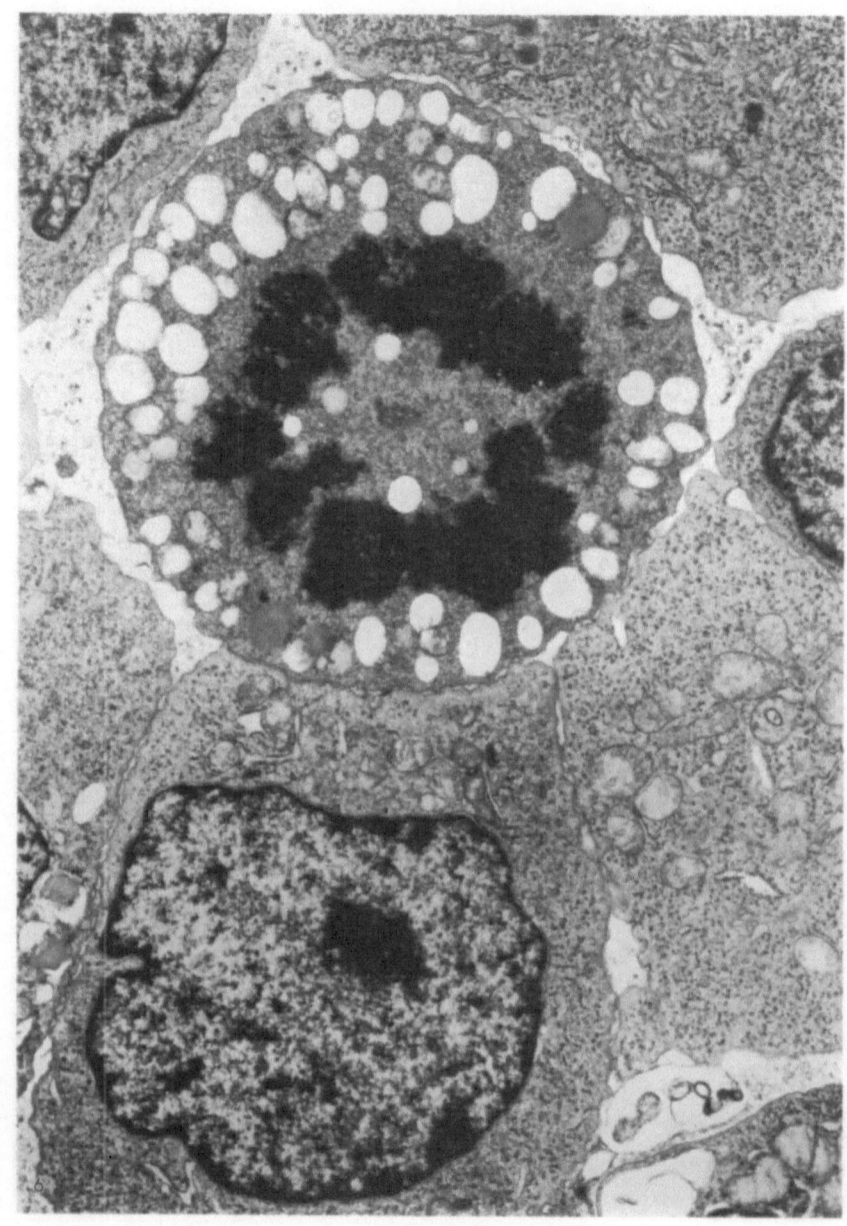

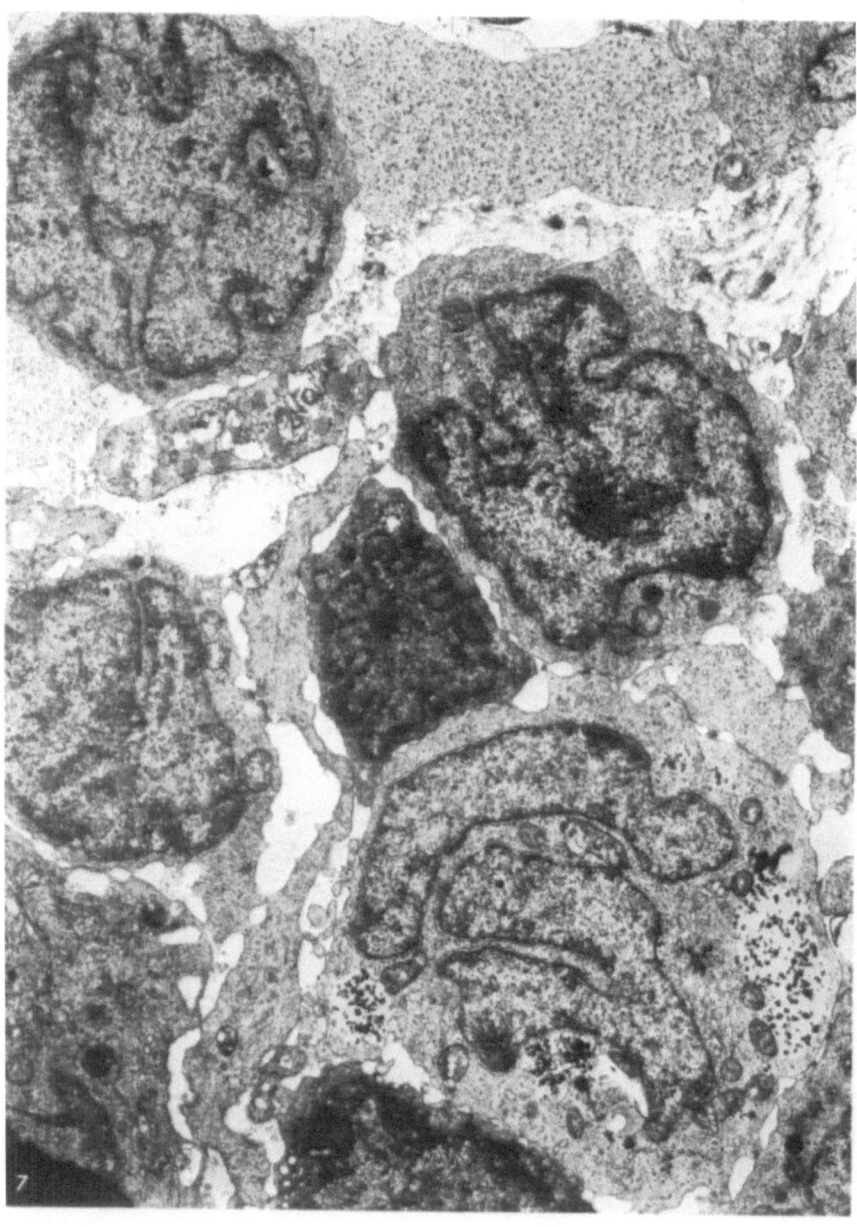

GANN Monograph on Cancer Research 28, 1982

HISTOCHEMICAL AND CYTOCHEMICAL OBSERVATIONS ON NORMAL AND NEOPLASTIC T LYMPHOCYTES

Atsuo Mikata,[*1] Hiroshi Suzuki,[*1] Shigeo Suzuki,[*1]
and Masanori Shimoyama[*2]

*Department of Pathology, Keio University School of Medicine[*1] and
Internal Medicine, National Cancer Center Hospital[*2]*

Enzyme histo- and cytochemical studies were performed on biopsy materials of reactive and lymphomatous lymph nodes, cell suspensions from these lymph nodes, and on peripheral blood lymphocytes of patients and healthy volunteers.

A dot-like reaction of β-glucuronidase (β-Gase), acid phosphatase, and non-specific esterase were found in most of the normal and neoplastic T-lymphocytes cytochemically. About 30% of the peripheral T-lymphocytes were always negative for β-Gase, while Meuller-Ranki's α-naphthyl acetate esterase at pH 5.4 (ANAE) method revealed positive reaction in more than 95% of the T-lymphocytes and 50% of the B-lymphocytes. Neoplastic T-lymphocytes were either positive or negative for ANAE and for α-naphthyl acetate esterase at pH 6.4 (αNE).

On sections, histochemically demonstrable αNE activity was more frequently seen in lymphoblastic lymphomas. Tumor cells of peripheral T-lymphomas were usually negative for αNE. Dot-like acid phosphatase and β-Gase reactions were also found in most T-lymphoma cells. β-Gase activities were more frequently seen in lymphoblastic and mixed cell types than in other histological subtypes.

Lymphomas of peripheral T-cells had a tendency to show reticular alkaline phosphatase activity of the neoplastic tissue.

Histochemistry and cytochemistry have been regarded as essential tools for the study of hematological diseases. In recent years, it was revealed that enzyme activities of the lymphocytes were related to their immunological characteristics (*2, 6, 19*). Thus, acid non-specific esterase and acid phosphatase were often described as cytochemical markers of T-cell lineage (*10, 12, 17*). Histochemical observations on malignant lymphomas in relation to their immunological and functional classification will provide new insight into the problems of lymphocytic neoplasms.

The present report is to characterize T-cell malignancies in the light of such enzyme histochemical and cytochemical findings and to corrleate the results with the differentiation and maturation of the lymphocytes.

[*1] Shinanomachi 35, Shinjuku-ku, Tokyo 160, Japan (三方淳男, 鈴木　裕, 鈴木繁生).
[*2] Tsukiji 5-1-1, Chuo-ku, Tokyo 104, Japan (下山正徳).

Histochemical and Cytochemical Staining

Biopsies of lymph nodes from various conditions with localized or generalized lymphadenopathy were subjected to multiparametric studies as described in previous papers (7, 15). For histochemical investigations, lymph nodes were fixed in 4% paraformaldehyde, and the methods of various researchers were utilized. Four μm sections were cut and stained for acid phosphatase (AcPase) by the method of Barka et al. (1), for β-glucuronidase (β-Gase) by Hayashi et al. (9), alkaline phosphatase (AlPase) by Burstone (4), 5′nucleotidase (5′Nase) and adenosine triphosphatase (ATPase) by Wachstein et al. (23), α-naphthyl acetate esterase at pH 6.4 (αNE) by Yam et al. (24) and in some cases at pH 5.4 (ANAE) (17) and α-naphthyl butyrate esterase (αNBE) by Li et al. (13). Cells with diffuse lysosomal activities over the entire cytoplasm were regarded as representing admixed non-neoplastic phagocytic cells. Lymphoid cells showed either large, dot-like, clustered or scattered, fine granular activities of these lysosomal enzymes. Lysosomal enzyme positive reaction was scored as ⧺ when shown by more than 75% of cells, ⧻ when 75% to 50% of the cells, + when 50% to 25% of the cells, and ± when less than 25% of the cells.

Lymph node stamp smears and cell suspension smears were fixed in Kaplow's fixative and studied for enzyme activities.

Peripheral blood mononuclear cells were prepared with Percoll sedimentation from 9 healthy males 20 to 30 years old. Smeared E (sheep red cells) and EAC (sheep erythrocyte antibody complex) rosette preparations were also fixed in Kaplow's fluid at 0°C for 1 min and stained for β-Gase (14), αNE (13), and for ANAE (17). Two hundred rosetted cells were studied for their enzyme reactions and reactive patterns. Reactive patterns were classified as: Localized, single dot or clustered fine granules; scattered, fine granular reactions more than 3 spots around the nuclei; and, a mixture of the two.

Normal Lymph Nodes and Peripheral Lymphocytes

Lymph node biopsy materials were examined histologically and those with lymphoid follicles and interfollicular areas that showed an ordinary degree of reactive change were judged as "normal." Histochemical findings of these lymph nodes were in agreement with earlier papers (17, 18, 22). In short, lymphocytes of the primary follicles and the perifollicular dark zone were strongly positive for ATPase, weakly so for 5′Nase and for uridine diphosphatase (UDPase). Very occasionally AlPase positive lymphocytes accumulated in this location. Cells of the germinal centers included a small number of ATPase positive cells. Fine granular AcPase positive cells were also occasionally present. Reticulum cells of the germinal centers were positive for 5′Nase. Large numbers of lymphocytes in the interfollicular or paracortical areas showed dot-like AcPase, β-Gase, αNE, and αNBE activity. ATPase positive lymphocytes were also present but in small number. Reticulum cells of the paracortex were positive for ATPase. In some cases, AlPase activity was very strong and widespread along the reticulum cells of the paracortex.

Normal peripheral lymphocytes showed various forms of AcPase, β-Gase, and esterase activity. These reactive patterns were divided into localized, localized and

TABLE I. Esterase and β-Gase Activities of Peripheral Lymphocytes

	EAC-rosetted cells	E-rosetted cells
Mueller-Ranki (ANAE) pH 5.4		
Positive		
Localized	48.3± 8.6%	70.3±10.3%
Localized and scattered	19.0± 9.2	20.3± 8.2
Negative	32.7±12.7	9.3± 2.6
Yam-Li (αNE) pH 6.4		
Positive		
Localized	36.7± 2.4%	57.7±10.7%
Localized and scatterd	2.7± 2.1	4.3± 1.3
Scattered	5.3± 4.3	17.3± 4.3
Negative	52.7± 3.4	19.7± 7.6
Hayashi et al. (β-Gase)		
Positive		
Localized	33.8± 5.2%	49.0± 8.0%
Localized and scattered	8.2± 2.7	10.8± 2.8
Scattered	28.1± 7.0	38.5± 8.3
Negative	29.3± 5.2	1.7± 1.5

$n=9$, 20 to 30 year old males. Mean±S.D.

scattered, and scattered forms (Photos 1, 2). As shown in Table I, approximately 30 and 50% of the EAC rosette lymphocytes were negative for β-Gase or esterase, while 95 and 75% of the E-rosette cells were positive for these enzymes, respectively. E-rosette cells showed more localized activity than EAC-rosette cells. Scattered patterns were also more frequently seen in E-rosette cells. With Mueller-Ranki's methods, scattered fine granular reactions blurred and were impossible to recognize. Approximately 30% and 50% of the EAC-rosette cells were negative for β-Gase and αNE reaction, respectively (Table I).

Neoplastic Lymph Nodes

Among 128 lymphomas studied with multiparameter methods, there were 30 T-cell lymphomas (Table II). Their histological types (27) were: diffuse large cell (DL), 11 cases; diffuse pleomorphic type (DPleo), 4; diffuse mixed cell type (DMx), 4; diffuse medium-sized cell type (DM), 5; lymphoblastic type (LBL), 4; and one case each of diffuse mixed and small cell type with abundant epithelioid cell contents (Lennert lesion). Three leukemic cases were diagnosed as adult T-cell leukemia (ATL); two of them showed a pleomorphic lymphomatous picture and one was of a diffuse mixed type.

ATPase was positive in a very moderate number of cells in 10 cases while the remaining 20 cases were completely negative except for blood vessels (Photos 3, 4). A few, usually smaller, cells were positive in 6 cases; 4 other cases contained ATPase positive cells which were difficult to separate from negative neoplastic cells on histochemical preparations. AlPase reaction showed positive deposits along the reticular fibers or reticulum cells in 14 cases (Photo 5). Eight of these were also judged ATPase

TABLE II. Enzyme Histochemical Findings of T-cell Lymphomas

Histology	Case		E	EACh	SIg	Ia	αT	OKT/TdT	ATP	AlP*	β-G	AcP	αNE	Others
DL	T. I.	50 M	36	9	18	−	+		−	−	−	−	−	
	S. D.	29 F	62	35	0	±			−	−	++	++	−	
	S. T.	71 M	51	0	0	−	+		−	−	++	+++	−	
	K. F.	54 M	65	44	6	−	+		−	−	++	++	−	
	J. H.	51 F	31	53	30				−	−	+++	+	±	
	K. T.	61 M	49	0	10	−			±	+	++	+++	+	
	T. M.	69 M	31	0	0	−			−	+	+	±	−	
	S. T.	F	85	0	0	+	+		−	−	+++	++	−	
	T. I.	67 M	98	13					−	−	+	+	−	Mycosis fungoides
	F. N.	43 F	34	9	13	−	+		−	−	±	±	±	
	Y. M.	41 M	66	44	0	−	+		+	+	+	++	±	Kyushu
DPleo	H. F.	68 F	34	8	6		+		−	±	±	±	−	ATL
	A. M.	56 M	63	1	2	−	+		±	±	++	++	−	ATL
	M. T.	57 M	6	1	0				−	±	++	++	±	
	K. Y.	53 F	38	8	0	−			±	+	+	++	±	
DMx	T. K.	67 M					+		±	+	++	+	±	Skin tumor
	G. O.	77 M	17	2			+		−	+	+	++	−	Mycosis fungoides
	S. H.	66 M	74	0	12	+	+	OKT 3+, 8+	±	+	++	+++	±	T s/c
	M. T.	53 F	57	15	0	+	+	OKT 3+, 4+	−	+	+	++	±	T i/h, ATL
DM	S. S.	23 M	37	12					−	−	++	+	+	
	N. T.	39 M	62	2	0	−			−	−	+	±	−	
	K. S.	33 F	33	8	0	±	+		−	±	+	+	−	
	K. Y.	39 M	55	14	11	+	+		+	±	++	++	−	
	K. F.	27 F					+		±	−	+	+	+	Skin tumor
LBL	K. O.	23 M	43	71	5		+	TdT +	−	−	+++	++	++	Thymic tumor
	M. M.	24 M	68	28	0	−	+	TdT ++	−	−	+++	++	−	
	Y. N.	34 M	21	4	0	+	+		−	−	+++	±	±	
	N. Y.	18 F	12	5	0	−			−	−	+++	+	++	
LNT	K. I.	41 M	57	8	0				±	−	+++	++	±	
	H. K.	66 M	95	3	0				±	±	+++	++	±	

a + and ± indicate strong and weak AlPase reaction of reticular pattern within the lymphomatous tissue.

Abbreviations: DL, diffuse large cell type; DPleo, diffuse pleomorphic type; DMx, diffuse mixed cell type; DM, diffuse medium-sized cell type; LBL, lymphoblastic type; LNT, lymphomas with Lennert lesion; EACh, SIg, percent of positive cells for C3b receptor and surface immunoglobulin; Ia, αT, cytotoxicity test for anti Ia-like antigen and anti T-cell antigen; TdT, terminal deoxynucleotidyl transferase; T s/c, suppressor cytotoxic T cell; T i/h, inducer helper T cell.

positive to some extent. All 4 cases of pleomorphic T-cell lymphoma showed a reticular AlPase pattern and contrasted well with the completely negative reaction of lymphoblastic cases (Photo 6).

AcPase and β-Gase were positive to varying degrees in 29 cases. The only exception was a case of a 50-year old man with large cell type. Tumor cells of this case showed reactivity to anti-T heterogenous serum, but did not form rosettes with either E or

TABLE III. Lysosomal Reactions in T-cell Lymphomas
(Frequency of AcPase or β-Gase Positive Tumor Cells)

Histology	AcP > β-G	AcP ≒ β-G	AcP < β-G
DL	3	3	3
DPleo	2	3	0
DMx	3	0	1
DM	0	3	2
LBL	0	1	3
LNT	0	1	1
Total	8	11	10

AcP > β-G indicates AcPase (dot-like) positive tumor cells were larger in number than β-Gase (dot-like) positive tumor cells.

EAC. AcPase positive cells were larger in number than β-Gase positive cells in 8 cases, they were approximately equal in number in 11 cases, and β-Gase positive cells occurred more frequently in 10 cases (Table III). There was a tendency for AcPase positive cells to be more frequently seen in diffuse large cell and pleomorphic types than in medium-sized cell or lymphoblastic types. Often the AcPase reaction of the larger tumor cells showed an ill-defined border of the positive dots. Strength of the reaction was also reduced.

On sections of malignant lymphomas, only very occasional cells showed dot-like activity of αNE or ANAE in 3 of DL, 2 of pleomorphic type, 3 of mixed cell type, 1 of LBL. and 2 cases with Lennert lesion. Most of the ANAE positive cells were smaller cells with dense nuclear chromatin. In cases of M.F. and T-cell lymphomas with cutaneous manifestations with Pautrier's microabscesses, cells within the abscess did not show αNE or ANAE reactivity (Photo 7).

Two cases of DM type were analyzed with the OKT series. One (S.H.) was OKT-3 and 8 positive and the other (M.T.) was OKT 3 and 4 positive. There were, however, no definite histochemical differences in regards to ANAE, AcPase, or β-Gase reactivities. Peripheral blood lymphocytes of the OKT 3 and 4 positive case (M.T.), including 20% tumor cells, contained both ANAE and αNE positive atypical cells. Larger atypical cells were, however, frequently negative (Photo 8). E-rosette forming lymphoma cells separated from a diseased lymph node of Case K.Y., a 53-year old female of the pleomorphic type, showed no αNE activity (Photo 9).

DISCUSSION

Ever since subclasses of lymphocytes were established, enzyme histochemical findings were correlated with immunological subclasses or even with functional subsets (6). Tamaoki and Essner (22) were the first in this sense to describe lysosomal activities of T-zone lymphocytes in animals and man. Mueller (17) reported non-specific esterase activity of Thy-1 positive mouse lymphocytes. Since then, ANAE has been regarded as a cytochemical marker for T-lymphocytes and their neoplasms (20). Knowles (12) recommended αNE reaction at pH 5.4 for 21 hr, and he obtained positive reaction in most of the T-cell lymphomas he tested. The method used by Knowles utilized three times more coupling agent than the method we used and the incubation time was too long for a reasonable enzyme reaction. Davey (5), using Yam-Li's method, as we did, found no meaningful difference between E and EAC rosetted cells; our results supported his findings (16). We also examined 30 T-cell lymphomas for esterase activity. A moderate number (75 to 50%) of the tumor cells showed the dot-like reaction in 2 cases of lymphoblastic lymphoma (T_1 lymphoma). Most of the peripheral T-cell tumors (T_2 lymphoma), including ATL and pleomorphic lymphomas, showed only occasional (less than 25%) positive cells. Moreover, these esterase positive cells were smaller than other neoplastic cells and often clustered together. Twelve out of 16 esterase positive cases were included in such histological types where medium-sized or small lymphocytes were essential constituents of the tumor. Therefore, differentiation of neoplastic and non-neoplastic cells on the histochemical preparation was often very difficult. These facts suggested that the cells with esterase activity represented remaining or admixed non-neoplastic cells. If we regard these cases as being actually esterase-negative in tumor cells, then we found only 2 positive cases of the lymphoblastic subtype. In normal human thymus, cortical thymocytes were positive for both β-Gase and AcPase but negative for esterase (αNE), while medullary thymocytes were occasionally positive for esterase. Dot-like lysosomal activities of T-lymphocytes were beautifully demonstrated in all 4 cases of lymphoblastic lymphomas (T_1 lymphoma) (Photo 10). Except for one case, cells with dot-like β-Gase reaction outnumbered those with AcPase reaction (Table III). In one case of acute lymphoblastic leukemia (ALL) with only OKI1+ and HLy2+ phenotype, not included in the present series, most of the tumor cells showed the dot-like reaction of AcPase, β-Gase, αNE, and of ANAE (pH 5.4). Although Bosso (3) reported that activities of β-Gase paralleled the maturation of T-lymphocytes, our observation suggested that tumors derived from immature T-lymphocytes tended to have more β-Gase and αNE activities than those from mature T-lymphocytes.

We have reported the possibility of histochemically demonstrable ATPase as a marker for B-cell lymphomas (8, 15). Kikuchi (11) reported that some of the T-cell lymphomas contained ATPase positive cells. Again, we were doubtful about their neoplastic nature. ATPase activity could be demonstrated on the cell membrane of the paracortical reticulum cells, histiocytes and epithelioid cells. In the present series, there were 10 lymphomas in which some of the constituent cells showed ATPase activity. Except for one case, the majority of cells were negative. Moreover, 8 out of 10 ATPase positive tumors also showed positive alkaline phosphatase reaction of reticular pattern. Two other cases contained a large number of phagocytic cells or epithelioid cells. When Mg^{2+} ion was omitted from the incubation medium, these ATPase reactions were not reduced in most cases (Photo 4). These observations suggested that ATPase positive cells were probably of a non-neoplastic component.

Positive alkaline phosphatase reactions of reticular pattern were found in T_2 lymphomas such as the pleomorphic or mixed type. This finding corresponded very well to the situation of T-zone reticulum cells in normal or reactive lymph nodes, and was in distinct contrast to the completely negative reaction, except for blood vessels, of AlPase in T_1 lymphomas.

Acknowledgment

This work was supported with Cancer Research Grant-in-Aid from Ministry of Education, Science, and Culture in Japan.

REFERENCES

1. Barka, T. and Anderson, P. J. Histochemical methods for acid phosphatase using hexazonium pararosanilin as coupler. *J. Histochem. Cytochem.*, **10**, 741–753 (1962).
2. Barr, R. D. and Perry, S. Lysosomal acid hydrolase in human lymphocyte subpopulation. *Br. J. Haematol.*, **32**, 565–572 (1976).
3. Bosso, G., Cocito, M. G., Semenzato, G., Pezzutto, A., and Zanesco, L. Cytochemical study of thymocytes and T lymphocytes. *Br. J. Haematol.*, **44**, 577–582 (1980).
4. Burstone, M. S. "Enzyme Histochemistry," 257 pp. (1962). Academic Press, New York and London.
5. Davey, F. R., Huntington, S. J., MacCallum, J., and McMath, J. M. Cytochemical reactions of normal and neoplastic lymphocytes. *J. Clin. Pathol.*, **30**, 653–660 (1977).
6. Grossi, C. E., Weff, S. R., Zicca, A., Lydyard, P. M., Moretta, L., Mingari, M. C., and Cooper, M. D. Morphological and histochemical analyses of two human T-cell subpopulations bearing receptors for IgM or IgG. *J. Exp. Med.*, **147**, 1405–1417 (1975).
7. Harigaya, K., Mikata, A., Suzuki, H., Ohishi, T., and Watanabe, S. Enzyme Cyto- and histochemical approach to lymphoreticular malignancies. *Recent Adv. RES Res.*, **17**, 79–96 (1977).
8. Harigaya, K., Mikata, A., Suzuki, H., Ohishi, T., Watanabe, S., and Kageyama, K. Mg^{2+} dependent adenosine triphosphatase as an enzyme histochemical marker for the lymphomas of B-cell origin. *Am. J. Pathol.*, **97**, 359–380 (1979).
9. Hayashi, M., Nakajima, Y., and Fishman, W. The cytologic demonstration of β-glucuronidase employing naphthol AS-BI glucuronide and hexazonium pararosanilin. *J. Histochem. Cytochem.*, **12**, 239–297 (1964).
10. Higgy, K. E., Burns, G. F., and Hayhoe, F.G.J. Discrimination of B, T, and null lymphocytes by esterase cytochemistry. *Scand. J. Haematol*, **18**, 437–448 (1977).
11. Kikuchi, M., Mitsui, T., Matsui, N., Sato, E., Tokunaga, M., Hasui, K., Ichimaru, M., Kinoshita, K., and Kamihira, S. T-cell malignancies in adults: Histopathological studies of lymph nodes in 110 patients. *Jpn. J. Clin. Oncol.*, **9** (Suppl.), 407–421 (1979).
12. Knowles, D. M., Halper, J. P., Machin, G. A., and Scherman, W. Acid α-naphthyl acetate esterase activity in human neoplastic lymphoid cells. *Am. J. Pathol.*, **98**, 257–271 (1979).
13. Li, C. Y., Lam, K. W., and Yam, L. T. Esterases in human leukocytes. *J. Histochem. Cytochem.* **21**, 1–12 (1973).
14. Machin, G. A., Halper, J. P., and Knowles, D. M. Cytochemically demonstrable β-glucuronidase activity in normal and neoplastic human lymphoid cells. *Blood*, **66**, 111–119 (1980).
15. Mikata, A., Harigaya, K., Suzuki, H., Ohishi, T., Tsutsumi, Y., Suzuki, S., Watanabe, S., and Kageyama, K. Enzyme histochemistry of non-Hodgkin's lymphomas. *Acta Pathol. Jpn.*, **29**, 739–753 (1979).
16. Mikata, A., Suzuki, H., Suzuki, S., and Kageyama, K. Enzyme activities of peripheral blood lymphocytes in resting and activated conditions. *J. Jpn. Soc. RES*, **21** (Suppl.), 129–136 (1981) (in Japanese).
17. Mueller, J., Brundel Re, Buerki, H., Keller, H., Hess, M. W., and Cottier, H. Non-

specific acid esterase activity; a criterion for differentiation of T and B lymphocytes in mouse lymph nodes. *Eur. J. Immunol.*, **5**, 270–274 (1975).

18. Meller-Hermelink, H. K. Characterization of the B-cell and T-cell regions of human lymphatic tissue through enzyme histochemical demonstration of ATPase and 5′-nucleotidase activities. *Virchow's Arch., B. Cell Pathol.*, **16**, 371–378 (1974).

19. Pengalis, G. A., Yataganas, X., and Fessas, P. H. β-Glucuronidase activity of lymph node imprints from malignant lymphomas and chronic lymphocytic leukemias. *J. Clin. Pathol.*, **30**, 812–816 (1977).

20. Ranki, A. Nonspecific esterase activity in human lymphocytes, histochemical characterization and distribution among major lymphocyte subclasses. *Clin. Immunol. Immunopathol.*, **10**, 47–58 (1978).

21. Suchi, T., Tajima, K., Nanba, H., Wakasa, H., Mikata, A., Kikuchi, M., Mori, S., Watanabe, S., Mohri, N., Shamoto, M., Harigaya, K., Itagaki, T., Matsuda, M., Kirino, Y., Takagi, K., and Fukunaga, S. Some problems on the histopathological diagnosis of non-Hodgkin's malignant lymphoma. A proposal for a new type. *Acta Pathol. Jpn.*, **29**, 755–776 (1979).

22. Tamaoki, N. and Essner, E. Distribution of acid phosphatase, β-glucuronidase and N-acetyl-β-glucosaminidase activities in lymphocytes of lymphatic tissues of man and rodents. *J. Histochem. Cytochem.*, **17**, 238–243 (1969).

23. Wachstein, M. and Meisel, E. Histochemistry of hepatic phosphatases at physiologic pH. *Am. J. Clin. Pathol.*, **27**, 13–23 (1957).

24. Yam, L. T., Li, C. Y., and Crosby, W. H. Cytochemical identification of monocytes and granulocytes. *Am. J. Clin. Phathol.*, **55**, 283–290 (1971).

EXPLANATION OF PHOTOS

PHOTO 1. β-Gase reaction of peripheral E-rosette lymphocytes. There is localized reaction in the left upper cell and scattered activity in the cell to the left of the picture. ×250.

PHOTO 2. αNE reaction of peripheral E-rosette lymphocytes. Coarse dot-like reactions may be seen. ×250.

PHOTO 3. ATPase reaction of a T-lymphoma case, S. H. 66-year old male, diffuse mixed type. ×400.

PHOTO 4. ATPase reaction without Mg^{2+} ion. Some of the cells remained positive. Same case as Photo 3. ×400.

PHOTO 5. AlPase activity of reticular pattern seen in lymphomas of peripheral T-lymphocytes, Y.M., 41-year old, diffuse large cell type. ×400.

PHOTO 6. Lymphomas of thymic T-lymphocytes showing completely negative AlPase reaction. Blood vessels were strongly positive, N.Y., 18-year old, lymphoblastic type. ×400.

PHOTO 7. Tumor cells in Pautrier's microabscess were negative for ANAE except on small cells. Dermis contained diffuse esterase positive histiocytes. ×400.

PHOTO 8. Peripheral blood smears from an ATL case, M.T., 53-year old female. Atypical cells were positive for αNE and ANAE. ×400.

PHOTO 9. E-rosetted tumor cells from a pleomorphic lymphoma case, K.Y., 53-year old female. αNE was negative. ×400.

PHOTO 10. β-Gase reaction of E-rosetted tumor cells separated from a T_1 lymphoma case, N.Y., 18-year old female, lymphoblastic type with thymic mass. ×400.

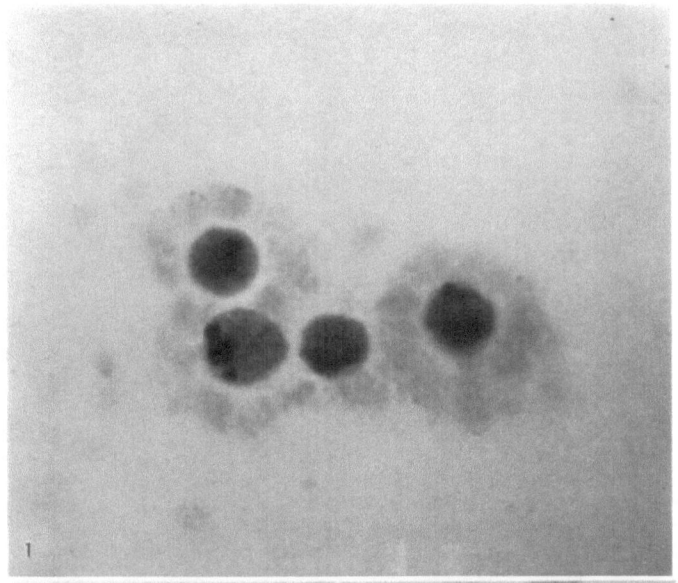

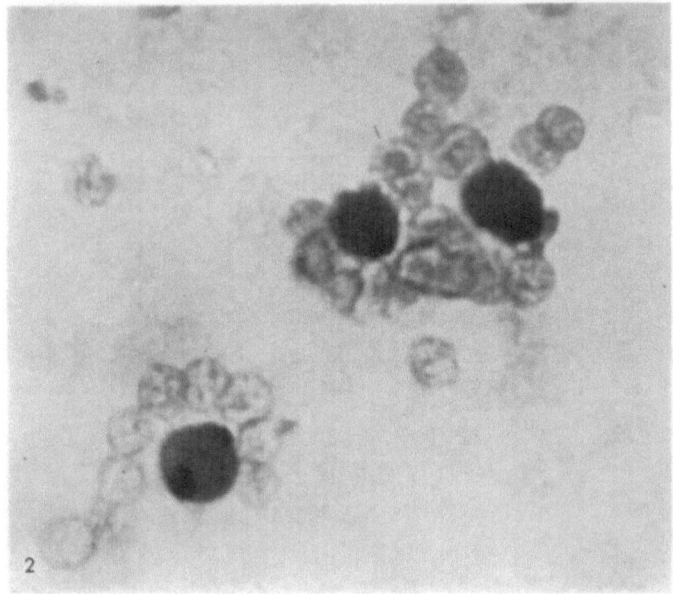

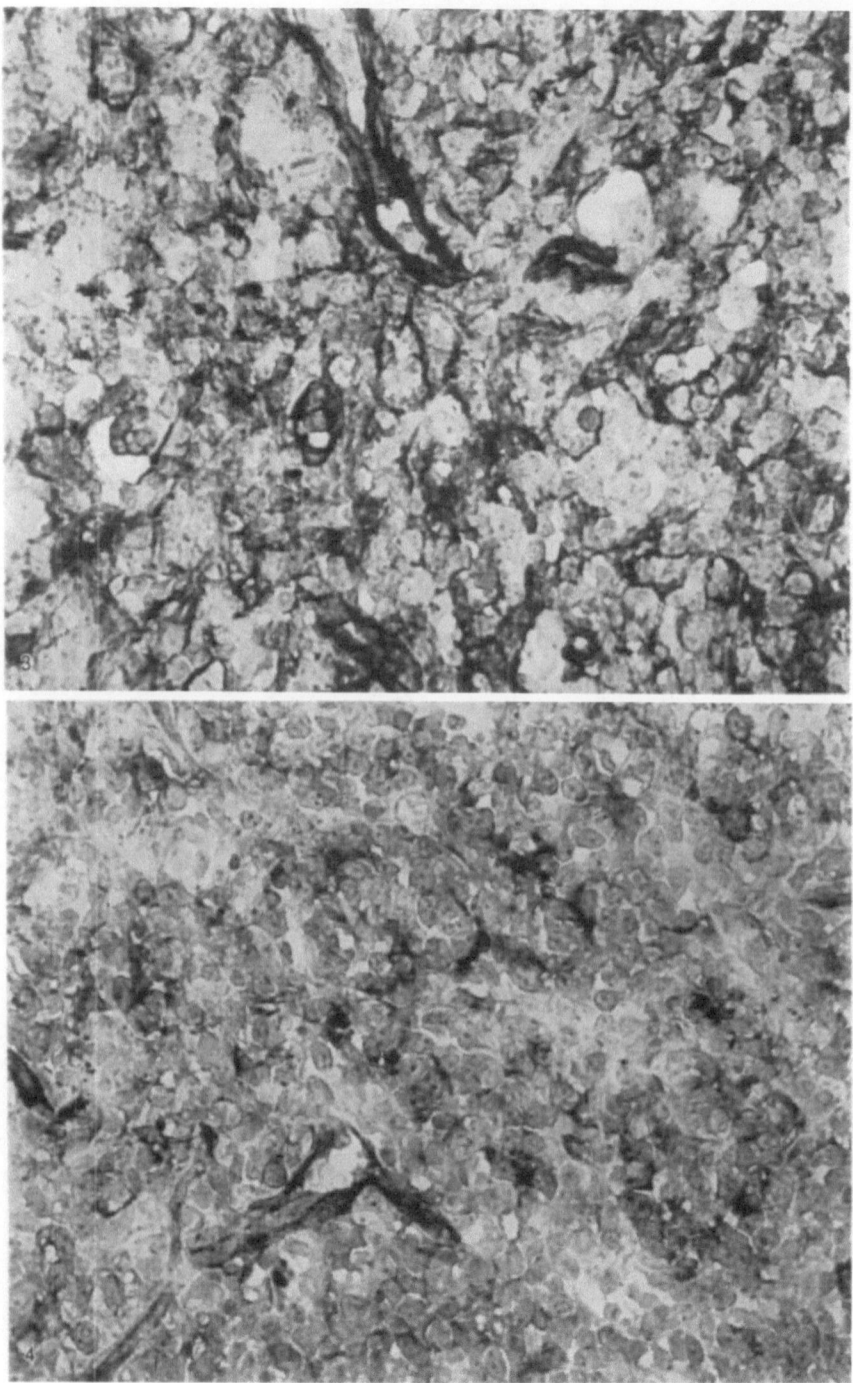

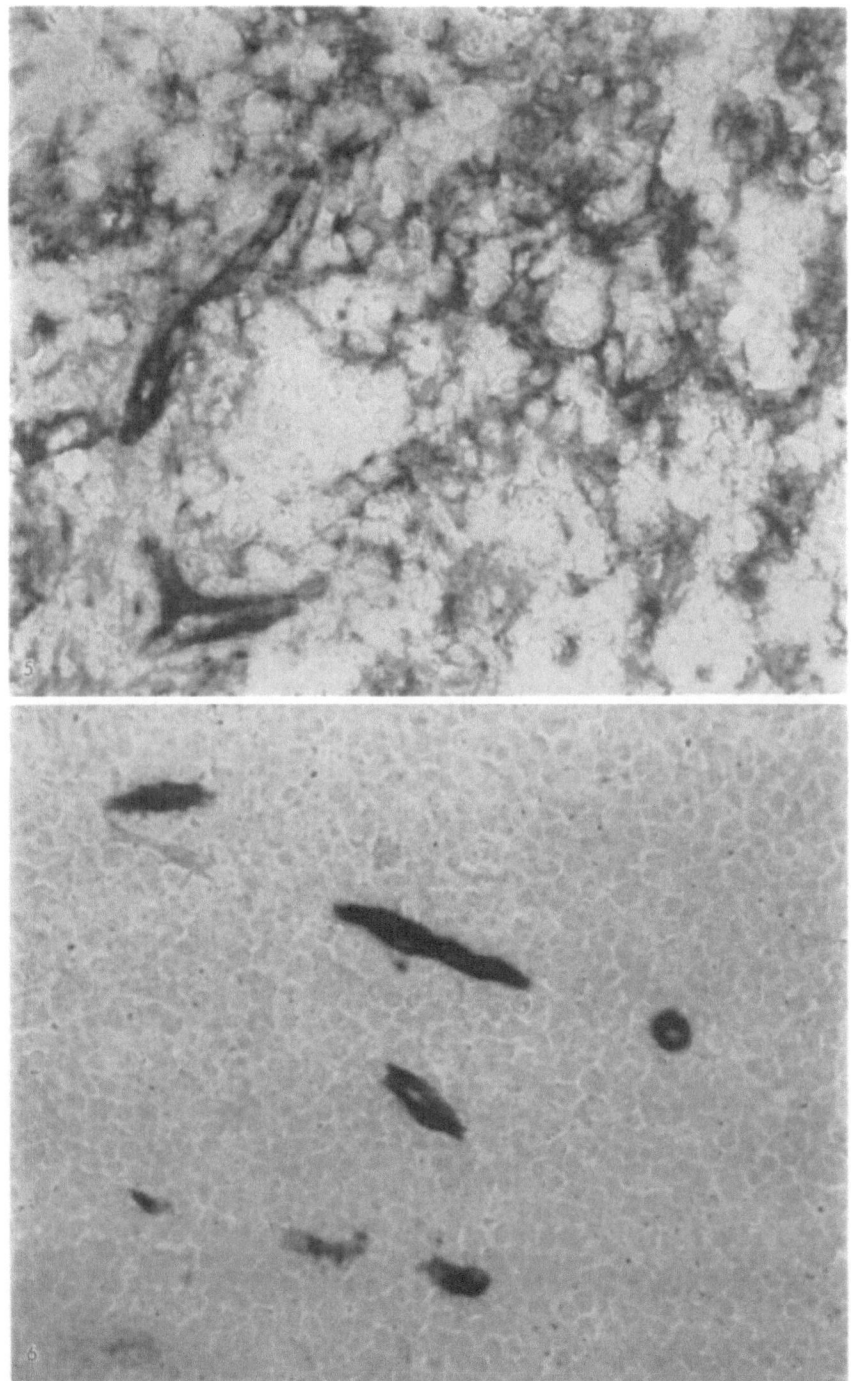

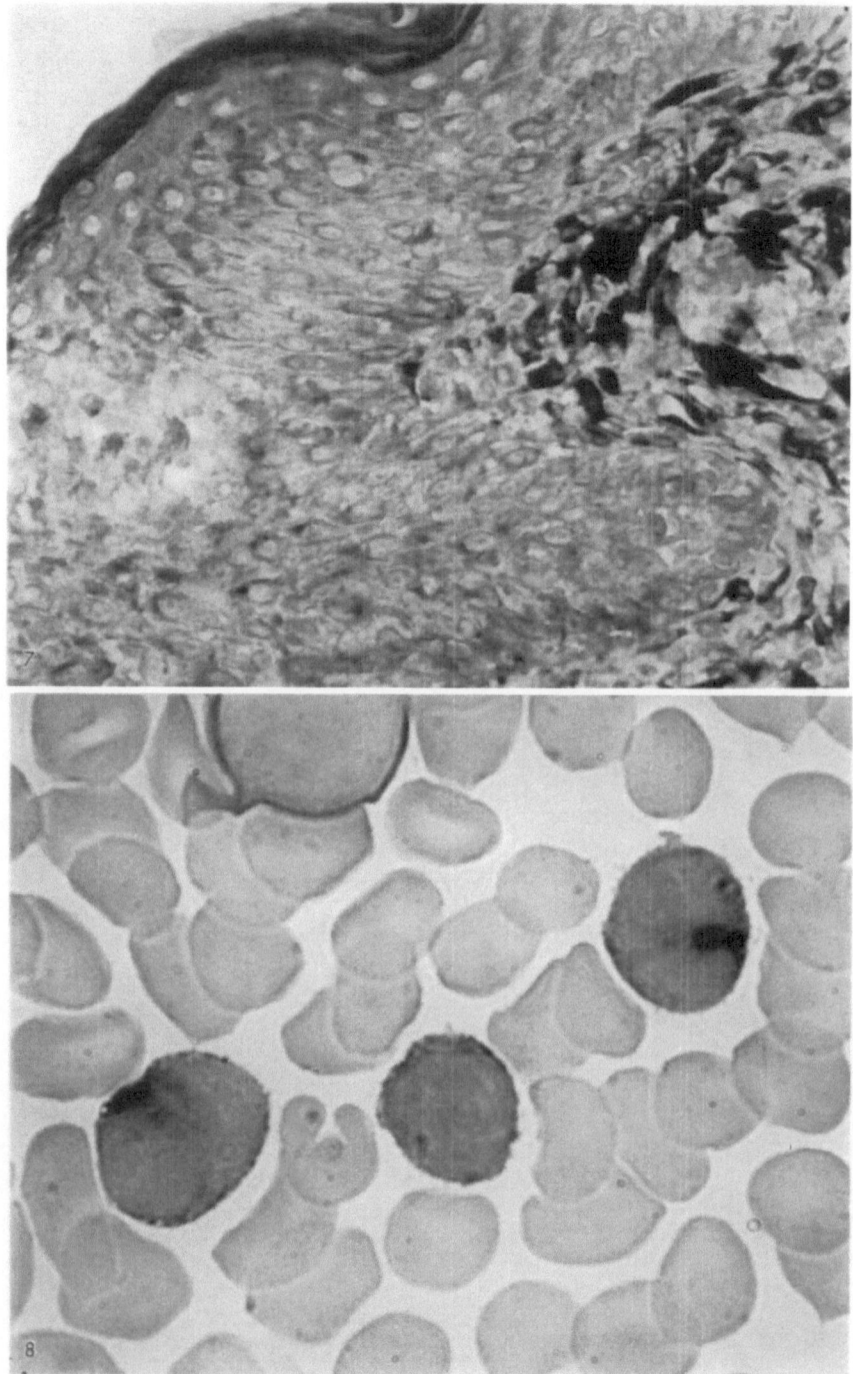

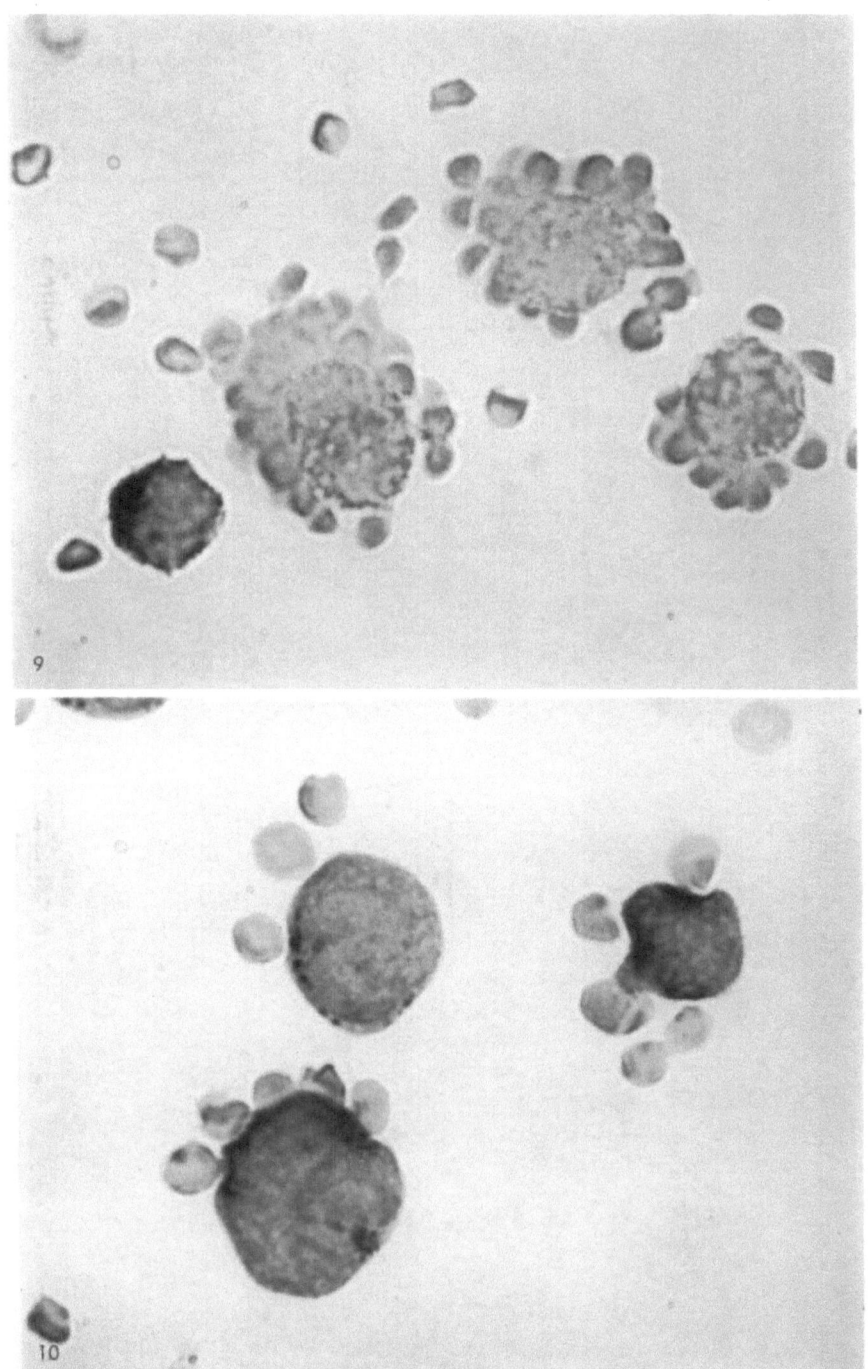

MALIGNANT LYMPHOMA AND LYMPHATIC LEUKEMIA; THEIR INTERRELATIONSHIP

Koji Nanba[*1] and Maso Hanaoka[*2]

*Department of Pathology, Kure Mutual Aid Hospital[*1] and Department
of Pathology, Virus Research Institute, Kyoto University[*2]*

The relationship between malignant lymphomas and lymphatic
leukemias has long been one of the great issues in hematopathology.
A theory that these are different diseases and can be differentiated
histologically has been popular in Japan. Recent advances in the knowledge of normal and neoplastic lymphocytes have enabled a re-evaluation
of the relationship of leukemia and lymphoma.

In the normal body, both T- and B-lymphocytes circulate between
the tissues and the blood. Their site of re-entry into the tissues is the
network of postcapillary venules, and they actively migrate through these
preferential areas before entering the lymphatics. These lymphocytes
are in a resting phase and are morphologically small and medium-sized
cells. After acceptance of ligand including antigens they enter the G_1
phase of the division cycle and become larger and cohesive. As they
approach the dividing phase their migratory properties decrease. These
two natures of the lymphocytes are reflected in the neoplastic cells.

Distinctions between lymphomas and lymphatic leukemias are
arbitrary, and are designations made according to the differences in
the number of neoplastic cells in the intravascular compartment. A leukemic change in Hodgkin's disease is extremely rare and probably non-
existent, although thoracic duct cannulation demonstrates the presence
of large atypical cells. Leukemic changes in non-Hodgkin's lymphomas,
on the other hand, are rather frequent and are classified into three types.
Type I is represented by small and medium-sized cell lymphomas. The
blood pictures are similar to chronic lymphocytic leukemia (CLL) and
they reflect physiological recirculatory properties of normal lymphocytes.
Type II is represented by lymphoblastic lymphomas and Burkitt's
lymphomas, and the blood picture is similar to acute lymphatic leukemia
(ALL). These cells are non-migratory, and mobilization into the blood
is based on "spilling over" of the neoplastic cells due to rapid growth.
Type III is typically seen in pleomorphic peripheral T-cell lymphomas
in Japan and the leukemic cells are a mixture of various sizes and shapes.

The relationship between malignant lymphomas and lymphatic leukemias has
long been one of the great issues among pathologists and hematologists. Originally
malignant lymphoma was defined as a neoplasm starting from a localized tumor of the
lymph node, which only secondarily involved systemic lymph nodes and other organs

[*1] Nishi-Chuoh 2-Chome, Kure 737, Japan (難波絋二).

[*2] Kawara-cho, Shogoin, Sakyo-ku, Kyoto 606, Japan (花岡正男).

TABLE I. Classic Concepts of the Histological Differences between Leukemias and Lymphomas

	Manner of proliferation	Nodal architecture	Extracapsular invasion	Tumor formation	Cellular atypism
Leukemia	Infiltrative	Preserved	Present	Absent	Minimal
Lymphoma	Destructive	Effaced	Absent	Present	Marked

and in which the appearance of many neoplastic cells in the peripheral blood (leukemic conversion) is not observable.

Sternberg (65), however, at the beginning of the century described a type of child-hood lymphoma starting with generalized lymphadenopathy and a thymic mass, which became leukemic during its clinical course. He named it "leucosarcomatosis" which, in retrospect, corresponded to malignant lymphoma, lymphoblastic (48) of the present day. After his report the question was immediately raised of the distinction between "leucosarcomatosis" and acute lymphatic leukemia (18). On the other hand, studies on leukemias have demonstrated the existence of cases in which leukemic cells are very few or absent in the peripheral blood in spite of clinical similarities to typical leukemia. These cases have been called subleukemic or aleukemic leukemias, respectively (8). In these cases the distinction of aleukemic lymphatic leukemias from generalized lymphomas or lymphosarcomatosis again became a problem. In contrast to a tendency to regard the malignant lymphoma and lymphatic leukemia as separate entities, theories have been forwarded in which the two diseases are interrelated and represented two extremes of a spectrum of the single disease, but they have remained in the minority until recently (1, 70).

The theory that lymphatic leukemias and malignant lymphomas are entirely different diseases and could be differentiated histologically was popular in Japan until some 10 years ago (21). Table I depicts this theory with its advocated criteria for differentiation. A fundamental idea underlying this theory is that leukemic cells proliferate within the tissue freely and infiltratively, whereas lymphosarcoma cells proliferate cohesively and destructively. It was particularly emphasized that lymphatic leukemia cells in contrast to lymphosarcoma cells preserve the structure of the lymph node and infiltrate the extracapsular soft tissue without destroying it. Morphological differences between lymphatic leukemia cells and leukemic lymphosarcoma cells have been also proclaimed (28).

The last decade saw a remarkable advancement in research for normal and pathological lymphocytes, stages of and significant new information has been accumulated with regard to kinetics, subpopulations, and maturation of normal lymphocytes as well as of lymphoma cells, to such an extent as to enable us to reconsider the relationship between leukemia and lymphoma.

Behavior of Lymphocytes in Vivo

The number of lymphocytes circulating through the peripheral blood in an adult human is on the order of 10^{10} and, together with those within the tissue, there are some 2×10^{12} lymphocytes in the human body (12). If these lymphocytes were collected to form a single mass, it would correspond in volume to organs such as the liver or the brain. These lymphocytes consist of separate systems of T- and B-cells which have differentiated at early stages of ontogeny, and there are almost equal numbers of lymphocytes belonging to each system within the body (15).

1. Lymphocytes in recirculation

The origin of T-and B-cells in ontogeny can be traced back to stem cells in the yolk sac. The stem cells migrate at an early stage of development to a primordial thymus and hematopoietic foci in other organs, and, after having differentiated into T- and B-cells, they leave these sitess for other target tissues for further differentiation and maturation. These fundamental behavioral patterns of lymphocytes in a developing body are maintained in the adult, and lymphocytes rotate as circulatory cells around the body from the tissue to the blood and then back to the tissue.

In the lymph node, T- and B-cells home separately, respectively, to the paracortex and the cortex after they have recirculated to the node mainly hematogenously *via* postcapillary venules (15, 63). They do not settle there, however; B-cells as well as T-cells pass through the paracortical area to enter at the medullary cord in the lymph sinus and are carried away by the lymph.

In the spleen, T- and B-cells come back from the blood to the white pulp at the marginal zone (46). They are remobilized into the venous sinuses from the area surrounding the central artery after following different routes for each system of cells. According to a study using the sex chromosome as a marker, intravenously administered lymphocytes reappeared in the thoracic duct about 10 hr later (51). In an another study using isotope-labeled lymphocytes, the minimal recirculation times of human lymphocytes were 1 and 2 hr for two patients with renal insufficiency (55). Recirculation times of lymphocytes are different for the two tyepes of cells. T-cells recirculate about 10 times faster than B-cells, and their lifespan is 3 to 4 times longer (15, 63). Continuous drainage of lymph nodes depletes most T-cells from the paracor-

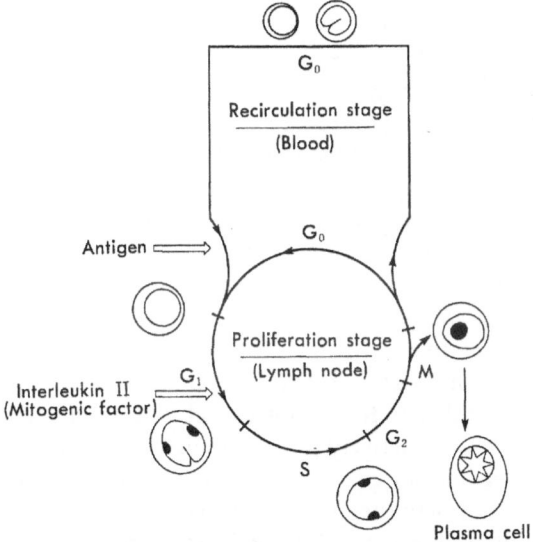

FIG. 1. Two physiological stages of lymphocytes.

tical areas, whereas B-cells are well preserved in the cortex, indicating a slow migration speed for B-cells in the tissue (63). These differences in property are contributory to the cells, variance in distribution; 80% of the blood lymphocytes are T-cells in contrast to a predominance of B-cells in the tissue (32). Both types, although differing in their circulation times, are constant travellers of the body, circulating ceaselessly within it without settling down permanently.

Most of the recirculating T- and B-cells belong to the resting (G_0) phase and assume the shape of "small or medium-sized lymphocytes" (Fig. 1). These lymphocytes are equipped with an avid migratory property as well as receptors for endothelial cells of the postcapillary venules and other specialized vessels (64), thus enabling themselves to be trapped by these special endothelial cells during blood circulation before entering the tissues through the interendothelial spaces. These properties explain the efficient recirculation of lymphocytes between the blood and the lymphatic tissues (15). Tissue factors responsible for migration of lymphocytes to the tissue across the blood vessels are known at present only in the inflammatory focus (26).

2. Lymphocyte in proliferative phase

According to animal experiments and *in vitro* studies of human cells, lymphocytes within the body are considered to divide and proliferate in the sequences described below:

Upon contact with antigens, resting lymphocytes change to large basophilic cells with prominent nucleoli (blastic trasnformation, rejuvenization), which are called "immunoblasts" or "lymphoblasts." Large lymphocytes now entering the G_1 phase receive as a second signal, just before the beginning of the S phase, the effect of interleukin II (mitogenic factor, MF) produced by T-cells activated by macrophages and others (34, 54). After 18 hr DNA synthesis begins and the lymphocytes are now in the S phase which eventually leads to cell division through the G_2 phase (Fig. 1). If antigens and interleukin II are consistently available, the lymphocytes repeat cell divisions, each time becoming smaller, until they reach the resting phase as small and medium-sized lymphocytes. These events take 4 to 5 days for completion (12, 15).

With the exception of prethymic and pre-B-cells and irrespective of maturational stages for T- and B-cells, lymphocytes are small and medium-sized cells in the resting phase and become large in the proliferation phase. Therefore, the expression that the large lymphocyte with a prominent nucleolus is immature and the small lymphocyte with condensed nuclear chromatin is mature or differentiated is inappropriate. The degree of maturity for lymphocytes cannot be directly measured by the morphology of the cells, a situation different from the case in myeloid cells.

As seen in allogenic mixed lymphocyte culture, *in vitro* lymphocytes which have become large and proliferative grow in a state in which the cells attach to each other. In other words, as the lymphocytes become larger, their migratory property decreases and they adhere to each other to form an islet and then eventually will divide. It may be said that lymphocytes can actively proliferate in a condition in which they are able to adhere to each other and an effective cellular interaction may be exerted, though this is not true in a state where they migrate freely.

In the lymph node proliferation of T- and B-cells begins around the postcapillary venules and in the cortex, respectively. B-cells at proliferation often form lymph follicles (germinal centers) together with dendritic cells, macrophages and a small number of T-cells (*19, 73*). B-cells transform into large cells within the follicles and afterwards move to the paracortex. The situation is similar for the other tissues. T-cells, on the other hand, do not form follicles but they are also in close association with mesenchymal cells such as macrophages and interdigitating cells in the proliferation focus in the paracortex. Such an actively proliferating focus occasionally assumes a nodular structure and is called a "tertiary follicle" (*53*).

Both large T- and B-cells which have started proliferation within the lymph node repeat cell division, while moving from the paracortex to the medullary cord, to again become cells of the resting phase which resume active migratory properties and enter the circulatory pathway. A maturing B-cell beyond this stage loses migratory properties, settles in the medullary cord without being mobilized and becomes a plasma cell as an end-stage cell. IgM-producing cells can be mobilized into the circulation not only in the form of small cells but also as large cells. IgA-producing cells are unique in their properties of selective migration to the lamina propria of the gastrointestinal tract (*27*). As for T-cells, any subsets of cells are mobilized in the form of lymphocytes of the resting phase, but some large T-cells with migratory properties can also be mobilized to enter the efferent lymphatics.

In short, there are two phases in the life cycle of the lymphocytes which correspond to their division cycle; in one phase lymphocytes are free cells with avid migratory properties and can easily appear in the peripheral blood from the tissues, and in the other phase they lose or decrease their migratory character owing to a tendency to form a mass and are not easily mobilized. This physiological biphasic nature of lymphocytes, retained even in neoplastic cells, makes the basis for a separation of lymphatic leukemias and malignant lymphomas in appearance.

Re-evaluation of the Relationship between Leukemia and Lymphoma

It is only in recent years that enough concrete data have been compiled to reconsider the relationship between leukemias and lymphomas. These are mainly brought by the following two ways approaches. First, widespread utilization of Rappaport's classification for non-Hodgkin's lymphomas (*52*) has enabled the accumulation of clinicopathological data on many lymphoma cases, which have clarified in a considerable degree the natural history of various histologic subtypes, including the frequency of leukemic conversion. Accordingly, the differences between lymphomas with a tendency toward leukemic change and those without have become increasingly apparent. Second, it has become possible in recent years to compare the cells of lymphomas and leukemias in detail, not only by morphological methods but also by immunological and cytochemical methods (*42, 61*).

1. Leukemic change in Hodgkin's disease

The present authors have not personally experienced any case of leukemic Hodgkin's disease. According to the literature, leukemias in Hodgkin's diseases can be separated into three categories. The first group consists of cases in which multinucleate Reed-Sternberg cells and/or mononuclear Hodgkin's cells were claimed to have been observed in the blood (*59, 71*). These could be called "true" leukemic Hodgkin's disease, although the reports are quite rare and not well-documented. In the terminal stage, neoplastic cells in Hodgkin's disease may reach the thoracic duct, thus enabling these cells to enter the subclavian vein (13). However, in a study involving a large series of cases the appearance of neoplastic cells in the peripheral blood was quite rare (0.2% of the cases) and was never frankly leukemic (4). Sequestration in the lung and spleen may play a role in the removal of neoplastic cells from the blood (43). To the second group belong rare cases in which transition to lymphatic leukemia has been observed. Sometimes a leukemia has been detected at the time of diagnosis of Hodgkin's disease (58). In retrospect, many such cases reported in Japan are considered in reality to have been leukemic type of pleomorphic T-cell lymphomas (25, 49). The need for stricter criteria for the diagnosis of Hodgkin's disease in Japan has been stressed (44). The relationship of terminal lymphatic leukemia to Hodgkin's disease remains to be elucidated, although one of the eight hitherto reported cases has been proved to be acute lymphatic leukemia (ALL) of T-cell nature (10).

Acute myelogenous leukemias following the treatment of Hodgkin's disease constitute the third group, and account for three quarters of the leukemias complicating Hodgkin's disease (58). These are treatment-related second malignancies and should not be included in the natural history of Hodgkin's disease (33). The significance of the reported vascular invasion in lymph nodes involved by Hodgkin's disease remains to be evaluated for the relation not only to leukemic change but also to hematogenous metastasis (33).

2. Leukemic change in non-Hodgkin's lymphomas

The leukemic change in malignant lymphomas was studied systematically for the first time by Gall and Mallory (16). According to their detailed study of 618 cases, leukemic change was observed in 48% of lymphocytic lymphomas and 38% of lymphoblastic lymphomas. Leukemic change in other types of lymphomas was rare. Rosenberg (56) studied 1,269 cases of non-Hodgkin's lymphomas and stated that leukemic changes were observed in 12.6% of lymphosarcomas in contrast to 8.6% and 2.4%, respectively, in follicular lymphomas and reticulum cell sarcomas. It has been known historically that more smaller cell lymphomas tend to become leukemic compared to large-celled ones.

Researchers' opinions are split with regard to how many neoplastic cells appearing in the peripheral blood should be called leukemic, and no consensus exists about this. Gall and Mallory as well as Rosenberg excluded cases which were leukemic at the time of diagnosis, and regarded those cases as leukemic conversion which were complicated during their course more than 30,000 white blood cells (WBC) in the peripheral blood or bone marrow involvement (16, 56). Lennert considers leukemic change as those with more than 1% neoplastic cells in the peripheral WBC (38). Shimoyama defines leukemia as having neoplastic cells in excess of 30% of the peripheral WBC count or with bone marrow involvement (61).

These distinctions are arbitrary and indicate that lymphatic leukemias and malignant lymphomas are a spectrum of diseases. They are designations according to differences in the quantity of neoplastic cells existing in the peripheral blood and bone marrow. We will review in the following the frequencies of leukemic changes in various types of non-Hodgkin's lymphomas according to Rappaport's and the Japanese Lymphoma Study Group (LSG) classifications (66), and will discuss the mechanism of leukemic conversion in lymphomas.

Leukemic change in follicular lymphomas was studied in detail by Rosenthal et al. (57) based on their own materials and the literature. According to their report, 7 cases (11.8%) out of their 59 studied turned out to be leukemic after careful review of the peripheral blood films, in contrast to 4% reported in the literature. The appearance of characteristic lymphocytes called "hematogones" was observed in the peripheral blood of all the leukemic cases (57). The "hematogone" corresponds to what is today called a notched nucleus cell or a small cleaved cell (39, 62). As for the relationship of leukemic change to histological types, the poorly differentiated lymphocytic (medium-sized cell) type tends to become leukemic compared to the histiocytic (large cell) type (31, 41).

Leukemic change in diffuse lymphomas is frequently observed in the small cell (well differentiated lymphocytic; WDL) type, medium-sized cell (poorly differentiated lymphocytic) type, lymphoblastic type, and pleomorphic type. The small cell lymphomas are regarded as a tissue manifestation of chronic lymphocytic leukemia (CLL) and their rates of leukemic change are reported to be as high as 44 to 66% (14, 50). These figures may be smaller than reality because the chances of lymph node biopsies are smaller when the peripheral blood involvement has been observed clinically. Leukemic change in medium-sized cell lymphomas, except lymphoblastic lymphomas, is reported to be 38% (69) or 33% (72), and 50% in Japanese cases (30). In many cases, leukemic cells are small cleaved cells.

Lymphoblastic lymphomas also tend to become leukemic and accompany ALL-like blood pictures. Nathwani et al. (48) observed leukemic conversion in 82% of their cases. Leukemic changes in Japanese cases are between 76 and 84% (11, 67). Leukemic changes in pleomorphic lymphomas are not paid much attention in Western countries, probably because of the rarity of these lymphomas. However, leukemic conversion as high as 84% was observed in Japanese cases (35). Peripheral blood pictures in these lymphomas are variable to a great extent from CLL-like ones to an admixture of large, medium-sized and small lymphocytes (23, 24). Although leukemic change in Burkitt's lymphomas has been considered a rare occurrence, a recent careful review of the issue has pointed out a conversion rate of 25% (40). Leukemic Burkitt's lymphomas are classified as ALL (L3) by the French-American-British Co-operative Group (FAB)-

TABLE II. Incidence of Leukemic Change in Non-Hodgkin's Lymphomas

	Japan		Western countries	
Follicular lymphoma	?		11.8%	(57)
Diffuse lymphoma				
Small cell	?		66%	(14)
Medium-sized cell	50%	(30)	33%	(72)
Mixed	?		?	
Large cell	30.7%	(30)	2.4%	(56)
Pleomorphic	84%	(35)	?	
Lymphoblastic	84%	(11)	82%	(48)
Burkitt's	?		25%	(40)

Notes: ? stands for data unavailable. The number in parenthesis refers to the literature.

classification of acute leukemias (2). Large cell (histiocytic) lymphomas become leukemic
only rarely, but when it occurs the blood picture is usually that of ALL. Table II
summarizes the rates of leukemic conversion for each subtype of lymphomas based on
the literature.

So far, we have discussed the mobilization of lymphoma cells into the peripheral
blood on the basis of the histologies of the lymphomas. This could also be viewed from
the opposite side. Dick et al., for example, studied the histologies of biopsied lymph
nodes for 41 patients whose peripheral blood pictures were those of typical CLL (i.e.,
predominantly small round lymphocytes (9)). In 54% of the cases, histologies corresponded to well differentiated lymphocytic lymphomas whereas 34% were poorly
differentiated lymphocytic, and 12% were mixed and histiocytic. This dissociation between the histology and blood picture is also often observed in pleomorphic lymphomas
in Japan (23). In the following considerations leukemic cells appearing in the peripheral
blood are divided, for convenience, into three categories and their mechanisms of leukemic conversion will be discussed.

Mechanism of Leukemic Conversion

1. Type I: small and medium-sized cells
The cells in the peripheral blood of this group are small lymphocytes with a diameter of less than 10 μm of medium-sized cells of 10 to 12 μm. They are relatively
monomorphic and mitoses are rare. Patients are mostly in middle or old age, and onsets
are insidious with gradual involvement of systemic lymph nodes and bone marrow.
The clinical couse is usually protracted. The tissue manifestation is usually diffuse
small cells (WDL), diffuse medium-sized (small cleaved) cell or follicular medium-sized
cell types. It is generally known that leukemic small cell lymphomas cannot be differentiated from CLL with regard to clinical symptoms, histologies and cellular morphologies. The surface marker studies demonstrate no differences between the two conditions
(5). Chronic lymphosarcoma cell leukemia (28, 60) and prolymphocytic leukemia (17)
correspond to diffuse or follicular medium-sized cell lymphomas (60). These are B-cells
with strong SIg and C3-receptors, and many of these cells are positive for alkaline phosphatase (47). The neoplastic cells are morphologically larger than CLL cells and their
nuclei are often indented. They have prominent single nucleoli and a moderate amount
of cytoplasm. There are several pieces of evidence indicating that the leukemic cells in
this group correspond phenotypically to normally recirculating B-lymphocytes. Small
round lymphocytes observed in CLL and diffuse small cell lymphomas are probably
equivalent to circulating memory B-cells after blastic trasnformation. Small cleaved
lymphocytes in medium-sized cell lymphomas are akin to prefollicular cells which are
normally observed in primary follicles and the mantle zone of germinal centers (20,
47). The latter are also known to belong to recirculating pool and most probably
represent virgin B-cells (3, 20). If we recognize these similarities between neoplastic
cells and normal lymphocytes with regard to morphologies and surface markers, it will
be reasonable to presume that these leukemic cells also express the migratory patterns
of their normal counterparts.

Bremer (6, 7) studied the recirculation of lymphocytes in B-CLL patients and
found that the reappearance of labeled CLL cells in the thoracic duct lymph was

significantly delayed compared to controls. This is not surprising because most of the lymphocytes in normal peripheral blood are T-cells with a recirculation time significantly shorter than that for B-cells (3, 63).

2. Type II: medium-sized cells and large cells

Neoplastic cells in this group are medium-sized to large, and are relatively monomorphic. The cell size is over 10 μm in blood films. The histological counterparts are lymphoblastic and Burkitt's lymphomas. Leukemic cells in this group are homogenous with regular nuclear shapes. They are morphologically primitive-looking "blasts," and correspond functionally to early T-cells or B-cells (42, 61). Both are histologically characterized by high mitotic rates reflecting their short doubling times (37). They frequently involve the bone marrow, a finding which may be related to the fact that pre-T and pre-B cells originate there.

The mechanism of leukemic change in this group seems to be different from that of group I. These cells decline active migratory properties. Lymph nodes or bone marrow biopsied in this group of lymphomas usually reveal abundant neoplastic cells in the medullary sinuses or in sinusoids. Increased tissue pressure resulting from high mitotic rates could drive these cells into the vascular channels. This mechanism is called "spilling over" or "overflow" and also explains the appearance of non-hematopoietic cells like cancer cells in the peripheral blood (43). The not infrequent appearance of these lymphoma cells in the serous cavities can also be explained on this basis. The other point to be considered is that in the thymus, which is often involved by lymphoblastic lymphomas, efferent lymphatics open directly into the veins without intercalating lymph nodes. This may facilitate the leukemic conversion of this type of lymphoma (48). Cell sizes also play an important role. The cells appearing in the blood are usually smaller than those in the tissue. This is applicable to rare cases of histiocytic (large cell) and plasma cell leukemias (29).

3. Type III: admixture of polymorphous cells

Neoplastic cells in the peripheral blood are heterogeneous, the ranging from small cells to large ones, and also occasional bizarre giant cells, although small and medium-sized ones usually predominate. Moreover, these cells characteristically demonstrate irregular, often lobulated nuclear shapes. They are neoplastic counterparts of peripheral T (T_2)-cells. Non-leukemic forms are called pleomorphic lymphomas (37, 66) and leukemic ones are collectively designated as adult T-cell leukemias (ATL) (22, 68). The tissue expression of many ATL is pleomorphic lymphoma which often resembles Hodgkin's disease, particularly mixed cellularity and lymphocyte depleted types, and malignant histiocytosis (23). Polymorphism of the leukemic cells in this group is a reflection of pleomorphism in the tissue, where lymphoma cells are in various stages of phenotypical activation as seen in the paracortical area of the non-malignant, activated lymph node. Leukemic changes are more frequent in those subtypes in which smaller lymphocytes predominate. However, there is not infrequently a dissociation between the cytology of the peripheral blood and that of the tissue as mentioned previously (23). This is partly because the smaller lymphocytes, which are probably the equivalent of normal small T-lymphocytes in the resting phase, are more easily mobilized into the blood through the efferent lymphatics. (36) A similar phenomenon was observed in CLL

TABLE III. Interrelationships of Malignant Lymphomas and Lymphatic Leukemias

Malignant lymphoma	Lymphatic leukemia
Small cell type ———————	CLL
Medium-sized cell type	Prolymphocytic leukemia (lymphosarcoma cell leukemia)
Mixed type	Large lymphoid cell leukemia
	Immunoblastic leukemia
Large cell type	"Histiocytic" leukemia
	"Leukemic reticuloendotheliosis"
Pleomorphic type ———————	ATL
Lymphoblastic type ———————	Lymphoblastic leukemia (ALL, L1)
Burkitt's type ———————	Burkitt's cell leukemia (ALL, L3)

(10). A histological study performed independently and based on clinical information demonstrated that the proliferation of postcapillary venules and the number of atypical small lymphocytes passing across their walls were intimately related to the leukemic picture of small cell predominance. When large or medium-sized cells are predominant in the peripheral blood, these features are not observed and instead, packing of neoplastic cells in the lymph sinuses as seen in group II lymphomas is conspicious (45). Apparently the mechanism of mobilization of lymphoma cells into the peripheral blood in group III is not singular. Phenotypical maturation of the lymphoma cells corresponding to normal recirculating small T-cells is responsible for the blood picture in many cases, but in others "spilling over" of the expanded clone may contribute to it. Bone marrow and thymus play only a limited roles if any, since these lymphomas usually do not involve them. The interrelationships of various lymphomas and lymphatic leukemias are briefly summarized in Table III.

CONCLUSION

There are no essential differencs between lymphatic leukemias and malignant lymphomas as have been emphasized in the past by some pathologists and hematologists. The relationships of the two categories of disease can be explained uniformly based on the two physiological properties of the lymphocytes. In the first place, lymphocytes are cells with a fate to circulate between the tissues and the blood. They actively migrate through the tissues to return to the blood, although some conditioning factors may be necessary. In the second place, lymphocytes in a resting phase with the shape of small and medium-sized cells become large and cohesive once they enter the G_1 phase of the division cycle. As they approach the dividing phase after passing through S and G_2 phases, their migratory properties decrease. These two characters are reflected in neoplastic lymphocytes and can explain the two mechanisms for the leukemic conversion of lymphomas. The first is the mobilization through migratory properties of neoplastic cells, which are probably similar to the physiological events. Leukemic change by this mechanism is often seen when the neoplastic cells are small or medium-sized cells. Leukemic change in the pleomorphic lymphomas is also largely due to this.

The second is a passive mobilization or "spilling over" of the neoplastic cells, which is caused by partial destruction of the tissue and/or increased tissue pressure. The mechanism is similar to that of the appearance of cancer cells in the peripheral blood, and even such actively dividing large and medium-sized cells that lose their migratory capacities can become leukemic. Lymphomas with high mitotic counts and short doubling times, such as lymphoblastic, Burkitt's and some large cell lymphomas, belong to this group. The relationships between lymphatic leukemias and malignant lymphomas can be summarized at present from a pathophysiological view point. However, leukemia is a stage IV systemic disease *ab initio* from a clinical point of view, and most of the malignant lymphomas are localized diseases in the beginning. They are clinically different diseases necessitating different modalities of treatment. However, these revised concepts of the relationships between the two diseases could be beneficial for the diagnosis, evaluation and treatment of malignant lymphomas, since they will give insight into the frequencies of leukemic changes or systematization according to their histological types.

REFERENCES

1. Apitz, K. Allgemeine Pathologie der menschlichen Leukämien. *Ergeb. Allg. Pathol. Anat.*, **35**, 1–104 (1940).
2. Bennett, J. M., Catovsky, D., Daniel, M. T., Flandrin, G., Galton, D.A.G., Gralnick, H. R., and Sultan, C. Proposal for the classification of the acute leukemias. French-American-British (FAB) Co-operative Group. *Br. J. Haematol.*, **33**, 451–458 (1976).
3. Bhan, A. K., Nadler, L. M., Stashenko, P., McCluskey, R. T., and Schlossman, S. F. Stages of B cell differentiation in human lymphoid tissues. *J. Exp. Med.*, **154**, 737–739 (1981).
4. Bouroncle, B. A. Sternberg-Reed cell in the peripheral blood of patients with Hodgkin's disease. *Blood*, **27**, 544–556 (1966).
5. Braylan, R. C., Jaffe, E. S., Burbach, J. W., Frank, M. M., Johnson, R. E., and Berard, C. W. Similarities of surface characteristics of neoplastic well-differentiated lymphocytes from solid tissues and from peripheral blood. *Cancer Res.*, **36**, 1619–1625 (1976).
6. Bremer, K., Fliedner, T. M., and Schick, P. Kinetic difference of autotransfused ^{3}H-cytidine labeled blood lymphocytes in leukemic and non-leukemic lymphoma. *Eur. J. Cancer*, **9**, 113–124 (1973).
7. Bremer, K., Wack, O., and Schick, P. Impaired recirculation of autotransfused blood lymphocytes *via* thoracic duct lymph in patients with chronic lymphoid leukemia. *Biomedicine*, **18**, 393–400 (1973).
8. Dameshek, W. and Gunz, F. "Leukemia," 2nd ed., pp. 16–27 (1964). Grune & Stratton, New York.
9. Dick, F. R. and Maca, R. D. The lymph node in chronic lymphocytic leukemia. *Cancer*, **41**, 283–292 (1978).
10. Dick, F. R., Maca, R. D., and Hankenson, R. Hodgkin's disease terminating in a T-cell immunoblastic leukemia. *Cancer*, **42**, 1325–1329 (1978).
11. Dohi, H., Okita, H., Saito, N., Kyo, S., Kamada, N., Okada, K., Kuramoto, J., Nanba, K., and Itagaki, T. Clinics of malignant lymphoma, lymphoblastic. *J. Jpn. Soc. RES*, **21**, 99 (1981) (in Japanese).
12. Douglas, S. D. Cells involved in immune responses. *In* "Basic and Clinical Immunology," 3rd ed., ed. H. H. Fudenberg, D. P. Stites, J. L. Caldwell, and J. V. Wells, pp. 96–114 (1980). Lange Med. Pub., Los Altos.
13. Engset, A., Höeg, K., Höst, H., Liverud, K., and Nesheim, A. Thoracic duct lymph cytology in Hodgkin's disease. *Int. J. Cancer*, **4**, 735–742 (1969).

14. Evans, H. L., Butler, J. J., and Youness, E. L. Malignant lymphoma, small lymphocytic type: A clinicopathologic study of 84 cases with suggested criteria for intermediate lymphocytic lymphoma. *Cancer*, **41**, 1440–1455 (1978).

15. Ford, W. L. Lymphocyte migration and immune responses. *Progr. Allergy*, **19**, 1–59 (1975).

16. Gall, E. A. and Mallory, J. B. Malignant lymphoma: A clinicopathologic survey of 618 cases. *Am. J. Pathol.*, **18**, 381–429 (1942).

17. Galton, D.A.G., Goldmann, J. M., Wiltshaw, E., Catovsky, D., Henry, K., and Goldenberg, G. J. Prolymphocytic leukaemia. *Br. J. Haematol.*, **27**, 7–23 (1974).

18. Goldberg, G. M. and Emanuel, B. A study of malignant lymphomas and leukemias. VII. Lymphogenous leukemia and lymphosarcoma involvement of the lymphatic and hemic bed with reference to differentiating criteria. *Cancer*, **17**, 277–287 (1964).

19. Gutman, G. A. and Weissman, I. L. Lymphoid tissue architecture: Experimental analysis of the origin and distribution of T-cells and B-cells. *Immunology*, **23**, 465–479 (1972).

20. Gutman, G. and Weissman, I. Homing properties of thymus-independent follicular lymphocytes. *Transplantation*, **16**, 621–629 (1973).

21. Hamazaki, Y. "Interpretation in Histopathology and Differential Diagnosis", pp. 71–72 (1972). Ishiyaku-Shuppan, Tokyo.

22. Hanaoka, M. Clinical pathology of adult T cell leukemia. *Acta Haematol. Jpn.*, **44**, 1131–1185 (1981).

23. Hanaoka, M., Sasaki, M., Matsumoto, H., Tankawa, Y., Yamabe, H., Tomimoto, K., Tasaka, C., Fujiwara, H., Uchiyama, T., and Takatsuki, K. Adult T cell leukemia: Histological classification and characteristics. *Acta Pathol. Jpn.*, **29**, 723–738 (1979).

24. Hanaoka, M., Shirakawa, S., Yodoi, J., Uchiyama, T., and Takatsuki, K. Adult T cell leukemia. Histological features of the lymphoid tissue. *In* "Function and Structure of the Immune System," ed. W. Müller-Ruchholts and H. K. Müller-Hermelink, pp. 613–621 (1979). Plenum Publ., New York.

25. Harada, R. Two cases complicating cryptococcal meningitis during the treatment of leukemia and Hodgkin's disease. *Nihon Kagaku-ryoho Gakkai-shi*, **22**, 302 (1974) (in Japanese).

26. Higuchi, Y., Honda, M., and Hayashi, H. Production of chemotactic factor for lymphocytes by neutral SH-dependent protease of rabbit PMN leucocytes from immunoglobulins, especially IgM. *Cell Immunol.*, **15**, 100–108 (1975).

27. Husband, A. J., Monié, H. J., and Gowans, J. L. The natural history of cells producing IgA in the gut. *In* "The Immunology of the Gut," Ciba Foundation Symposium, Vol. 46, pp. 29–54 (1977). Elsevier, Amsterdam.

28. Isaacs, R. Lymphosarcoma cell leukemia. *Ann. Intern. Med.*, **11**, 657–662 (1937).

29. Isobe, T., Ikeda, Y., Imura, H., and Ohta, H. Plasma cell leukemia. A clinical study of 13 cases, with a demonstration of small-sized plasma cells. *Acta Haematol. Jpn.*, **10**, 529–540 (1977).

30. Itoyama, S., Shimamine, T., Mori, S., Imamura, T., Saito, H., and Mohri, N. On the appearance of neoplastic cells in the peripheral blood with malignant lymphomas. *Trans. Soc. Pathol. Jpn.*, **69**, 299 (1980).

31. Jones, S. E., Rosenberg, S. A., and Kaplan, H. S. Non-Hodgkin's lymphomas. 1. Bone marrow involvement. *Cancer*, **29**, 954–960 (1972).

32. Jønsson, V. and Cristensen, B. E. Distribution of B. T., and O lymphocytes in blood and tissues of normal humans reflecting a kinetic model. *Scand. J. Haematol.*, **18**, 185–196 (1977).

33. Kaplan, H. S. Hodgkin's disease: Biology, treatment, prognosis. *Blood*, **57**, 813–822 (1981).

34. Kawano, M., Namba, Y., and Hanaoka, M. Regulatory factors of lymphocyte-lymphocyte interaction. 1. Con A-induced mitogenic factor acts on the late G_1 stage of T cell proliferation. *Microbiol. Immunol.*, **25**, 505–515 (1981).

35. Kikuchi, M., Mitsui, T., Matsui, N., Sato, E., Tokunaga, M., Hasui, K., Ichimaru, M., Kinoshita, K., and Kamihira, S. T-cell malignancies in adults: Histopathological studies of lymph nodes in 110 patients. *Jpn. J. Clin. Oncol.*, **9** (Suppl.), 407–421 (1979).

36. Kinoshita, K., Kamihira, K., Ikeda, S., Yamada, Y., Oyakawa, K., Yoshioka, A., Muta, T., Kitamura, T., and Ichimaru, M. Surface marker study of malignant lymphomas. III. On maturation, differentiation and mechanism of leukemic change of malignant lymphoma, T-cell type as seen from the morphology of neoplastic cells in the peripheral blood. *J. Jpn. Soc. RES*, **19**, 295–304 (1979) (in Japanese).

37. Kojima, M., Iijima, S., Hanaoka, M., and Suchi, T. (eds.) "Atlas of Malignant Lymphomas Based on New Classifications," pp. 73–77 (1981). Bunko-do, Tokyo.

38. Lennert, K. "Histopathology and Diagnosis of Non-Hodgkin's Lymphoma, pp. 54–89 (1980). Springer-Verlag, New York.

39. Lukes, R. J. and Collins, R. D. Immunological characterization of human malignant lymphomas. *Cancer*, **34** (Suppl.), 1488–1503 (1974).

40. Magrath, I. T. and Ziegler, J. L. Bone marrow involvement in Burkitt's lymphoma and its relationship to acute B-cell leukemia. *Leukemia Res.*, **4**, 33–59 (1979).

41. McKenna, R., Bloomfield, C. D., and Brunning, R. Nodular lymphoma—bone marrow and blood manifestations. *Cancer*, **36**, 428–440 (1975).

42. Minato, K. and Shimoyama, M. Immunological surface characteristics of malignant hematopoietic tumor cells. *Recent Adv. RES Res.* **17**, 116–132 (1977).

43. Myerowitz, R. L., Edwards, P. A., and Sartiano, G. P. Carcinocythemia (carcinoma cell leukemia) due to metastatic carcinoma of the breast. Report of a case. *Cancer*, **40**, 3107–3111 (1977).

44. Nanba, K. and Itagaki, T. On the incidence of Hodgkin's disease in Japan. *Trans. Soc. Pathol. Jpn.*, **69**, 298 (1980).

45. Nanba, K., Itagaki, T., Kinoshita, K., Kamihira, K., Ikeda, S., and Ichimaru, M. On the histological predictability of leukemic conversion of peripheral T-cell lymphomas. Abstr. 18th Int. Congr. Hematol., p. 1219 (1980).

46. Nanba, K., Itagaki, T., Ono, T., Hara, H., and Iijima, S. Comparative morphology of spleens of birds and mammals: A study by scanning and transmission electron microscopes, vascular corrosion cast, gelatinized carbon injection and enzyme histochemistry. *Recent Adv. RES Res.*, **19**, 15–42 (1980).

47. Nanba, K., Jaffe, E. S., Braylan, R. C., Soban, E. J., and Berard, C. W. Alkaline phosphatase-positive malignant lymphoma: A subtype of B-cell lymphomas. *Am. J. Clin. Pathol.*, **68**, 535–542 (1977).

48. Nathwani, B. N., Kim, H., and Rappaport, H. Malignant lymphoma, lymphoblastic. *Cancer*, **38**, 964–983 (1976).

49. Oshima, Y. A case of Hodgkin's sarcoma with the appearance of atypical lymphocytes of T-cell nature in the peripheral blood. *Acta Haematol. Jpn.*, **40** 383 (1977).

50. Pangalis, G. A., Nathwani, B. N., and Rappaport, H. Malignant lymphoma, well differentiated lymphocytic. Its relationship with chronic lymphocytic leukemia and macroglobulinemia of Waldenström. *Cancer*, **39**, 999–1010 (1977).

51. Perry, S., Irvin, G. L., III, and Whang, J. Studies of lymphocyte kinetics in man. *In*

"The Lymphocyte in Immunology and Hematopoiesis," ed. J. M. Yoffey, pp. 99–107 (1967). E. Arnold Publisher Ltd., London.

52. Rappaport, H. "Tumor of the Hematopoietic System," Altas of Tumor Pathology Sect. III, Fasc. 8 (1966). A.F.I.P., Washington, D. C.

53. Ree, H. and Fanger, H. Paracortical alteration in lymphadenopathic and tumor-draining lymph nodes: Histological study. *Human Pathol.*, **6**, 363–372 (1975).

54. Reinhertz, E. O., Kung, P. C., Breard, J. M., Goldstein, G., and Schlossman, S. F. T cell requirements for generation of helper factors in man. Analysis of the subsets involved. *J. Immunol.*, **124**, 1883–1887 (1980).

55. Revillard, J. P., Brochier, J., Durix, A., Bernhard, J. P., Byron, P. A., Archmbaud, J. P., Fries, D., and Taeger, J. Drainage du canal thoracique avant transplantation chez des malades atteints d'insuffisance rénale chronique. *Nouv. Rev. Franc. Hematol.* **8**, 585–602 (1968).

56. Rosenberg, S. A., Diamond, H. D., Jaslowitz, B., and Craver, L. F. Lymphosarcoma: A review of 1269 cases. *Medicine*, **40**, 31–84 (1961).

57. Rosenthal, N., Dreskin, O. H., Vural, I. L., and Zak, F. G. The significance of hematogenes in blood, bone marrow and lymph node aspiration in giant follicular lymphoblastoma. *Acta Haematol.*, **8**, 368–377 (1952).

58. Rosner, F. and Grunwald, H. Hodgkin's disease and acute leukemia. Report of eight cases and review of the literature. *Am. J. Med.*, **58**, 339–353 (1975).

59. Scheerer, P. P., Pierre, R. V., Schwartz, D. L., and Linman, J. W. Reed-Sternberg cell leukemia and lactic acidosis: Unusual manifestation of Hodgkin's disease. *N. Engl. J. Med.*, **270**, 274–278 (1964).

60. Schnitzer, B., Loesel, L. S., and Reed, R. E. Lymphosarcoma cell leukemia. A clinicopathological study. *Cancer*, **26**, 1082–1096 (1970).

61. Shimoyama, M. and Kimura, K. Clinics of leukemia. B. Acute and chronic lymphatic leukemias. *In* "Nihon Ketsueki-gaku Zensho," 6-II, pp. 365–397 (1979). Maruzen, Tokyo (in Japanese).

62. Spiro, G., Galton, D.A.G., Wiltshaw, E., and Lohmann, R. C. Follicular lymphoma: A survey of 75 cases with special reference to the syndrome resembling chronic lymphocytic leukaemia. *Br. J. Cancer*, **31** (Suppl. II), 60–72 (1975).

63. Sprent, J. Circulating T and B lymphocytes of the mouse. 1. Migratory properties. *Cell. Immunol.*, **7**, 10–39 (1973).

64. Stamper, H. B. and Woodruff, J. J. An *in vitro* model of lymphocyte homing. 1. Characterization of the interaction between thoracic duct lymphocytes and specialized high-endothelial venules of lymph nodes. *J. Immunol.*, **119**, 772–780 (1977).

65. Sternberg, C. Leukosarkomatose und Myeloblastenleukämie. *Beitr. Pathol.*, **61**, 75–100 (1916).

66. Suchi, T., Tajima, K., Nanba, K., Wakasa, H., Mikata, A., Kikuchi, M., Mori, S., Watanabe, S., Mohri, N., Shamoto, M., Harigaya, K., Itagaki, T., Matsuda, M., Kirino, Y., Takagi, K., and Fukunaga, S. Some problems on the histopathological diagnosis of non-Hodgkin's malignant lymphoma:A proposal of a new type. *Acta. Pathol. Jpn.*, **29**, 755–776 (1979).

67. Tajima, K. and Suchi, T. On clinicopathological and enzyme cytochemical characteristics of malignant lymphoma, lymphoblastic. *Trans. Soc. Pathol. Jpn.*, **70**, 242 (1981).

68. Takatsuki, K., Uchiyama, T., Ueshima, Y., and Hattori, T. Adult T-cell leukemia. Further clinical observations and cytogenetic and functional studies of leukemic cells. *Jpn. J. Clin. Oncol.*, **9** (Suppl.), 317–323 (1979).

69. Toksforf, G., Stein, H., and Lennert, K. Morphological and immunological definition of a malignant lymphoma derived from germinal-centre cells with cleaved nuclei (centrocytes). *Br. J. Cancer*, **41**, 168–182 (1980).
70. Türk, W. Ein System der Lymphomatosen. *Wien. Klin. Wochenschr.*, **16**, 1073–1085 (1903).
71. Varadi, S. Reed-Sternberg cells in the peripheral blood and bone-marrow in Hodgkin's disease. *Br. Med. J.*, **1**, 1239–1243 (1960).
72. Weisenburger, D. D., Nathwani, B. N., Diamond, L. W., Winberg, C. D., and Rappaport, H. Malignant lymphoma, intermediate lymphocytic type: A clinicopathologic study of 42 cases. *Cancer*, **48**, 1415–1425 (1981).
73. Yanaginuma, Y. Immunocytochemical study of the cells composing secondary follicles. *J. Jpn. Res. RES*, **19**, 165–191 (1979) (in Japanese).

T CELL LYMPHOMAS IN RELATION TO SUBPOPULATION OF T LYMPHOCYTES

Shaw Watanabe, Takashi Nakajima, and Masanori Shimoyama

Pathology Division and Clinical Laboratory, National Cancer Center Research Institute and Hospital*

Histologic characteristics of peripheral T-cell lymphoma were described based upon different stainability for monoclonal antibodies. OKT4 and Leu3a positive lymphomas consisted of 3 diffuse large cell types, 2 diffuse medium-sized cell types, and OKT8 and Leu2a positive lymphomas consisted of 1 so-called Lennert's lymphoma, and 3 immunoblastic lymphadenopathy (IBL)-like T-cell lymphomas.

Histiocytic infiltration was analyzed based upon the hypothesis of the existence of two histiocytic cell lineages; one was S100 protein positive, nonspecific cross reacting antigen with carcinoembryonic antigen (NCA) negative, and the other was S100 protein negative, NCA positive.

Lymphoma and leukemia of peripheral T-lymphocyte origin are frequent in Japan compared to the United States and Europe (7, 8, 15, 22–26). In the National Cancer Center, 40% of the lymphoma and lymphoid leukemia cases are of T-cell origin, and the these 65% are peripheral T-cell type (34). The most well known neoplasms belonging to that category are mycosis fungoides, Sézary syndrome, and adult T-cell leukemia (ATL) or pleomorphic T-cell lymphoma/leukemia. ATL was originally reported by Takatsuki and his associates, and high incidence has been reported in Kyushu and Okinawa in the southern part of Japan (6, 26). Recent work on materials from patients with this lymphoma/leukemia revealed the presence of antibodies (anti-ATL antigen; ATLA) and further work succeeded in isolating a new type of retrovirus as the causative agent. The pathology of ATL has received much attention in the last few years, and it has been shown to have a pleomorphic appearance, composed of large and small cells (8, 32).

Other peripheral T-cell lymphomas also have a mixed cell composition of large and small cells, but their relationship to the ATL-type lymphoma is still obscure (16). We previously suggested that research using monoclonal antibodies against T-cell subsets would clarify these problems (32). Diffuse lymphoblastic lymphoma and acute lymphoblastic leukemia has been studied by these methods (1, 7). In this manuscript we deal with 11 cases of T-cell lymphoma in adults, with special reference to whether peripheral T-cell lymphoma could be subdivided by their surface antigens and whether they could have subset-associated histologic characteristics.

---

* Tsukiji 5-1-1, Chuo-ku, Tokyo 104, Japan (渡辺　昌, 中島　孝, 下山正徳).

T-cell Subsets in Reactive Lymph Nodes and Thymoma

Three reactive lymph nodes, three dermatopathic lymphadenopathies, and one Castleman's tumor were studied in terms of the composition of T-cell subsets, for comparison with the results of peripheral T-cell lymphomas. The methods of detection for surface receptors and surface immunoglobulins were described in a previous paper (22). To determine subpopulations of T-lymphocytes, monoclonal antibodies against human T-cells were used: OKT3 (21) or Leu1 (28) for all T-lymphocytes, OKT4 (20) or Leu3a (4) for inducer/helper T-lymphocytes, OKT8 (19) or Leu2a (12) for suppressor/cytotoxic T-lymphocytes, OKT6 (2) and/or 036 for immature T-lymphocytes. The OKT series was purchased from Ortho Pharmaceutical Co. U.S.A., the Leu series from Becton-Dickinson, U.S.A., and 036 from Sera Lab, U.K. FITC-labeled anti-mouse Ig rabbit IgG (Cappel, U.S.A.) was applied for indirect immunofluorescence studies. This second antibody was used after absorption with human spleen cells (1:1 in volume) to exclude occasional non-specific cross reaction. Fluorescent staining was evaluated by a fluorescent microscope (Olympus Optical Co., Japan) and some by the fluorescence activated cell sorter (FACS IV, Becton-Dickinson, U.S.A.). Some materials were frozen sections, acetone fixed and stained with monoclonal antibody by the peroxidase-anti-peroxidase (PAP) method (DAKOPATTS, Denmark) for histologic observation (18, 29).

The distribution of T-cell subsets within the lymph nodes was studied with subset specific antibodies. OKT3 and Leu1, OKT4 and Leu3a, and OKT8 and Leu2a showed the same comparable stainability, respectively. Most of the small lymphocytes in the paracortical area and some in the germinal centers positively stained for inducer/helper antigen, and suppressor/cytotoxic T-lymphocytes were scattered in the paracortical area but were very rare in the reactive follicles (Photo 1). Dendritic cells in the paracortical area were diffusely stained by OKT6 and/or 036. They were also S100 protein positive and constituted a family of T-zone histiocytes, which are independent of the monocyte-macrophage system (30). This will be dealt with later.

An increased ratio of inducer/helper T-cells was observed in dermatopathic lymphadenopathy. S100+ histiocytic infiltration was marked both in the paracortical area and in the lymphatic sinuses. In Castleman's tumor, the decreased paracortical area was occupied by vascular proliferation and plasma cells, and many germinal centers containing vessels with hyperplastic endothelial cells were noted. A decreased ratio of T-lymphocytes was noted, mainly due to decreased helper T-cells which resulted in a relatively increased ratio of suppressor T-cells.

Lymphomas with Inducer/helper T-cell Antigen

It is well known that cutaneous T cell lymphoma belongs to this category because of the work of Kung *et al.* (11), Broder *et al.* (3), and others. Neoplastic cells possess a helper function in the Ig synthesis of pokeweed mitogen (PWM)-stimulated B-lymphocytes. Leukemic cells of ATL were also reported to have inducer/helper T-cell antigens, whereas they functionally acted as suppressor cells on Ig synthesis (27). Therefore, their nature was considered to be a suppressor T- inducer, but the precise *in vivo* mechanism was not known.

TABLE I. T-cell Lymphoma with Inducer/helper T-antigen
and Adult Diffuse Lymphoblastic Lymphoma

Case No.	Age	Sex	Diagnosis	Surface phenotype
1	69	M	Diffuse large cell type	En+, OKT4+
2	48	F	Diffuse large cell type	OKT3+, OKT4+
3	58	M	Diffuse large cell type and mixed cell type	En+, OKT3+, OKT4+
4	34	M	Diffuse medium-sized cell type	En+, OKT3+, OKT4+
5	62	F	Diffuse medium-sized cell type	En+, OKT4+
6	35	F	Diffuse lymphoblastic type	En+, OKT3+
7	30	M	Diffuse lymphoblastic type	En+, OKT3+, OKT4+

Five lymphoma cases in this series revealed phenotypes of inducer/helper T-cells (Table I). Some cases showed the same helper/suppressor ratio as that of reactive lymph nodes, but cytologic observation confirmed the positive reaction of atypical cells to be OKT4 or Leu3a positive. Monomorphic composition of large cells permitted easy recognition of malignancy. Histologically they consisted of three large cell type diffuse lymphomas and two medium-sized cell type diffuse lymphomas. The large cell type diffuse lymphoma was composed of large cells with vesicular nuclei, distinct nucleoli of various sizes and moderate amounts of rather pale cytoplasm (Photo 2). The nuclear figure was irregular compared to that of B-immunoblasts. Intermingled small cells were not as conspicuous. The diffuse medium-sized cell type in this category was more monomorphic compared to the large cell type (Photo 3). Two diffuse lymphoma lymphoblastic types showed some maturation toward peripheral type, compared to the typical thymic T-lymphoma in children. They lost immature T-cell antigen and occasionally suppressor T-antigen. Histology revealed diffuse proliferation of convoluted cells and numerous mitotic figures, which satisfied the criteria of diffuse lymphoblastic lymphoma. However, in some parts there were foci of cells with more condensed nuclei and clear cytoplasm (Photo 4). Remaining peripheral parts of the biopsy specimen revealed infiltration of neoplastic cells in the T-zone, which was composed of larger cells with vesicular nuclei (Photo 5).

Histologic appearances in this group as a whole gave the impression of relatively monomorphic proliferation (or less pleomorphic composition) compared to the typical pleomorphic type. Vascular proliferation, histiocytic aggregates and infiltration of eosinophils were not conspicuous.

Lymphomas with Suppressor/cytotoxic T-cell Antigen

Neoplastic cells from four cases revealed dominancy of expression of suppressor/cytotoxic T-cell antigen (Table II). This group of lymphomas showed varied histologic finding compared to the former group. The first biopsy of Case 8 was actually considered to be Hodgkin's diseases, with lymphocyte predominance, because of the presence of multinuclear giant cells, histiocytic infiltration and no atypism of small lymphocytes in the background (Photo 6). The second biopsy performed 5 months later yielded a diagnosis of Lennert's lymphoma, because of numerous histiocytic aggregates, no diagnostic Reed-Sternberg cells and atypical lymphocytes between

TABLE II. T-cell Lymphoma with Suppressor/cytotoxic T-antigen

Case No.	Age	Sex	Diagnosis	Surface phenotype
8	62	M	Lennert's lymphoma	En⁺, OKT3⁺, OKT8⁺
9	50	M	IBL-like T-cell lymphoma	En⁺, OKT3⁺, OKT8⁺ Leu1⁺, Leu2a⁺ (autopsy material)
10	65	M	IBL-like T-cell lymphoma	En⁺, OKT3⁺, OKT8⁺ (LN1) En⁺, OKT3⁺, OKT8⁺ (PB) Leu1⁺, Leu2a⁺ (LN2)
11	36	M	IBL-like T-cell lymphoma	En⁺, OKT3⁺, OKT8⁺

LN, lymph node; PB, peripheral blood.

the small granulomas (Photo 7). He died of the tumor 12 months after the onset and the autopsy material revealed more pleomorphic composition of cells with decreased histiocytic infiltration (Photo 8). Coexistence of multiple small hepatomas was also found.

This patient revealed polyclonal hypergammaglobulinemia: IgG 3,000 mg/dl, IgA 566 mg/dl, and IgM 159 mg/dl. Kim et al. (9) reported 25 cases with so-called Lennert's lymphoma and 29% of them showed polyclonal hypergammaglobulinemia. Their cases were not determined their immunologic markers, but Lukes et al. (15) and others (5, 17) reported lymphoepithelioid cellular lymphomas (Lennert's lymphoma) with T-cell markers. Lennert et al. (13) reported that 40% of T-zone lymphoma cases showed polyclonal hypergammaglobulinemia, and Levine et al. (14) also reported that 41% of T-immunoblastic sarcoma revealed polyclonal hypergammaglobulinemia. Certain T-cell lymphomas were considered to stimulate B-lymphocytes to secrete immunoglobulins by non-specific stimulation.

Polyclonal hypergammaglobulinemia is more conspicuous in cases with immunoblastic lymphadenopathy (IBL)-like T-cell lymphoma. Histologic characteristics were common in Cases 9, 10, and 11. They revealed vascular proliferation, many perivascular plasma cells, and foci of pale cells and mixed composition of atypical cells (Photo 9). These findings coincided with IBL-like T-cell lymphoma (24, 33). The relative abundance of OKT4⁺ cells in the first biopsy of Case 12 was probably due to remnants of normal lymphocytes because neoplastic cells after leukemic change and from the second biopsy were almost completely composed of different sizes of monoclonal OKT8⁺ and Leu2a⁺ (Photo 10).

We formerly considered that IBL-like T-cell lymphoma derived from helper T-cells. As the inducer/helper T-cell character of ATL caused suppression of Ig synthesis of B-lymphocytes, there is a discrepancy between the expression of suppressor/cytotoxic T-antigen on proliferating neoplastic cells and laboratory findings of hypergammaglobulinemia. The in vitro activity of the neoplastic cells has not been examined. Decreased helper/suppressor ratio in Castleman's disease may be suggestive on this point. One possible hypothesis is that the neoplastic cells secrete T-cell replacing factor (TRF) (10) which promotes B-lymphocytes to the secretory phase, or else that they have impaired suppressor activity on B-lymphocytes. We pointed out the resemblance of the clinical manifestations and prognosis of these three histologically separable Lennert's lymphoma, T-zone lymphoma, and IBL-like T-cell lymphoma, which suggested a close relationship (34). Some reported cases showed histologic change. Although the number of cases was limited, characterization of T-cell subsets in these cases also indicated their similarity.

Histiocytic Reaction in T-cell Lymphomas

As previously described, malignant lymphomas having inducer/helper T-cell antigen were composed of relatively monomorphic neoplastic cells and the formation of histiocytic granuloma was rare, even though histiocytic infiltration was conspicuous. In contrast, suppressor/cytotoxic T-cell lymphoma revealed complicated histology with various modifications such as vascular proliferation, infiltration of eosinophils, proliferation of plasma cells, and histiocytic aggregates.

We noticed histiocytic infiltration in T-cell lymphoma, because it is rare in lymphoblastic lymphoma and common in peripheral type T-cell lymphoma. Histiocytes are usually considered to be derived from blood monocytes, but we recently found another histiocytic cell lineage, independent of the monocyte-macrophage system (30). They are characterized by stainability with anti-S100 protein antibody, but non-stainability with either anti-NCA or anti-lysozyme IgG (Photo 11). Langerhans cells in the skin and interdigitating cells in the T-zones of various lymphoid organs belong to this histiocytic cell lineage, and are tentatively termed T-zone histiocytes. They were also stained with monoclonal antibody OKT6 and 036 (18).

The number of S100+ T-zone histiocytes was significantly greater in helper T-cell lymphoma compared to suppressor/cytotoxic T-cell lymphoma (Table III). Even mitotic figures of histiocytes were present (Photo 12). The early phase of cutaneous T-cell lymphoma also contained numerous S100+ T-zone histiocytes, so it may be said that proliferation of T-zone histiocytes is closely associated with helper T-lymphocytes. On the contrary, histiocytic aggregates, which were frequently present in suppressor/cytotoxic T-cell lymphoma, were mainly composed of lysozyme+ NCA+ histiocytes (macrophages probably derived from monocytes).

The histiocytes may be activated by lymphokine or lymphokine-like substances from neoplastic cells. The immunological cell-to-cell interaction has not been studied but as these markers for histiocytes were stable, application of these in immunohistochemical staining studies would make possible classification of cells in the biopsy specimen for accurate interpretation.

CONCLUSION

There has been no systematic subclassification of peripheral T-cell lymphomas and leukemias. We have tried to categorize T-cell lymphoma/leukemia based on cytolo-

TABLE III.   Number of Histiocytes in T-lymphoma

Diagnosis	T-zone histiocyte	NCA+ macrophage
DLB	78±39	6±8
OKT4+ lymphoma	105±26	20±18
OKT8+ lymphoma	27±24	11±10

Number of positive cells were counted per ten unit areas. DLB, diffuse lymphoblatic lymphoma.

gical, histological and some immunologic markers (32–34). In this study it was evident that peripheral T-cell lymphomas expressed surface antigen of either inducer/helper T-lymphocytes or suppressor/cytotoxic T-lymphocytes. Suppressor/cytotoxic T-cell lymphoma showed a relatively distinct category including so-called "Lennert's lymphoma" and IBL-like T-cell lymphoma. T-zone lymphoma may be a probable candidate for inclusion in this category, because of the clinicopathologic similarity and morphologic transition between the sequential biopsies.

However, the relationship between lymphomas with inducer/helper markers in this study and the established category of cutaneous T-cell lymphoma with helper activity and ATL with suppressor activity on Ig synthesis of B-lymphocytes is unclear. Case 5 showed leukemic change as well as multiple skin eruptions. This case may relate to ATL, however, other cases had neither superficial skin involvement nor leukemic change.

Prognosis was very poor in both groups. Despite the short follow-up period, two of the helper/inducer T-cell tumors and three of the suppressor/cytotoxic T-cell lymphomas died within one year. Complications due to other coexisting malignant diseases seemed high in peripheral T-cell lymphoma. In this series although autopsy was carried out in only four of the five cases, Case 1 was recognized to have squamous cell carcinoma shortly before lymphoma, and Case 8 was found to have multiple small hepatoma at the autopsy.

Further accumulation of cases is necessary to appropriately clarify the role of this factor in the subclassification of peripheral T-cell lymphoma/leukemia.

Acknowledgments

A part of this work was supported by a Grant-in-Aid for Cancer Research (No 56-S1) of the Ministry of Health and Welfare. The authors would like to express their appreciation to Mr. Y. Sato for technical assistance, to Mr. E. Nishizaki for his photographic work, and to J. C. Barron, Associate Professor of St. Marianne Univ. Medical School for English revision.

REFERENCES

1. Bernard, A., Boumsell, L., Reinherz, E. L., Nadler, L. M., Ritz, J., Coppin, H., Richard, Y., Valensi, F., Dansset, J., Flandrin, G., Lemerle, J., and Schlossman, S. F. Cell surface characterization of malignant T-cells from lymphoblastic lymphoma using monoclonal antibodies: Evidence for phenotypic differences between malignant T cells from patients with acute lymphoblastic leukemia and lymphoblastic lymphoma. *Blood*, **57**, 1105–1110 (1981).

2. Bhan, A. K., Reinherz, H. L., Poppema, S., McClusky, R. T., and Schlossman, S. F. Location of T cell and major histocompatibility complex antigens in the human thymus. *J. Exp. Med.*, **152**, 771–782 (1980).

3. Broder, S. and Bunn, P. A. Cutaneous T cell lymphomas. *Semin. Oncol.*, **7**, 310–331 (1980).

4. Engleman, E. G., Warnke, R., Fox, R. I., and Levy, R. Studies of a human T lymphocyte antigen recognized by a monoclonal antibody. *Proc. Natl. Acad. Sci. U.S.*, in press.

5. Han, T., Barcos, M., Yoon, J. M., Rakowski, I., and Minowada, J. Malignant lymphoma

with a high contect of epithelioid histiocytes: Report of a T cell variant of so-called Lennert lymphoma and review of the literature. *Med. Pediatr. Oncol.*, **8**, 227–236 (1980).

6. Hanaoka, M., Sasaki, M., Matsumoto, H., Tankawa, H., Yamabe, H., Tomimoto, K., Tasaka, C., Fujiwara, H., Uchiyama, T., and Takatsuki, K. Adult T-cell leukemia-Histological classification and characteristics. *Acta Pathol. Jpn.*, **29**, 723–738 (1979).

7. Janossy, G., Tomas, J. A., Pizzolo, G., Granger, S. M., McLanghlin, J., Habeshaw, J. A., Stansfeld, A. G., and Sloane, J. Immuno-histological diagnosis of lymphoproliferative diseases by selected combinations of antisera and monoclonal antibodies. *Br. J. Cancer*, **42**, 224–242 (1980).

8. Kickuchi, M., Mistui, T., and Matsui, N. T cell malignancies in adults: Histopathological studies of lymph nodes in 110 patients. *Jpn. J. Clin. Oncol.*, **9** (Suppl.), 407–422 (1979).

9. Kim, H., Nathwani, B. N., and Rappaport, H. So-called "Lennert's lymphoma": Is it a clinicopathologic entity? *Cancer*, **45**, 1379–1399 (1980).

10. Kindred, B., Beosing-Schneider, R., and Corley, R. B. *In vivo* activity of a nonspecific T cell-replacing factor. *J. Immunol.*, **122**, 350–354 (1979).

11. Kung, P. C., Berger, C. L., Goldstein, G., LoGerfo, P., and Edelson, R. L. Cutaneous T cell lymphoma: Characterization by monoclonal antibodies. *Blood*, **57**, 261–266 (1981).

12. Ledbetter, J. A., Evans, R. L., Lipinski, M., Cunningham-Rundles, G., Good, R. A., and Herzenberg, L. A. Evolutionary conservation of surface molecules that distinguish T lymphocyte helper/inducer and cytotoxic/suppressor subpopulations in mouse and man. *J. Exp. Med.* **153**, 310–323 (1981).

13. Lennert, K. T-zone lymphoma. *In* "Malignant Lymphomas Other Than Hodgkin's Disease," pp. 196–209 (1978). Springer-Verlag, New York-Heidelberg-Berlin.

14. Levine, A. M., Taylor, C. R., Schneider, D. R., Koehler, S. C., Forman, S. J., Lichtenstein, A., Lukes, R. J., and Feinstein, P. I. Immunoblastic sarcoma of T-cell *versus* B cell origin: 1. Clinical features. *Blood*, **58**, 52–61 (1981).

15. Lukes, R. J., Parker, J. W., Taylor, C. R., Tindle, B. H., Cramer, A. D., and Lincoln, T. L. Immunological approach to non-Hodgkin lymphomas and related leukemias. Analysis of the results of multiparameter studies of 425 cases. *Semin. Hematol.*, **15**, 322–351 (1978).

16. Palutke, M., Tabaczka, P., Weise, R. W., Axelrod, A., Palacas, C., Margolis, H., Khilanani, P., Patanatharathorn, V., Piligian, J., Pollard, R., and Husain, M. T-cell lymphomas of large cell type. A variety of malignant lymphomas: "Histiocytic and mixed lymphocytic-histiocytic." *Cancer*, **46**, 87–101 (1980).

17. Palutke, M., Varadachari, C., Weise, R. W. Lennert's lymphoma, a T-cell neoplasm. *Am. J. Clin. Pathol.*, **69**, 643–646 (1978).

18. Poppema, S., Bhan, A. K., Reinherz, E. L., McCluskey, R. T., and Schlossman, S. F. Distribution of T cell subsets in human lymph nodes. *J. Exp. Med.*, **153**, 30–41 (1981).

19. Reinherz, E. L., King, P. C., Goldstein, G., Levey, R. H., and Schlossman, S. F. Discrete stages of human intrathymic differentiation: Analysis of normal thymocytes and leukemic lymphoblasts of T cell lineage. *Proc. Natl. Acad. Sci. U.S.*, **77**, 1588–1592 (1980).

20. Reinherz, E. L., Kung, P. C., Goldstein, G., and Schlossman, S. F. Further characterization of the human inducer T-cell subset defined by monoclonal antibody. *J. Immunol.*, **123**, 2894–2896 (1979).

21. Reinherz, E. L. and Schlossman, S. F. The differentiation and function of human T-lymphocytes. *Cell*, **19**, 821–827 (1980).

22. Shimoyama, M. Cellular origin, differentiation and classification of leukemia and lymphoma cells as based on surface marker analysis. *Acta Haematol. Jpn.*, **42**, 897–998 (1979).

23. Shimoyama, M. and Minato, K. Clinical, cytological and immunological analysis of T-cell type lymphoid malignancies. *Jpn. J. Clin. Haematol.*, **20**, 1056–1069 (1979).

24. Shimoyama, M., Minato, K., Saito, H., Takenaka, T., Watanabe, S., Nagatani, T., and Naruto, M. Immunoblastic lymphadenopathy (IBL)-like T-cell lymphoma. *Jpn. J. Clin. Oncol.*, **9** (Suppl.), 347–356 (1979).

25. Stein, R. S., Cousar, J., Flexner, J. M., and Collins, R. D. Correlation between immunologic markers and histopathologic classification: Clinical implications. *Semin. Oncol.*, **7**, 244–254 (1980).

26. T and B-cell Malignancy Study Group. Statistical analysis of immunological, clinical and histopathologic data on lymphoid malignancies in Japan. *Jpn. J. Clin. Oncol.*, **11**, 15–38 (1981).

27. Tobinai, K., Hirose, M., Yamada, H., Minato, K., and Shimoyama, M. Cellular origin of human lymphoid malignancies as based on immunologic analysis of membrane differentiation antigens. *Jpn. J. Clin. Oncol.*, **12**, 73–90 (1982).

28. Wang, C. T., Good, R. A., Ammirati, P., Dymbort, G., and Evans, R. L. Identification of a p 69, 71 complex expressed on human T cells sharing determinants with B-type chronic lymphatic leukemia cells. *J. Exp. Med.*, **151**, 1539–1548 (1980).

29. Warnke, R. and Levey, R. Detection of T and B cell antigens with hybridoma monoclonal antibodies: A biotin-avidin-horseradish peroxidase method. *J. Histochem. Cytochem.*, **28**, 771–787 (1980).

30. Watanabe, S., Nakajima, T., Sato, Y., Shimamura, K., and Sakuma, H. T-zone histiocytes with S100 protein: Development and distribution in human fetuses. *Acta Pathol. Jpn.*, in press.

31. Watanabe, S., Nakajima, T., Shimosato, Y., Sato, Y., and Shimizu, K. Malignant histiocytosis and Letterer-Siwe disease. Neoplasms of T-zone histiocyte with S100 protein. *Cancer*, in press.

32. Watanabe, S., Nakajima, T., Shimosato, Y., Shimoyama, M., and Minato, K. T-cell malignancies: Subclassification and interrelationship. *Jpn. J. Clin. Oncol.*, **9** (Suppl.), 423–442 (1979).

33. Watanabe, S., Shimosato, Y., Shimoyama, M., Minato, K., Suzuki, M., Abe, M., and Nagatani, T. Adult T cell lymphoma with hypergammaglobulinemia. *Cancer*, **46**, 2472–2482 (1980).

34. Watanabe, S., Shimosato, Y., Shimoyama, M., and Minato, K. Studies with multiple markers on malignant lymphomas and lymphoid leukemias. *Cancer*, **50**, in press.

EXPLANATION OF PHOTOS

Photo 1. Reactive lymph node stained with monoclonal antibodies, Leu3a and Leu2a. Left: Leu3a positive cells are numerous in the paracortical area (lower area), scattered in the germinal center, and some are clustered in the corona region (top). Right: Leu2a positive cells scattered in the paracortical area, but not in the germinal center. Leu3a or Leu2a, anti-mouse rabbit IgG, anti-rabbit IgG swine IgG, PAP, and then 3,3′-diaminobenzidine (DAB) reaction. ×330.

Photo 2. T-diffuse lymphoma, large cell type (Case 1). Large cells with vesicular nuclei and pale cytoplasm are noted. Contour of the nuclei is irregular. Hematoxylin-eosin (H-E) staining, ×330.

Photo 3. T-diffuse lymphoma, medium-sized cell type (Case 4). Diffuse proliferation of medium-sized cells with somewhat twisted nuclei is noted. H-E, ×160.

Photo 4. T-diffuse lymphoma, lymphoblastic type (Case 7). Diffuse proliferation of convoluted cells faces to focus composed of more maturated cells with condensed small nuclei and pale cytoplasm. H-E, ×160 (inset; ×330).

Photo 5. Lymph node metastasis in Case 7. Large cells with vesicular nuclei and pale cytoplasm infiltrate the paracortical area. H-E, ×160.

PHOTO 6.   The first biopsy of Case 8. This was diagnosed as Hodgkin's lymphoma, lymphocyte predominant type. Note multinuclear giant cells and small lymphocytes without atypism. H-E, ×330.

PHOTO 7.   The second biospy of Case 8. Typical histiocytic aggregates and absence of diagnostic Reed-
Sternberg cells are consistent with so-called Lennert's lymphoma. H-E, ×160.

PHOTO 8.   Autopsy material of Case 8. Pleomorphic composition of neoplastic cells is noted. H-E, ×330.

PHOTO 9.   a) Vascular proliferation of IBL-like T-cell lymphoma. H-E and silver impregnation, ×160.
b) Perivascular plasma cells and mixed cell population with pale cells of various sizes are noted.
H-E, ×330.

PHOTO 10.   Fluorescent microphotographs and their analysis by fluorescence activated cell sorter
(FACS) IV (Case 10). Leu2a brightly stains variously sized neoplastic cells (left). Leu3a positive
cells are very few (right upper). Three dimensional analysis shows variously sized Leu3a positive
cells. Horizontal axis: cell size, longitudinal axis: fluorescence intensity, height: histogram.

PHOTO 11.   Interdigitating cells in the reactive lymph node. Immunohistochemical stain with anti-
S100 protein IgG stains brown (left), whereas that with anti-NCA IgG does not (right, arrow).
PAP stain, ×660.

PHOTO 12.   Histiocytes in the periphery of T-cell lymphoma (Case 6). T-zone histiocytes stained brown,
proliferate and extend their cytoplasm (left) intermingled with NCA+ macrophages, also stained
brown (right). Both stains permit accurate observation of the degree of non-neoplastic histiocytic
reaction. PAP stain, ×330.

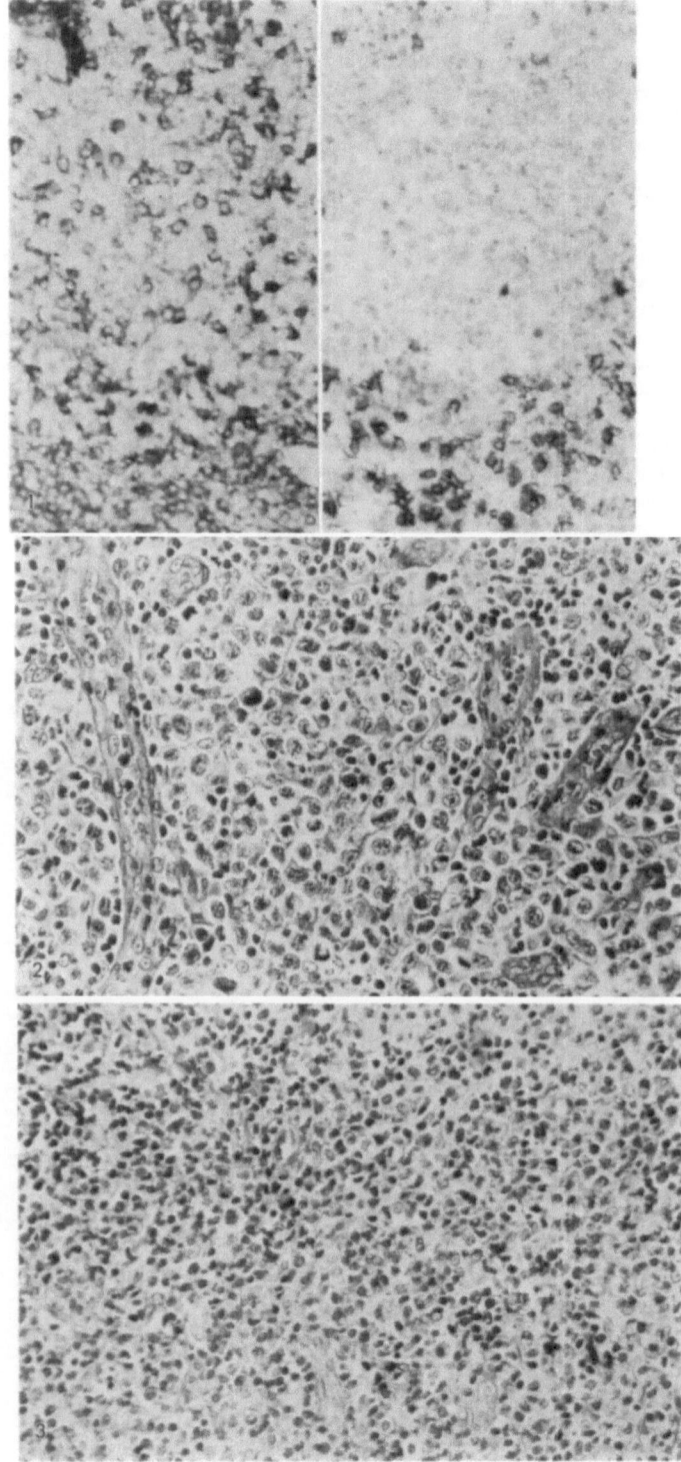

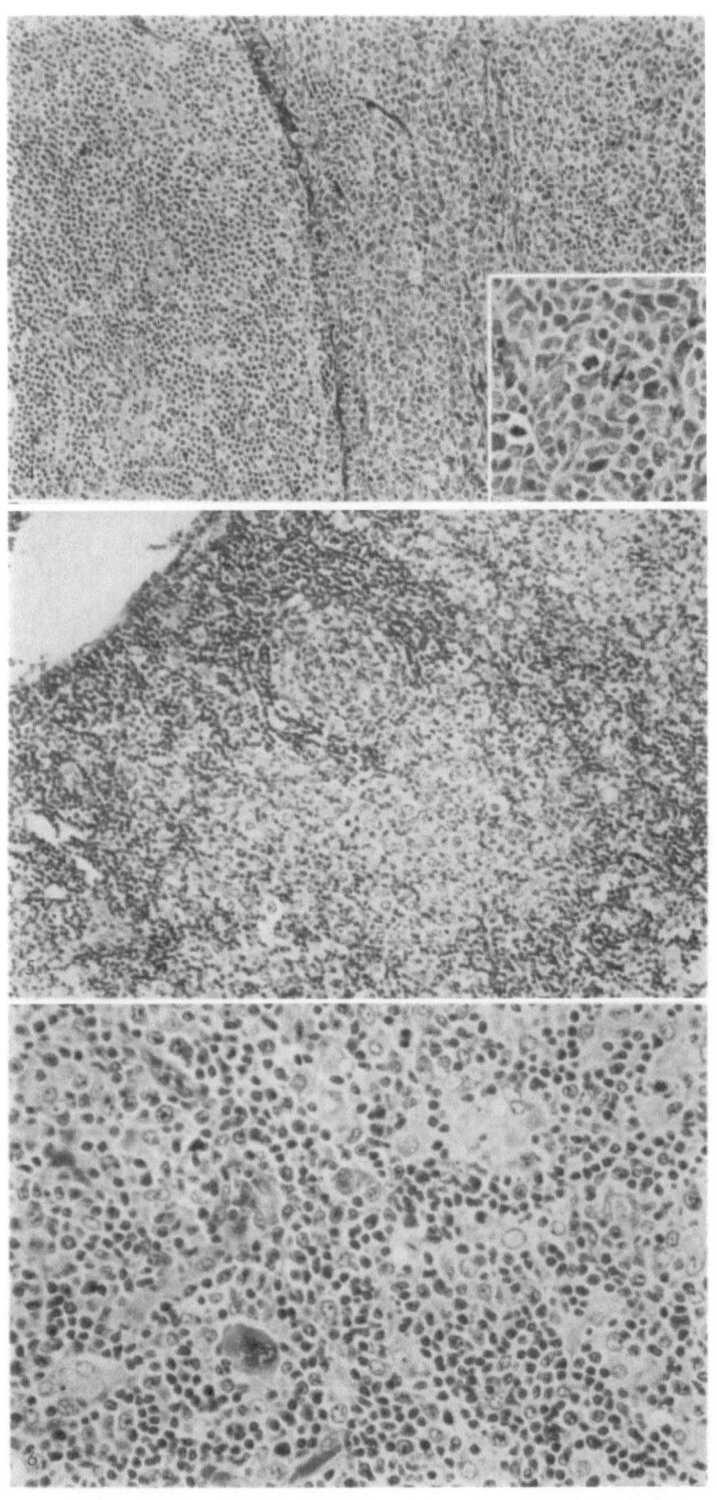

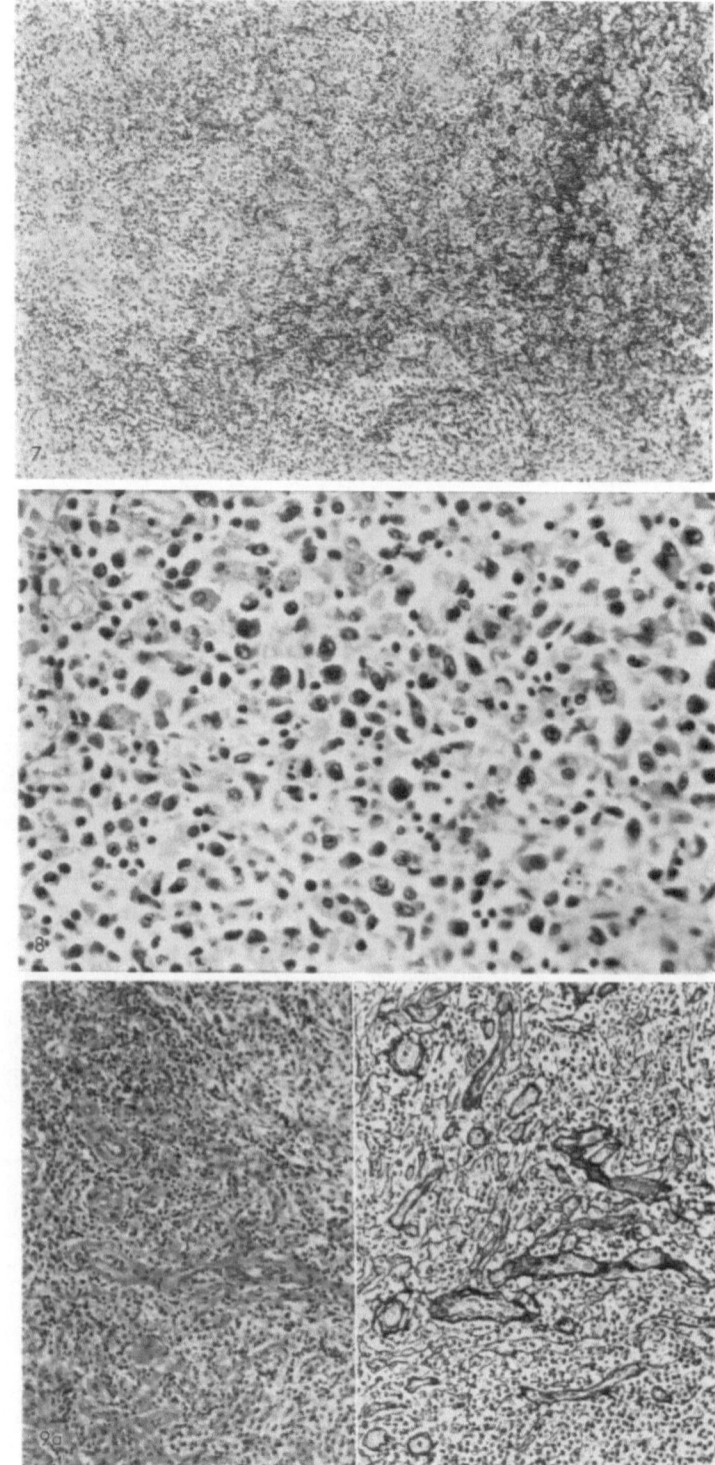

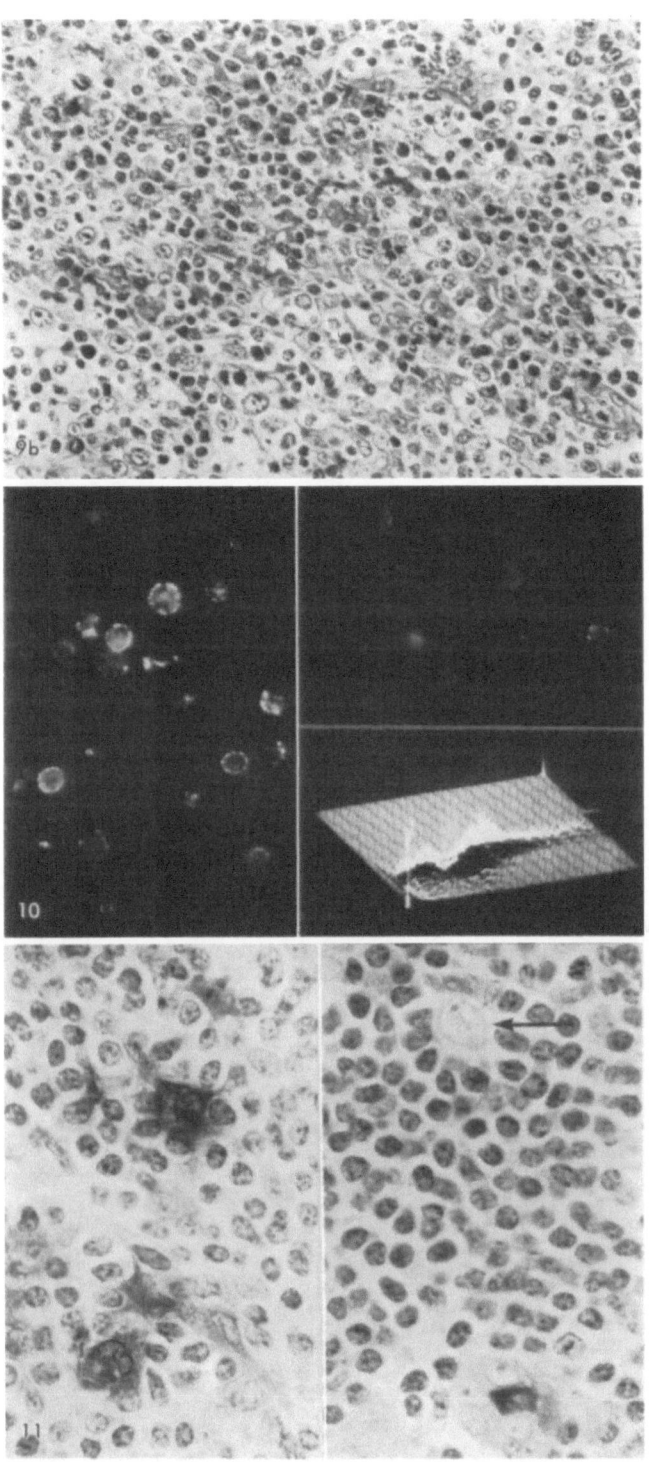

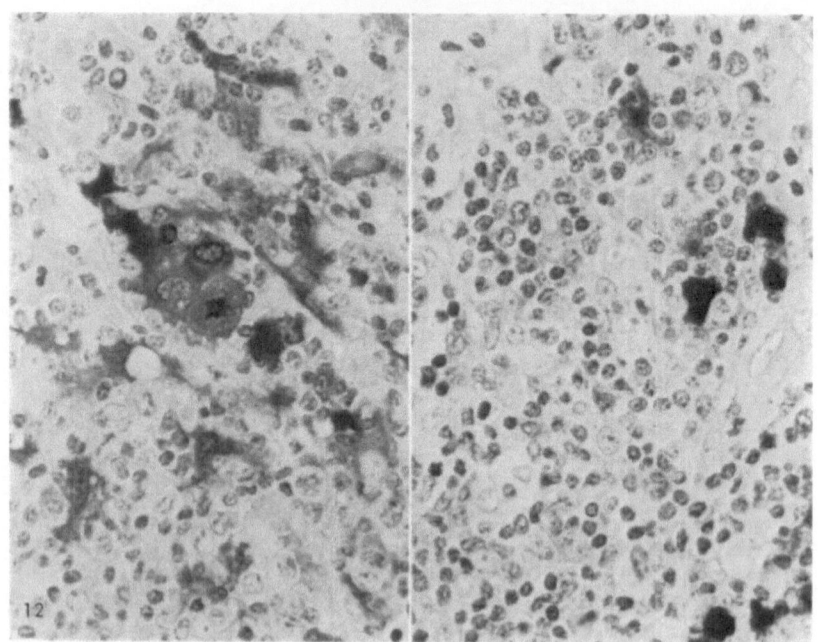

IMMUNOBLASTIC LYMPHADENOPATHY (IBL)-LIKE T CELL LYMPHOMA

Masanori SHIMOYAMA,*1 Kensei TOBINAI,*1 Keisuke MINATO,*1 and Shaw WATANABE*2

*Departments of Clinical Laboratory and Internal Medicine, National Cancer Center Hospital*1 and Pathology Division, National Cancer Center Research Institute*2*

We proposed a new disease entity called "Immunoblastic lymphadenopathy (IBL)-like T-cell lymphoma" in 1979. The present study represents an analysis of 14 cases. IBL-like T-cell lymphoma, although its clinical and morphological findings resemble immunodysplastic disease, IBL, angioimmunoblastic lymphadenopathy with dysproteinemia, lymphogranulomatosis x and polyclonal immunoblastosis, is a distinct peripheral T-cell lymphoma with suppressor/cytotoxic T-cell phenotype in adult; it is completely different from adult T-cell leukemia-lymphoma. The characteristics of this disease are summarized as follows: 1) the disease usually starts with generalized lymphadenopathy, frequently associated with high fever, skin rash and weakness; 2) lymphadenopathy is partially regressed by steroid hormone therapy, especially in the early phases of the disease; 3) frequent involvement of hepatosplenomegaly, but infrequent leukemic change and no thymic involvement; 4) poor prognosis; 5) marked male predominance; 6) polyclonal hypergammaglobulinemia; 7) Coombs test sometimes positive, occasionally associated with autoimmune hemolytic anemia and pure red cell aplasia; 8) elevation of various anti-virus titer (measles, rubella, varicella, and Epstein-Barr virus (EBV)), and/or of anti-toxoplasma titer; 9) leucocytosis with neutrophilia, lymphocytopenia and atypical plasmacytoid cells; 10) no endemic distribution of the patients' birthplace; 11) multifocal or diffuse neoplastic proliferation of immunoblasts, large lymphoid cells and/or so-called "pale cells" with angioimmunoblastic and granulomatous lesions, zonal proliferation of plasma cells, disappearance of germinal center, deposition of amorphous acidophilic interstitial material and depletion of small lymphocyte; the patient is often diagnosed as IBL or angioimmunoblastic lymphadenopathy (AILD) at initial biopsy, so serial examinations must be indicated; 12) neoplastic cells express the T-cell nature of suppressor/cytotoxic T-cell phenotype; 13) surface and cytoplasmic immunoglobulins of lymph node cells are not monoclonal, but polyclonal. It is necessary to disclose why IBL-like T-cell lymphoma is frequently associated with variegated and brilliant clinical manifestations such as fever, skin rash, polyclonal hypergammaglobulinemia, elevation of various anti-virus titer and autoimmune

*1,*2 Tsukiji 5-1-1, Chuo-ku, Tokyo 104, Japan (下山正徳, 飛内賢正, 湊　啓輔, 渡辺　昌).

mechanism, and granulomatous lesions in lymph nodes, despite the
tumor cells having suppressor/cytotoxic T-cell phenotype.

It is known that there are patients with more or less generalized lymphadenopathy
whose disease is not properly diagnosed histopathologically despite the fact that the
process is often fatal. In Japan, these conditions have been variously called "idiopathic
reticulosis or Hodgkinoid type (7)" and "specific granulomatosis (8)" without a definite
disease entity. Recently, however, it has been noticed that an immunoproliferative
disorder associated with hypergammaglobulinemia is present among these diseases,
and some of these disorders have been characterized as chronisches pluripotentielles
immunoproliferatives syndrome (36), immunodysplastic disease (32), angioimmunoblastic lymphadenopathy (AILD) (2, 3), immunoblastic lymphadenopathy (IBL) (19),
and lymphogranulomatosis x (26, 16).

As the disease entity of IBL proposed by Lukes and Tindle in 1975 (19) is the
most distinct and attractive, case reports of IBL have been presented in Japan since
then as a morphologically definite disease entity. Kojima (15) reviewed 26 cases of IBL
reported in Japan before 1978 and pointed out that only four of them corresponded
completely to the IBL proposed by Lukes and Tindle (19). As he noted, however, the
histologic findings of the rest of the cases suggested hyperimmune proliferation probably of the B-cell system; he proposed the disease as polyclonal immunoblastosis (15).
It is considered, however, that these disorders are probably the same disease entity
although there are some differences in histopathological observations and conceptual
pathogenesis. The basic process of these diseases has been thought to be an abnormal
immune condition of unknown etiology, in principle, a non-neoplastic hyperimmune
proliferation of the B-cell system, but a kind of prelymphomatous state which occasionally converts to malignant lymphoma of the immunoblastic type (15, 16, 19, 25).

During our studies on patients diagnosed histologically as having IBL, "Hodgkinoid" or so-called Lennert's lymphoma (10, 11, 17), despite their having progressive
generalized lymphadenopathy associated with polyclonal hypergammaglobulinemia
and often a fatal outcome, we found that the proliferating atypical lymphoid cells such
as immunoblasts and the so-called "pale cells" in their lymph nodes had a T-cell nature.
Serial cytological and immunologic examinations revealed during the follow-up study
that these atypical cells of T-cell nature showed neoplastic proliferation (27–29). We
summarized an initial eight cases and reported them as IBL-like T-cell lymphoma (29),
whose clinical and morphological characteristics appeared to be completely different
from adult T-cell leukemia-lymphoma. Since then, we have experienced 15 more patients with IBL-like T-cell lymphoma and found that six of them whose tumor cells
were examined for immunologic phenotype all had suppressor/cytotoxic T-cell phenotype (6, 30, 31, 33, 34). Since IBL-like T-cell lymphoma is also completely different
in this aspect from adult T-cell leukemia-lymphoma whose tumor cells have inducer/
helper T-cell phenotype (4, 30, 31, 33), it is therefore considered to be a new, distinct
disease entity. We report here on 14 patients with IBL-like T-cell lymphoma whose
clinical and morphological data are available and summarize the characteristics of the
disease.

Morphological Characteristics

As already described (*29, 35*), the lymph nodes in IBL-like T-cell lymphoma exhibited disappearance of germinal centers, proliferation of arborizing blood capillaries (Fig. 1), zonal or focal proliferation of plasma cells along the vessels, and focal or diffuse neoplastic proliferation of immunoblasts and/or so-called "pale cells" with moderate amounts of pale cytoplasm and round nuclei (Fig. 2a, b). In most cases, the initial histological diagnosis of swollen lymph nodes was AILD, IBL, or Hodgkinoid type, but repeated histological, cytological and immunologic examinations of swollen lymph nodes revealed the neoplastic proliferation of immunoblasts and/or so-called "pale cells," which were found to have T-cell markers. In some cases, cytologic examination was useful to identify tumor cells.

Cytologic examination of touch smears of biopsied lymph nodes or smears of aspirated swollen lymph nodes revealed that large basophilic immunoblasts, plasmacytoid immature cells, plasma cells and large to medium-sized atypical "pale cells" were present. Small lymphocytes were also present in variable numbers (Fig. 3a–c). Generally, basophilic atypical immunoblasts or large atypical cells can be easily cytologically recognized as tumor cells. In peripheral blood, a few atypical plasmacytoid lymphocytes were occasionally seen (Fig. 3d).

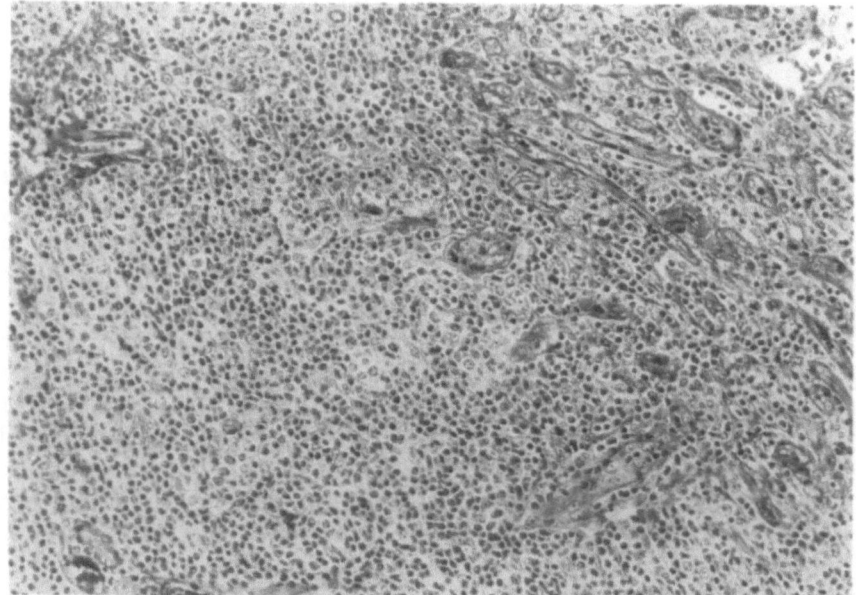

Fig. 1. Histology of IBL-like T-cell lymphoma. Lymphoid follicles completely disappeared in the enlarged lymph node and vascular proliferation was conspicuous. Both capillaries and postcapillary venules were noticed and mature plasma cells and their immature type were present around the vessels Hematoxylin-eosin (H-E), ×330.

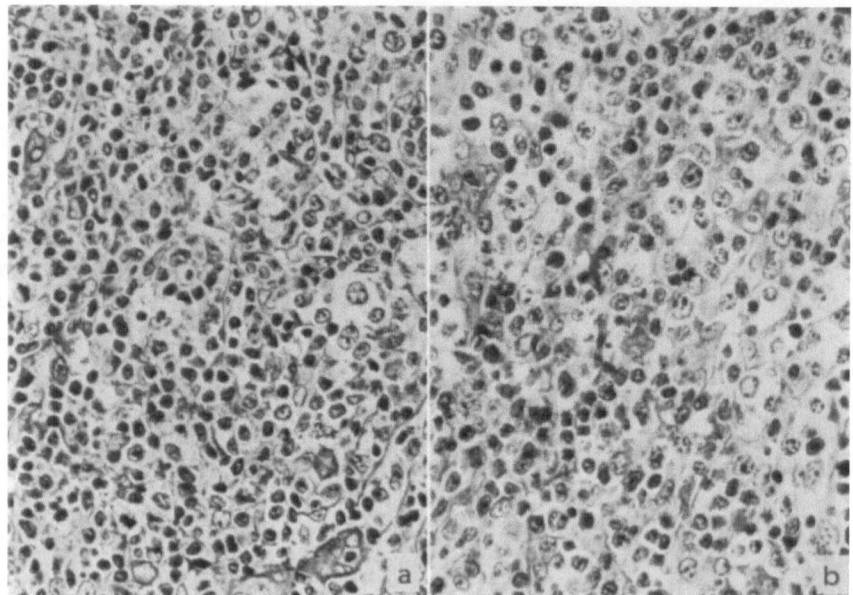

FIG. 2. Focal proliferation of atypical cells. a) Focus of medium-sized atypical cells with irregular nuclei of chromatin condensation and relatively abundant clear cytoplasma. b) Large immunoblast with vesicular nuclei and conspicuous nucleoli, medium-sized pale cell. Plasma cell and plasmacytoid cells are also found. H-E, ×660.

Immunological Properties

The immunological profiles of cells obtained from biopsied lymph nodes of the 14 patients are summarized in Table I. The basophilic immunoblasts as well as large to medium-sized atypical cells from all 14 patients were found to be E-rosette formers as shown in Fig. 4. Human T-lymphocyte antigen or pan T-cell antigen was detected in these atypical large cells as well as in 50 to 80% of the lymph node cells. Ia-like antigen was also found in the large cells of four patients. C3-receptor, Fcγ-receptor and monoclonal surface immunoglobulins were never detected in the large cells. As shown in a previous report (29) and elsewhere in this book (page 32, Table V), surface immunoglobulins and cytoplasmic immunoglobulins were detected only in small to medium-sized cells which comprised about 20 to 40% of the lymph node cells, but they were always polyclonal. Subset analysis of large to medium-sized cells by several monoclonal antibodies revealed that these cells were OKT3 and OKT8 positive, but OKT4 and OKT6 negative, indicating that they had suppressor/cytotoxic T-cell phenotype. TdT activity of the lymph node cells was not detected in seven cases tested.

Clinical Observations

The clinical and laboratory data are summarized in Tables II to IV. Patients with IBL-like T-cell lymphoma were middle-aged or older. The range in age was from

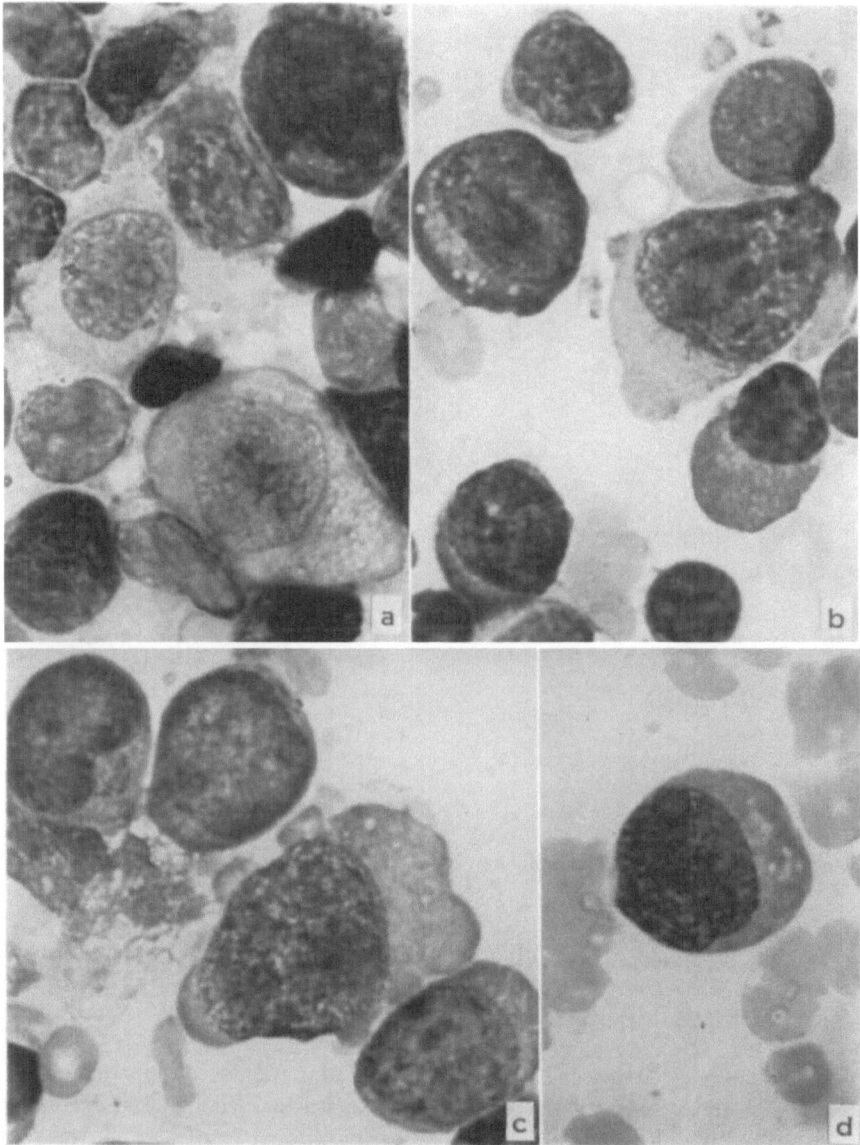

FIG. 3. Cytological observations. a–c) So-called pale cell, atypical basophilic immunoblast, large lymphoid cell, plasma cell and plasmacytoid cells in lymph node. d) Atypical plasmacytoid cell in peripheral blood.

36 to 80 years. Males markedly predominated with 13 males to one female. There was no special geographical distribution of the patients' birthplace, as shown in Table II. Nine patients died, with a median survival of 8.5 months, ranging from 3 to 153 months after diagnosis. Five patients were alive 3 to 13 months after diagnosis.

Signs and symptoms of the patients are shown in Table III. As initial symptoms, lymphadenopathy was observed in all 14 individuals, fever in eight, skin rash in seven,

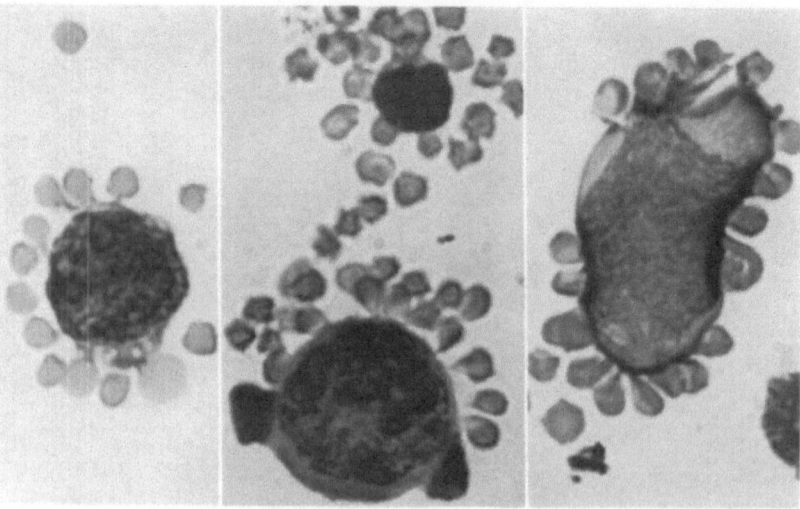

FIG. 4.   Cells with rosette-forming capacity with sheep erythrocytes.

TABLE I.   Surface Markers of Tumor Cells

No. of cases	14
ERFC[a]	14
T-lymphocyte antigen[b]	14
Ia-like antigen[c]	9
C3-R	0
Fcγ-R	0
Monoclonal S-Ig[d]	0/12 (All polyclonal)
TdT[e]	Negative (0/7)
Subset analysis by monoclonal antibody	OKT3+, OKT8+, OKT4−, OKT6− (6/6)

[a] ERFC, rosette forming capacity with sheep erythrocyte.
[b] Detected by specific heteroantisera against T-lymphocyte and/or monoclonal antibodies (9.6 and 10.2).
[c] Detected by specific heteroantisera against Ia-like antigen and/or monoclonal antibody (OKI1).
[d] S-Ig, surface immunoglobulins.
[e] TdT, terminal deoxynucleotidyl transferase.

fatigue in three and edema in two patients. In 11 patients, lymphadenopathy was associated with fever and/or skin rash, and in two was associated with edema.

Generalized lymphadenopathy was the most prominent feature and it was partially regressed by treatment with steroid hormone in six patients, although they later did have the progressive disease. Hepatosplenomegaly was also frequently found, and leukemic manifestation was seen in four patients, but the degree was not as severe. Skin rash was observed in 10 of the 14 studied. It seems likely that in four of them this was a hypersensitivity reaction induced by antibiotics and/or antipyretica. The rash of the other six, however, was associated with progression of the disease. Skin involvement of the T-cell lymphoma cells was observed in one patient. Fever was an common symptom of this disease; eight patients had fever as an initial symptom, and this usually fluctuated in accordance with the progression and remission of the disease, suggesting a sort of tumor fever.

TABLE II. Data on 14 Patients with IBL-like T-cell Lymphoma

Case		Age	Sex	Birthplace	Survival (months)	
1	W. J.	55	M	Tokyo	18	Dead
2	K. Y.	69	M	Tokyo	3	Dead
3	S. K.	41	M	Ibaragi	153	Dead
4	S. T.	43	M	Tokyo	6	Dead
5	O. H.	45	M	Hokkaido	10	Dead
6	W. E.	62	F	Tokyo	5+	Alive
7	A. K.	51	M	Hokkaido	3+	Alive
8	I. T.	47	M	Yamagata	24	Dead
9	S. R.	50	M	Hokkaido	6	Dead
10	H. K.	80	M	Kanagawa	8+	Alive
11	Y. I.	36	M	Saitama	13+	Alive
12	S. R.	71	M	Tokyo	7	Dead
13	S. N.	49	M	Gunma	11+	Alive
14	K. T.	60	M	Saitama	12	Dead

TABLE III. Signs and Symptoms

Case		Fever >38°C	Skin rash	Lymph node swelling	Hepato-megaly	Spleno megaly	Initial symptoms
1	W. J.	$(+)^f$	$(+)^{a,f}$	Generalized[b]	−	$(+)^f$	Anorexia, fatigue, lymphadenopathy
2	K. Y.	+	+	Generalized	+	−	Rash, fever, lymphadenopathy
3	S. K.	−	−	Generalized	−	$(+)^f$	Lymphadenopathy
4	S. T.	−	+	Neck, tonsil (→ generalized)	$(+)^f$	$(+)^{d,f}$	Lymphadenopathy, rash
5	O. H.	$(+)^f$	−	Generalized	$(+)^f$	−	Lymphadenopathy
6	W. E.	+	+	Generalized[c]	+	+	Fever, rash, lymphadenopathy
7	A. K.	+	$(+)^f$	Generalized[c]	+	+	Fever, lymphadenopathy
8	I. T.	+	$+^a$	Generalized	+	$+^{d,e}$	Back pain, lumbago, fever, rash, lymphadenopathy
9	S. R.	+	$(+)^f$	Generalized[c]	+	$+^d$	Fever, edema, lymphadenopathy, anemia, fatigue
10	H. K.	+	−	Generalized	+	$−^{d,g}$	Fever, lymphadenopathy
11	Y. I.	+	$+^a$	Generalized[c]	+	+	Fever, lymphadenopathy, rash, fatigue
12	S. R.	$(+)^f$	$+^a$	Generalized[c]	−	−	Lymphadenopathy, edema, rash
13	S. N.	−	+	Inguinal[c] → generalized	−	−	Lymphadenopathy, rash
14	K. T.	+	−	Axillary → generalized	+	−	Fever, edema, lymphadenopathy

[a] Drug induced.
[b] Regressed after antibiotic therapy.
[c] Partially regressed after steroid hormone therapy.
[d] Bone marrow involvement.
[e] Skin involvement (erythroderma).
[f] ( ) indicates later signs and symptoms.
[g] Leukemic conversion.

The signs and symptoms of the patients were variegated and gaudy. A typical example (Case No. 9) of fluctuation of these signs and symptoms is shown in Fig. 5. The patient is a 50 year old male and his disease started with edema of neck and shoul-

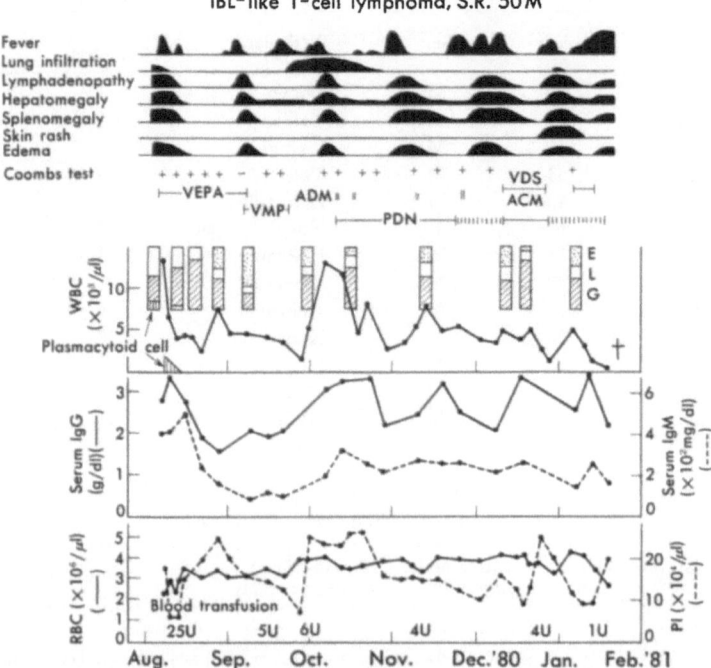

FIG. 5. Clinical course of a patient with IBL-like T-cell lymphoma (Case No. 9). Abbreviations: VEPA, VEPA therapy (20); VMP, vincristine, methotrexate, and prednisolone; ADM, adriamycin; PDN, prednisolone; VDS, vindesine; ACM, aclacinomycin A; E, erythropoiesis; L, lymphocyte; G, granulopoiesis; WBC, white blood cell; RBC, red blood cell; pl, platelet.

der, generalized lymphadenopathy, weakness associated with high fever and progressive anemia. Physical and chest X-ray examinations revealed that he had hepatosplenomegaly and lymphangitic infiltration of the lung. Laboratory examination disclosed polyclonal hypergammaglobulinemia, Coombs positive hemolytic anemia and pure red cell aplasia. He was treated with VEPA therapy (20) with complete remission, but the disease completely relapsed during the consolidation with VEPA therapy. The startling fluctuation of these signs, symptoms and laboratory data associated with progression or remission of the disease related to the treatment can be seen in Fig. 5. Skin rash observed in the late stage of this patient is shown in Fig. 6. This appeared along with progression of the disease and disappeared with regression of the tumor.

Laboratory data are summarized in Table IV. Definite polyclonal hypergammaglobulinemia was recorded in 13 patients at onset of the disease. In one patient the abnormality was recorded as a diffuse polyclonal hypergammaglobulinemia, in five as an increase in both IgG and IgA, IgG and IgM or IgA and IgM, in four as IgA, in two as IgG and in one as IgM. Only one patient showed polyclonal hypergammaglobulinemia at relapse. The level of immunoglobulins usually increased as the disease progressed. The Coombs test was positive in two of the 13 patients tested. Anemia was observed in one patient who had Coombs positive hemolytic anemia and pure red cell aplasia. Leucocytosis (more than 10,000/μl) was observed in six patients, one of whom

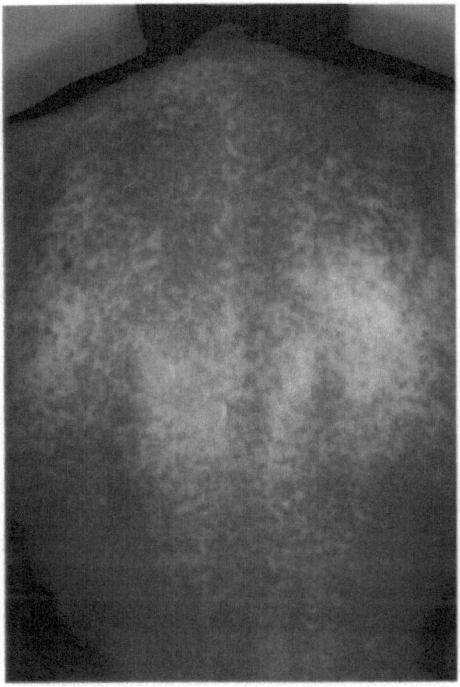

FIG. 6. Skin rash observed in a patient with IBL-like T-cell lymphoma (Case No. 9).

TABLE IV. Laboratory Findings before Therapy

Case		Immunoglobulins			Coombs test	LDH (IU)	WBC /μl	Lympho-cytes (%)	Eosino-philes (%)
		IgG	IgA (mg/dl)	IgM					
1	W. J.	1,700	362	394	—	341	8,100	15	1
2	K. Y.	1,500	610	48	—	366	8,800	14	5
3	S. K.	1,266	408	192	—	405	17,200	13	1
4	S. T.	4,200	464	167		202	11,800	25	3
5	O. H.	1,160 (→ 3,750)	157	191	—(→ +)	300	6,400	13	4
6	W. E.	3,500	153	560	—	635	16,100	5	29
7	A. K.	1,092	468	192	—	133	5,300	21	3
8	I. T.	2,970	969	450	—	275	8,900	11	6
9	S. R.	2,836	269	488	+[a]	966	13,000	11	1
10	H. K.	2,100	298	290	—	553	26,800[b]	3	1
11	Y. I.	4,560	202	240	—	429	6,500	40	0
12	S. R.	1,677	471	255	—		10,900	39	5
13	S. N.	1,720	656	681	—	322	9,200		
14	K. T.	2,618	566	109	—	1,062	6,100	19	2

[a] Autoimmune hemolytic anemia and jaundice.

[b] Leukemic cell 67%.

showed leukemic manifestation. Lymphocytopenia of less than 1,500 μl was observed in 10 patients. An increase in the serum lactic acid dehydrogenase (LDH) level was observed in five patients.

In a few patients, serum titer against various viruses was examined. In Case No. 10 (H.K.), serum titers against varicella virus and measles virus proved elevated to 1: 1,020 and 1: 2,048, respectively. In Case No. 11 (Y.I.), anti-rubella virus titer amounted to 1: 256, anti-EBVCA (Epstein-Barr virus capcid antigen) and anti-EBNA (Epstein-Barr virus nuclear antigen) titers were elevated to 1: 2,560 and 1: 40, respectively. In Case No. 13 (S.M.), this anti-virus titer was not increased. Elevated serum titer against various viruses decreased rapidly to normal level at remission induced by anticancer chemotherapy, indicating that these high serum titers were non-specifically elevated. Anti-ATLA antibody (antibody against adult T-cell leukemia cell associated antigen) (5) was not detected in any of the five patients tested (Case Nos. 9, 10, 11, 12, 14). Against toxoplasma, only one (Case No. 1) of three patients tested (Case Nos. 1, 2, 4) had high titer (1: 512→1: 8,192) and the other two were found to have usual titers. The Paul-Bunnel test was used on four patients (Case Nos. 1, 5, 9, 14) and proved not elevated. Cold aggultinatinin titers were done on four patients (Case Nos. 3, 5, 9, 14) and found to be elevated (1: 258) in only one (Case No. 5).

Relation between IBL-like T-cell Lymphoma and Its Related Disorders

As mentioned above, clinical manifestation and morphological characteristics of IBL-like T-cell lymphoma are almost the same as malignant lymphoma arising in AILD or IBL (16, 19, 25, 26). The immunoproliferative diseases which were diagnosed histologically as immunodysplastic disease, AILD, IBL, lymphogranulomatosis x or polyclonal immunoblastosis with often fatal outcome were also found to have almost the same clinical manifestation as IBL-like T-cell lymphoma. The clinical characteristics of IBL-like T-cell lymphoma, which is also commonly seen in its related disorders (1–3, 9, 12, 14–16, 19, 21, 25, 26), are summarized as follows:
1) The disease starts with generalized lymphadenopathy, frequently associated with high fever, skin rash and weakness, and occasionally with edema.
2) Lymphadenopathy is partially regressed by steroid hormone at an early phase of the disease.
3) Progressive disease with fatal outcome.
4) Frequent involvement of hepatosplenomegaly but infrequent leukemic conversion and no thymic involvement.
5) Polyclonal hypergammaglobulinemia is observed in most patients even at onset of the disease.
6) Coombs test sometimes positive, occasionally associated with hemolytic anemia. Pure red cell aplasia is observed in the patient.
7) Non-specific elevation of various anti-virus titer (measles, rubella, varicella, EBV) and of anti-toxoplasma titer.
8) Presence of a small population of basophilic or plasmacytoid atypical cells in peripheral blood or bone marrow.
9) Leukocytosis with neutrophilia and lymphocytopenia.
10) Marked male predominance.

11) Occurrence in adulthood.

12) No special geographical distribution of patients' birthplace or dwelling place.

In the morphological examination of these cases, common morphological characteristics were also observed, although there were some differences between them. These common characteristics may be summarized as follows:

1) Proliferation of arborizing blood capillaries.

2) Proliferation of immunoblasts and/or so-called pale cells.

3) Zonal proliferation of plasma cells along the vessels.

4) In principle, diffuse involvement, disappearance of germinal center, deposit of an amorphous, acidophilic interstitial material and depletion of small lymphocytes.

The morphological difference between IBL-like T-cell lymphoma or malignant lymphoma arising in AILD or IBL is dependent upon whether or not multifocal or diffuse neoplastic proliferation of immunoblasts, so-called "pale cells" and/or atypical large lymphoid cells are observed. Cytological examination of swollen lymph nodes by aspiration or touch smear is also useful to identify neoplastic cells as shown in Fig. 2. In order to make accurate diagnosis of IBL-like T-cell lymphoma, it is necessary to identify tumor cells morphologically, to prove T-cell markers on these tumor cells, and to disclose polyclonal immunoglobulin production in proliferated plasma cells and plasmacytoid cells of B-cell lineage. On the other hand, the basic process of immuno-dysplastic disease, AILD, IBL, lymphogranulomatosis x and polyclonal immunoblastosis has been considered to be hyperimmune proliferation of the B-cell system in a pre-lymphomatous state (15, 16, 25, 26, 32). Nevertheless, among immunoblastic sarcoma (IBS) arising in AILD, IBL or lymphogranulomatosis x, only a few cases have been proved to have B-cell marker, namely, monoclonal immunoglobulin on their tumor cells (9, 12, 25). Most cases have been reported to have polyclonal immunoglobulins in lymph node cells (15, 25). Recently, several case reports have been presented in which IBL or AILD had T-cell marker on its tumor cells (6, 13, 14, 22–24, 27–29, 34). Besides this, IBS with polyclonal hypergammaglobulinemia has been found to be of T-cell nature, but not of B-cell nature (18). These facts suggest that IBL-like T-cell lymphoma and most of IBS arising in AILD or IBL and IBS of T-cell nature are the same disease.

Multifocal or diffuse proliferation of large to medium-sized lymphoid cells resembling immunoblast or so-called "pale cell" is considered to be a diagnostic criteria for IBS arising in AILD by Nathwani et al. (25). However, this criteria is controversial; Lennert et al. (16) reported that multifocal proliferation of large to medium-sized cells can be seen in a certain virus infection, and therefore these morphological characteristics are not always specific for IBS. Kojima (15) and Abe (1) reported that polyclonal immunoblastosis is so-called cataplastic hyperplasia which is in between reactive and neoplastic hyperplasias.

Although the morphological criteria of malignant transformation in IBL, AILD, polyclonal immunoblastosis or lymphogranulomatosis x have not been agreed upon, chromosome abnormalities have been found in these cases, strongly suggesting that most of these diseases are malignant lymphoma. Immunological phenotypic analysis of lymph node cells should be conducted in future to resolve the relationship between IBL-like T-cell lymphoma and its related disorders with poor prognosis such as AILD, IBL, lymphogranulomatosis x and polyclonal immunoblastosis.

We also found that tumor cells of IBL-like T-cell lymphoma expressed the sup-
pressor/cytotoxic T-cell phenotype (*30, 31, 33*). However, it is necessary to determine
why IBL-like T-cell lymphoma is frequently associated with granulomatous lesions,
polyclonal hypergammaglobulinemia and sometimes autoimmune disorders despite
its having suppressor/cytotoxic T-cell phenotype on its tumor cells.

Acknowledgments

The following doctors gave us the opportunity to examine biopsied lymph nodes and to
obtain clinical information. We are deeply grateful for their cooperation: Tazuko Ibuka,
M. D., Yukio Ozaki, M. D., Tetsuo Nagatani, M. D., Haruhisa Nagoshi, M. D., Hisashi
Yamada, M. D., Takeaki Takenaka, M. D., and Naoto Inada, M. D.

REFERENCES

1. Abe, M. Pathological study on polyclonal immunoblastosis. *J. Jpn. Soc. RES*, **19**,
    145–163 (1979) (in Japanese).
2. Frizzera, G., Moran, E. M., and Rappaport, H. Angio-immunoblastic lymphadenopathy
    with dysproteinemia. *Lancet*, **i**, 1070–1073 (1974).
3. Frizzera, G., Moran, E. M., and Rappaport, H. Angio-immunoblastic lymphadenopathy,
    diagnosis and clinical course. *Am. J. Med.*, **59**, 803–818 (1975).
4. Hattori, T., Uchiyama, T., Tobinai, T., Takatsuki, K., and Uchino, H. Surface pheno-
    type of Japanese adult T-cell leukemia cells characterized by monoclonal antibodies.
    Blood, **58**, 645–647 (1981).
5. Hinuma, T., Nagata, K., Hanaoka, M., Nakai, M., Matsumoto, T., Kinoshita, K.,
    Shirakawa, S., and Miyoshi, I. Adult T-cell leukemia: Antigen in an ATL cell line and
    detection of antibodies to the antigen in human sera. *Proc. Natl. Acad. Sci. U.S.*, **78**,
    6476–6480 (1981).
6. Inada, N., Oyamada, K., Shimoyama, M., Minato, K., Tobinai, K., and Watanabe, S.
    A case report of IBL-like T-cell lymphoma. *J. Jpn. Soc. RES*, **21**, 91 (1981) (in
    Japanese).
7. Isobe, T. and Kato, T. Immunologic aberrations in idiopathic reticulosis. *Recent Adv.
    RES Res.*, **9**, 53–64 (1969).
8. Kageyama, K., Mikata, A., and Watanabe, S. Hodgkin's disease in Japan. *GANN
    Monogr. Cancer Res.*, **15**, 239–252 (1973).
9. Kaneto, A., Yoshitake, M., Ikejiri, N., Koga, T., Shimokawa, Y., and Tanikawa, K.
    A case of immunoblastic lymphadenopathy: Evolution into immunoblastic sarcoma
    associated with polyclonal hypergammaglobulinemia. *Jpn. J. Clin. Hematol.*, **22**, 1463–
    1468 (1981) (in Japanese).
10. Kim, H., Jacobs, C., Warnke, R. A., and Dorfman, R. F. Malignant lymphoma with
    a high content of epitheloid histiocytes: Distinct clinicopathologic entity and a form of
    so-called "Lennert's lymphoma." *Cancer*, **41**, 620–635 (1978).
11. Kim, H., Nathwani, B. N., and Rappaport, H. So-called "Lennert's lymphoma." Is it
    a clinicopathologic entity? *Cancer*, **45**, 1379–1399 (1980).
12. Kimoto, M., Morinaga, S., Yamaguchi, H., Asai, I., Tsukada, T., Nozawa, Y., and
    Kamiyama, R. Immunoblastic lymphadenopathy terminating in immunoblastic sarcoma.
    Report of a case. *Jpn. J. Clin. Hematol.*, **21**, 416–420 (1980) (in Japanese).
13. Kinoshita, K. Personal communication.
14. Kita, K., Tatsumi, E., Nasu, K., Takiuchi, Y., Shirakawa, S., Takatsuki, K., and

Uchino, H. A case of T-cell lymphoma associated with M-component. *Jpn. J. Clin. Hematol.*, **22**, 1809–1814 (1981) (in Japanese).

15. Kojima, M. Immunoblastic lymphadenopathy (Lukes & Tindle)—Proposal of polyclonal immunoblastosis—. *Jpn. J. Clin. Hematol.*, **19**, 412–417 (1978) (in Japanese).

16. Lennert, K., Knecht, H., and Burkert, M. Vorstadien maligner lymphome: Prelymphomas. *Verh. Dtsch. Ges. Pathol.*, **63**, 170–196 (1979).

17. Lennert, K. and Mestdagh, J. Lymphogranulomatosen mit konstant hohem epitheloid Zell gehalt. *Virchows Arch.*, *Abt. A Pathol.*, **344**, 1–20 (1968).

18. Levine, A. M., Taylor, C. R., Schneider, D. R., Koehler, S. C., Forman, S. J., Lichtenstein, A., Lukes, R. J., and Feinstein, D. I. Immunoblastic sarcoma of T-cell *versus* B-cell origin: I. Clinical features. *Blood*, **58**, 52–61 (1981).

19. Lukes, R. J. and Tindle, B. H. Immunoblastic lymphadenopathy: A hyperimmune entity resembling Hodgkin's disease. *N. Engl. J. Med.*, **292**, 1–8 (1975).

20. Lymphoma study group. Combination chemotherapy with vincristine, cyclophosphamide (Endoxan), prednisolone and adriamycin (VEPA) in advanced non-Hodgkin's lymphoid malignancies: Relation between T-cell or non-T-cell phenotype and response. *Jpn. J. Clin. Oncol.*, **9** (Suppl.), 397–406 (1979).

21. Mannoji, M., Shimada, M., Koresawa, S., Yamada, O., Togawa, A., Yawata, Y., Umemura, H., and Kozuru, M. A case of angioimmunoblastic lymphadenopathy with dysproteinemia associated with autoimmune hemolytic anemia and pure red cell aplasia — with special references to its pathogenesis—. *Jpn. J. Clin. Hematol.*, **22**, 1751–1758 (1981) (in Japanese).

22. Matsumoto, T. Personal communication.

23. Mizoguchi, H. Personal communication.

24. Nagatani, T. Personal communication.

25. Nathwani, B. N., Rappaport, H., Moran, E. M., Pangalis, G. A., and Kim, H. Malignant lymphoma arising in angioimmunoblastic lymphadenopathy. *Cancer*, **41**, 578–606 (1978).

26. Radaszkiewicz, T. and Lennert, K. Lymphogranulomatosis X: klinisches Bild, Therapie und Prognose. *Dtsch. Med. Wochenschr.*, **100**, 1157–1163 (1975).

27. Shimoyama, M. and Minato, K. Clinical, cytological and immunological analysis of T-cell type lymphoid malignancies—a classification of T-cell type lymphoid malignancy —. *Jpn. J. Clin. Hematol.*, **20**, 1056–1069 (1979) (in Japanese).

28. Shimoyama, M., Minato, K., Saito, H., Nagatani, T., Ozaki, Y., and Watanabe, S. T-cell lymphoma histologically diagnosed as immunoblastic lymphadenopathy-like, Hodgkinoid type or lymphogranulomatosis. *Jpn. J. Clin. Hematol.*, **21** (Suppl. 1), 65 (1979) (in Japanese).

29. Shimoyama, M., Minato, K., Saito, H., Takenaka, T., Watanabe, S., Nagatani, T., and Naruto, M. Immunoblastic lymphadenopathy (IBL)-like T-cell lymphoma. *Jpn. J. Clin. Oncol.*, **9** (Suppl. 1), 347–356 (1979).

30. Shimoyama, M., Tobinai, K., Hirose, M., and Minato, K. Cellular origin of T-cell malignancies. This volume, pp. 23–35 (1982).

31. Shimoyama, M., Tobinai, K., and Minato, K. Immunological, clinical and prognostic characteristics of Japanese T-cell lymphomas. In "Leukemia Markers," ed. W. Knapp, pp. 525–528 (1981). Academic Press, London.

32. Suchi, T. A typical lymph node hyperplasia with fatal outcome. A report on the histopathological, immunological and clinical investigations of the cases. *Recent Adv. RES Res.*, **14**, 13–34 (1974).

33. Tobinai, K., Hirose, M., Yamada, H., Minato, K., and Shimoyama, M. Cellular origin

of human lymphoid malignancies as based on immunologic analysis of membrane differentiation antigens. *Jpn. J. Clin. Oncol.*, **12**, 73–90 (1982).

34. Tobinai, K., Minato, K., Yamada, H., Hirose, M., Shimoyama, M., and Watanabe, S. A case report of IBL-like T-cell lymphoma with suppressor/cytotoxic T-cell phenotype (OKT3+, OKT8+). *Jpn. J. RES Syst.*, **21**, 91 (1981) (in Japanese).
35. Watanabe, S., Shimosato, Y., Shimoyama, M., and Minato, K. Adult T-cell lymphoma with hypergammaglobulinemia. *Cancer*, **46**, 2472–2483 (1980).
36. Westerhausen, M. and Oehlert, W. Chronisches pluripotentielles immunproliferatives Syndrom. *Dtsch. Med. Wochenschr.*, **97**, 1407–1413 (1972).

MACROSCOPICAL AND HISTOPATHOLOGICAL ANALYSES ON CUTANEOUS LYMPHOMATOUS LESIONS OF PERIPHERAL T CELL NATURE

Testuji Mitsui,[*1] Taizan Suchi,[*2] and Masahiro Kikuchi[*1]

*Department of Pathology, Fukuoka University School of Medicine,[*1] and
Department of Pathology and Clinical Laboratories,
Aichi Cancer Center Hospital[*2]*

1.   Histopathological analysis of 36 pairs of skin and lymph node sections of various T-cell malignancies with cutaneous manifestations revealed that mycosis fungoides, Sézary syndome (SS) and the rapidly progressive lymphoma/leukemia group have fairly clear-cut tendencies distinctly different from each other in each category of their mode of neoplastic cell proliferation and infiltration in the two organs.

2.   Thirty-six cases of skin lesions were found among 70 cases of peripheral T-cell lymphoma with known survival. These were 5 cases of primary cutaneous lymphoma including SS and "classical" mycosis fungoides (CMF), and 31 cases of node-based lymphoma composed mostly of adult T-cell leukemia-lymphoma (ATLL). Histologically, skin biopsies of the primary cutaneous lymphomas disclosed the typical feature of SS-CMF. However, such a histologic picture was also found in 56% of the node-based lymphomas with cutaneous infiltration. Moreover, immunological surface markers and cytochemistry of the tumor cells in node-based lymphoma demonstrated inducer/ helper T-cell characters similar to those of SS-CMF. Macroscopically, however, both lesions were strikingly different; *i.e.*, cases of node-based lymphoma chiefly showed generalized papular eruptions (48%), whereas SS was characterized by erythrodermia and CMF by tumor-in-plaque eruptions. Besides this type of cutaneous change, node-based lymphoma showed tumorous (19%), papulonodular (16%), plaque (13%), and ulcerative (3%) eruptions, which resemble those of "D'emblee" type mycosis fungoides. We suggest that macroscopic analysis is valuable in distinguishing primary cutaneous lymphoma from cutaneous infiltration of node-based lymphoma, and believe that many of the cases reported as "D'emblee" type in Japan may indeed belong to ATLL.

A type of rapidly progressive peripheral T-cell malignancy with cutaneous infiltration, which largely corresponds to the so-called adult T-cell leukemia/lymphoma (ATLL) is frequently encountered in Japan. This type of T-cell malignancy has many common characteristics with Sézary syndrome (SS) and the mycosis fungoides group in cutaneous histology (epidermotropism and convoluted lymphoid cell infiltration)

[*1] Nanakuma 34, Jonan-ku, Fukuoka 814-01, Japan (三井徹次, 菊池昌弘).
[*2] Kanokoden 81-1159, Tashiro-cho, Chikusa-ku, Nagoya 464, Japan (須知泰山).

and immunological phenotype of the tumor cells (inducer/helper T-cells). Although Lutzner (8) categorized cutaneous T-cell lymphoma as one clinicopathological entity, ATLL with cutaneous infiltration should be differentiated by its short clinical course and poor therapeutic response. In this report we have demonstrated that detailed macroscopic analysis of the skin lesions is indispensable in differentiating the two groups.

Comparative Analysis of Skin and Lymph Node Histology

The purpose of this report is to see if there is any tendency in histological appearances of either skin or lymph nodes to reflect more or less their clinical features among the various forms of peripheral T-cell neoplasms with cutaneous manifestations.

Used for the study were hematoxylin and eosin stained histological sections of skin and lymph nodes contributed from the dermatology department of five university hospitals within Japan, three of which are located in Kyushu, the endemic area of the rapidly fatal T-cell malignancy. All cases have been investigated for immunological characterization of tumor cells by various methods employed at the respective institutions, and have proven to be of T-cell nature. The cases in which both skin and lymph node sections were available numbered 36 among 60 cases of peripheral T-cell malignancy with cutaneous manifestations.

Mode of Infiltration of Neoplastic Cells and Clinical Diagnosis

The mode of infiltration and/or proliferation of neoplastic cells in the skin and in the nodes showed, a widely varied range, but they can be roughly divided into a number of types. Epidermotropism, mostly with Pautrier's microabscesses, was seen in the great majority of the cases and the dermal infiltration can be categorized into 3 types, namely, 1) superficial diffuse, 2) perivascular aggregation, and 3) massive, as described in the next section. The lymph node histology can be divided into 6 types, namely, 1) minimal or no involvement; 2) a dermatopathic lymphadenitis pattern with atypical cells in enlarged paracorteces (Photo 1) (10); 3) diffuse scattering of neoplastic cells in single cells and/or in small clusters (malignant histocytosis-like distribution, Photo 2); 4) T-zone distribution of neoplastic cells with sparing of follicles (Photo 3); 5) angioimmunoblastic lymphadenopathy (AIBL)-like pattern (Photo 4); and 6) diffuse lymphoma.

Clinical diagnoses accompanying these slides were roughly divided into the following categories, 1) mycosis fungoides (MF); 2) SS; 3) malignant lymphoma; and 4) leukemia. Most cases in the latter two categories belonged to the rapidly progressive T-cell malignancy prevailing in the southwest part of Japan (ATLL).

Individual cases are plotted in Fig. 1 according to the mode of infiltration in the skin on one axis and that in the lymph node on the other, with their diagnostic categories by respective marks. Although the cases included in a category of "clinical diagnosis" in a collection of cases from different sources do not constitute a purely homogeneous group, nor is a biopsy taken arbitrarily at one time during the course necessarily a representative histology of the individual disease, yet the figure seems to show that the cases of MF, those of SS and those of the lymphoma/leukemia group

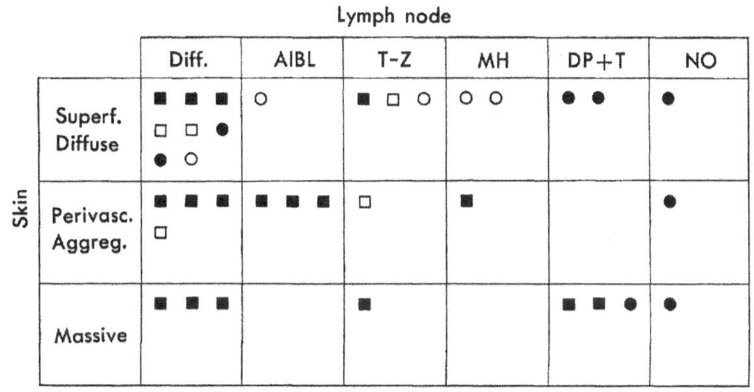

Lymph node

	Diff.	AIBL	T-Z	MH	DP+T	NO
Superf. Diffuse	■ ■ ■ □ □ ● ● ○	○	■ □ ○	○ ○	● ●	●
Perivasc. Aggreg.	■ ■ ■ □	■ ■ ■	□	■		●
Massive	■ ■ ■		■		■ ■ ●	●

(left side label: Skin)

FIG. 1. Mode of infiltration in lymph nodes and skin by various "clinical diagnoses." Diff., diffuse lymphoma; AIBL, angioimmunoblastic pattern; T-Z, T-zone distribution; MH, malignant histiocytosis-like infiltration; DP+T, dermatopathic lymphadenitis with tumor cells in paracortex; NO, no or minal infiltration of tumor cells; Superf. Diffuse, superficial diffused infiltration in upper dermis; Perivasc. Aggreg., perivascular aggregation of tumor cells; Massive, diffuse massive infiltration. ■ ML; □ leukemia; ● MF; ○ Sézary syndrome.

are fairly clearly distinguished from each other in their behavioral characters. Moreover, the MF appears to display the feature of primary cutaneous lymphoma most clearly, whereas the SS seems somewhat more like T-chronic lymphocytic leukemia (CLL) with specific affinity to the skin. The findings in this study indicate the importance of lymph node biopsy in the diagnosis of lymphoid malignancy with skin manifestation, and also appear to justify the criteria set for "primary cutaneous lymphoma" in next section.

Skin Lesions of Peripheral T-cell Malignancies

In this section, immunopathological and macroscopic characters of cutaneous infiltration of node-based lymphomas are documented and compared with those of primary cutaneous lymphomas.

The file of the Department of Pathology of Fukuoka University situated on Kyushu island in southwestern Japan, was reviewed for the period from April 1977 through

TABLE I. Age and Sex of Patients with Cutaneous Infiltration

Histological type	Number of cases	Age (Median)	Sex (M/F)
Small cell	2	37–53 (45)	2/0
Medium-sized cell	10	41–78 (57)	8/2
Large cell	5	39–79 (62)	3/2
Pleomorphic	11	33–74 (49)	5/6
T-ML with AIBL	3	43–83 (71)	2/1
Primary cutaneous	5	27–72 (62)	2/3
Total	36	27–72 (57)	22/14

June 1981. Cutaneous infiltration was found in 36 out of 70 cases of peripheral T-cell lymphoma, which had immunological, clinicopathological work-up and follow-up studies. The cases with skin lesions were divided into 31 of node-based lymphoma which had been histologically classified by biopsied lymph node and 5 of primary cutaneous lymphoma. The age and sex of the cases are described in Table I.

1. Macroscopic analysis

The skin lesions in the peripheral T-cell lymphomas showed some variations in size, appearance and distribution (localized or generalized) of individual eruptions. According to these macroscopic varieties the skin lesions were divided into 7 types, which are schematically drawn in Fig. 2 and tabulated in comparison with histologic types in Table II.

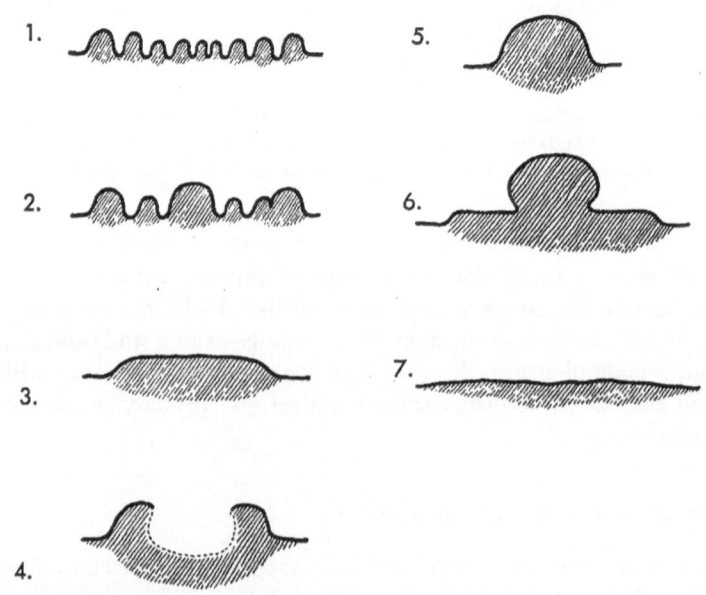

Fig. 2. Type of macroscopic appearances of skin lesion. 1, Generalized-papular; 2, papulo-nodular; 3, infiltrative plaque; 4, ulcerative lesion; 5, localized tumor; 6, tumor in plaque; 7, erythroderma.

TABLE II. Macroscopic Type of Skin Lesion and Leukemic Changes

Histological type	Number of cases	Leukemic changes (%)	Papular	Papulo-nodular	Plaque	Ulcerative	Tumor	Tumor in plaque	Erythrodermic
Small cell	2	2 (100.0)	2	0	0	0	0	0	0
Medium-sized cell	10	7 (70.0)	7	1	2	0	0	0	0
Large cell	5	0 (0.0)	0	1	0	1	3	0	0
Pleomorphic	11	11 (100.0)	6	2	1	0	2	0	0
T-ML with AIBL	3	3 (100.0)	0	1	1	0	1	0	0
Primary cutaneous ML	5	3 (60.0)	0	2	0	0	0	1	2
Total	36	26 (72.2)	15	7	4	1	6	1	2

1) Generalized papular type (15 cases)

In this type, the eruptions were distributed over the whole body and consisted of solid, erythematous papules which varied in size from pin-head to pea. These eruptions may give suggest leukemia cutis to dermatologists (Photo 5). In two cases the papules caused confusion with toxic eruptions of drug or viral origin because of their small size and mixed appearance with erythemas (Photo 6), but the eruptions always disappeared within one or 2 weeks. Cases of this type were composed of node-based lymphoma of medium-sized cell type (7 cases), pleomorphic type (6 cases), and small cell type (2 cases).

Hematologically, 13 cases were leukemic, and one of the remaining 2 cases showed bone marrow infiltration.

2) Generalized papulo-nodular type (7 cases)

The eruptions were those of a generalized papular type with solid nodules up to finger tip size, which occasionally showed secondary ulceration (Photo 7). In this type there were 2 cases of primary cutaneous lymphoma and 5 cases of node-based lymphoma (2 of pleomorphic type, and one each of medium-sized cell type and T-malignant lymphoma (T-ML) with AILBL). Leukemic pictures were found in one of the 2 cases of primary cutaneous lymphoma, and 4 of the 5 cases of node-based lymphoma.

3) Infiltrative plaque type (4 cases)

The eruptions were distributed rather generally and consisted of circumscribed, elevated, erythematous induration with a size slightly larger than a thumb. In one case, the extensive and confluent eruption resembled erythrodermia but the lack of or only minimal scaling with residual normal skin excluded this (Photo 8). Leukemic pictures were found in all but one case. This type consisted of 2 medium-sized cell type, and one each of pleomorphic type and T-ML with AIBL.

4) Ulcerative type (1 case)

The single case of this type (non-leukemic large cell type) showed large ulcers with well demarcated granular margins and was about the size of a handteller (Photo 9).

5) Localized tumor type (6 cases)

This type had one or several tumors with some satellite nodules which were dark-red or purple in color, occasionally showing central ulcerations (Photo 10). There were 3 cases of the non-leukemic large cell type, 2 of the pleomorphic type with leukemic changes and one of T-ML with AIBL.

6) Tumor in infiltrative plaque type (1 case)

Several soft mushroom-like tumors arising from brown-colored, scaly, infiltrative plaques were scattered on the arms with other infiltrative plaques and scaly patches (Photo 11). The patient had a 2.5 year history of chronic eczematous eruption. This case was considered to be classical mycosis fungoides (CMF).

7) Erythrodermic type (2 cases)

The erythematous and exfoliative eruptions covered the entire body with no normal appearing skin (Photo 12). Hyperkeratosis of the palms and soles together with onychodystrophy was observed. Both patients had had such eruptions for several years, and demonstrated a typical leukemic picture of SS.

2. Histological analysis

Five cases of primary cutaneous lymphoma demonstrated typical histologic pictures

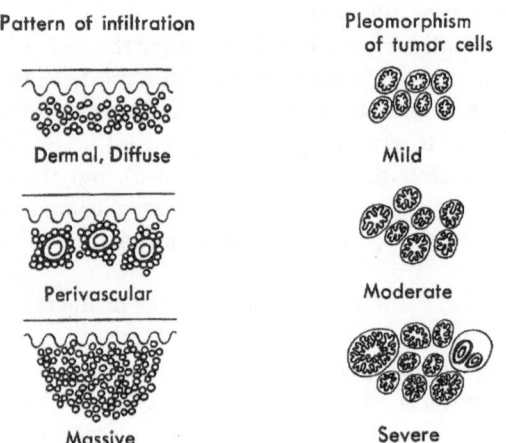

FIG. 3.   Histology of skin lesion.

of SS-CMF. In accordance with the purpose of this study, histological characteristics of cutaneous infiltration of node-based lymphomas are chiefly described.

Skin lesions from 25 of 31 cases of node-based lymphomas were examined for: 1) Epidermotropism, including Pautrier's microabscess; 2) features of tumor cells in the skin, compared with those in the lymph node; 3) pleomorphism of tumor cells; and 4) dermal distribution of infiltrates, which are schematically described in Fig. 3.

1)   Epidermotropism of tumor cells

Epidermotropism of the tumor cells was demonstrated in 14 cases (56%), including 11 with Pautrier's microabscesses (Photo 13). This was found in all 5 histological types of node-based lymphoma.

2)   Comparison with tumor cells in lymph node

Nineteen cases demonstrated a population of tumor cells similar to that of biopsied lymph nodes. In the remaining 6 cases prevalence of medium-sized cells in the skin was noted.

3)   Pleomorphism of tumor cells

In 6 cases chiefly composed of the tumor type, the pleomorphism was more prominent in the cutaneous infiltrates than in those of biopsied lymph nodes. In such cases, bizarre nucleated giant cells superimposed on the cutaneous infiltrates were seen

TABLE III.   Histology of Cutaneous Infiltration

Histological type	Number of cases	Epidermotrophism (%)	Pattern of dermal infiltrates		
			Perivas-cular	Superficial diffuse	Massive
Small cell	2	1 (50.0)	0	2	0
Medium-sized cell	7	3 (42.9)	3	3	1
Large cell	5	4 (80.0)	0	2	3
Pleomorphic	9	5 (55.6)	1	6	2
T-ML with AIBL	2	1 (50.0)	1	1	0
Total	25	14 (56.0)	5	14	6

(Photos 14 a, b). On the other hand, pleomorphism was milder in 8 cases of the leukemic, generalized papular type.

4) *Distribution of dermal infiltrates*

There were 5 cases (20%) of the perivascular type, 14 cases (56%) of the superficial diffuse type, and 6 cases (24%) of the massive type. A comparison of the distribution of infiltrates and macroscopic types showed that the generalized papular type corresponded chiefly to the perivascular and superficial diffuse types, and the papulonodular, infiltrative plaque, and tumor types chiefly to the massive distributed type. In other words, distribution of the dermal infiltrates correlates with the macroscopic appearances of the skin lesions.

Summary of the histologic analysis is shown in Table III.

3. *Cytochemistry and monoclonal antibody*

Cytochemical analysis was performed on 3 cases of primary cutaneous lymphoma and 18 cases of node-based lymphoma. All cases examined demonstrated dot-like or nuclear capped pattern of positivities for both acid phosphatase and acid α-naphthyl acetate esterase. The latter is considered to be a marker enzyme of helper T-lymphocytes (4). Many cases demonstrated membranous positivity for adenosine triphosphatase.

Immunofluorescent assays for cell surface antigens were performed using OR-THOCLON's monoclonal antisera against T-lymphocytes (9) in one case of primary cutaneous lymphoma and 7 cases of node-based lymphoma. All cases showed high values of OKT-3 and OKT-4 (inducer/helper T-cell).

4. *Prognosis*

Patients other than those with CMF, SS, and small cell type showed a rapid

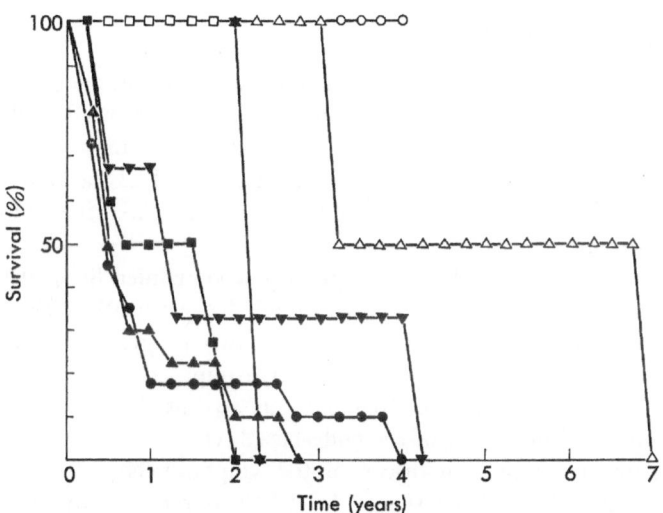

FIG. 4. Survival of patients with each histologic type. ○ MF-classical type (1); □ small T-CLL (2); △ SS (2); ● pleo (11); ■ large (5); ▲ medium-sized (10); ▼ T-ML+AIBL (3); ★ cutaneous ML (2).

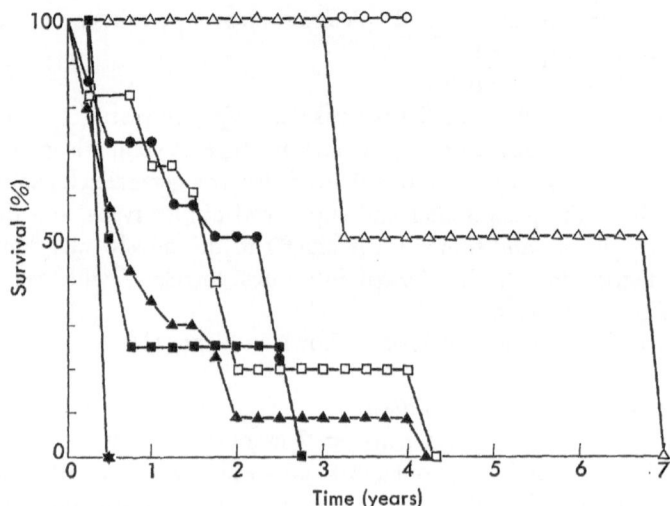

Fig. 5. Survival of patients with each macroscopic type. ○ tumor in plaque (1);
△ erythrodermic (2); □ tumor (6); ▲ papular (15); ■ plaque (4); ● nodulo-
papular (7); ★ ulcer (1).

clinical course, those with pleomorphic and medium-sized cell types having the worst
prognosis in this series (Fig. 4).

With regard to macroscopic types, patients with generalized paular, and infiltrative
plaque types had the highest malignancy with a rapidly fatal course of within one year.
On the other hand, patients with tumor-in-plaque and erythrodermic types had low
grade malignancy with a slowly progressive course (Fig. 5).

Cutaneous T-cell Lymphoma and ATLL

In Western countries, where T-cell malignancies are low in incidence, lymphomatous lesions of the skin consist mostly of primary cutaneous lymphomas such as
SS-CMF, a peripheral T-cell neoplasm of low grade malignancy. In Japan, however,
lymphomatous skin lesions are usually associated with ATLL, a kind of node-based
T-cell lymphoma. The cutaneous infiltration is frequently extensive and may be found
as an initial symptom.

In our series, node-based T-cell malignancy accompanied 86% of the cases with
cutaneous lymphomatous lesions in contrast to only 8% with SS-CMF. The latter was
so regarded by the unique skin manifestation and slowly progressive course as originally
described (*1, 11*). On the other hand, the former, composed mostly of ATLL, showed
variable manifestations on the skin, frequently as an initial symptom.

In cutaneous histology, 56% of the node-based lymphomas demonstrated a superficial diffuse or massive infiltration of convoluted lymphoid cells with epidermotropism,
which was indistinguishable from that of SS-CMF as reported by Hanaoka (*5*). The
picture seemed to be not a hallmark of SS-CMF but a cutaneous manifestation common to the peripheral T-cell malignancy as suggested by Leong *et al.* (*7*). Moreover,
examination using monoclonal anti-human T-cell antisera as well as cytochemical

studies revealed that node-based lymphomas with cutaneous infiltration possessed peripheral inducer/helper T-cell characters as shown for SS-CMF (2, 6). Therefore, in Japan, cutaneous histology or an immunological method for cell surface marker may not be very usueful in distinguishing between SS-CMF and cutaneous infiltration of node-based lymphomas.

However, the two groups should be differentiated because they have different prognoses and therapeutic effects. Especially, it is important to make a distinction between adult T-cell leukemia (ATL) with cutaneous infiltration and SS. In our series, ATL with cutaneous infiltration chiefly showed generalized papular eruptions but no erythrodermia, which was confined to cases of SS. Even if cutaneous infiltration of ATL were extensive, a distinction between the two groups was possible based on the precise macroscopic criterion of erythrodermia (generalized exfoliative eruption without sparing normal skin). Recently, Uchiyama et al. (12) reported that the leukemic cells of ATL showed a suppressor function for pokeweed mitogen (PWM)-induced transformation of normal B-cells in cocultivation. The fact seemed to be an important clue to separating ATLL from SS-CMF.

On the other hand, we had 8 cases of non-leukemic node-based lymphomas, composed mostly of the large cell type. They showed skin manifestations, such as tumor, plaque, and ulcerative lesions; these might be confused with the "D'emblee" type of mycosis fungoides because they demonstrated many common histologic and macroscopic characters. From our results, the "D'emblee" type seemed to be not a clinico-pathological entity but heterogenous lymphomatous lesions which included the cutaneous infiltration of ATLL. Therefore, we consider that the name "mycosis fungoides (MF)" should be given only to the "classical" type, which demonstrates a unique skin manifestation of tumor-in-plaque eruption, clearly different from other lymphomatous skin lesions.

CONCLUSIONS

The results of this study suggest macroscopic analysis is more valuable than skin histology and the immunological method to separate ATLL from SS-CMF. In Japan, as lymphomatous skin lesion consists mostly of a cutaneous infiltration of ATLL occasionally noticed as the initial sign and which showed the same histological and immunological characters, Lutzner's proposal of cutaneous T-cell lymphoma (CTLL) and Edelson's amplified concept of CTLL (3) may be incomplete. Our proposal of a classification of skin lymphomatous lesion as listed in Table IV seems to be more practical in Japan.

TABLE IV. Skin Lymphomatous Lesion of Peripheral T-cell Malignancies

A) Low-grade malignancy
    1) Cutaneous infiltration of T-CLL (small cell type)
    2) Sézary syndrome (SS)
    3) " Classical " mycosis fungoides (CMF)
    4) Primary cutaneous lymphoma except SS-CMF
B) High-grade malignancy
    1) Cutaneous infiltration of ATLL
    2) Cutaneous infiltration of node-based lymphomas except ATLL

Acknowledgments

The cases used for Part I of this study were generously contributed from the following institutions to which the authors' sincere gratitude is due: Department of Dermatology, University of Yamaguchi (Prof. E. Fujita), Department of Dermatology, University of Kagoshima (Prof. M. Tashiro), Department of Dermatology, University of Kumamoto (Prof. T. Arao), Department of Dermatology, University of Nagasaki (Prof. H. Yoshida), and Department of Dermatology, Yokohama City University (Prof. R. Nagai).

REFERENCES

1. Bluefarb, S. M. Mycosis fungoides. Granuloma fugoides. *In* "Cutaneous Manifestations of the Malignant Lymphomas," ed. A. C. Curtis, pp. 7–12 (1959). C. C. Thomas, Springfield.
2. Broder, S., Edelson, R. L., Lutzner, M. A., Nelson, D. L., MacDermott, R. P., Durm, M. E., Goldman, C. K., Meade, B. D., and Waldmann, T. A. The Sézary syndrome: A malignant proliferation of helper T cells. *J. Clin. Invest.*, **58**, 1297–1306 (1976).
3. Edelson, R. L. Cutaneous T cell lymphoma: Mycosis fungoides, Sézary syndrome, and other variants. *J. Am. Acad. Dermatol.*, **2**, 89–106 (1980).
4. Grossi, C. E., Webb, S. R., Zicca, A., Lydyard, P. M., Moretta, L., Mingari, M. C., and Cooper, M. D. Morphological and histochemical analysis of two human T-cell subpopulations bearing receptors for IgM or IgG. *J. Exp. Med.*, **147**, 1405–1417 (1978).
5. Hanaoka, M., Sasaki, M., Matsumoto, H., Tankawa, H., Yamabe, H., Tomimoto, K., Tasaka, C., Fujiwara, H., Uchiyama, T., and Takatsuki, K. Adult T-cell leukemia. Histological classification and characteristics. *Acta Pathol. Jpn.*, **29**, 723–738 (1979).
6. Kung, P. C., Berger, C. L., Goldstein, G., LoGerfo, P., and Edelson, R. L. Cutaneous T-cell lymphoma: Characterization by monoclonal antibodies. *Blood*, **57**, 261–266 (1981).
7. Leong, A. S.-Y., Sage, R. E., Kinnear, G. C., and Forbes, I. J. Preferential epidermotropism in adult T-cell leukemia-lymphoma. *Am. J. Surg. Pathol.*, **4**, 421–430 (1980).
8. Lutzner, M., Edelson, R., Schein, P., Greene, I., Kirkpatric, C., and Ahmed, A. Cutaneous T-cell lymphoma: The Sézary syndrome, mycosis fungoides and related disorders. *Ann. Intern. Med.*, **83**, 534–552 (1975).
9. Reinherz, E. L. and Schlossman, S. F. The differentiation and function of human T lymphocytes. *Cell*, **19**, 821–827 (1980).
10. Scheffer, E. and Meijer, C.J.L.M. Early involvement of lymph nodes in mycosis fungoides. *In* "Malignant Lymphoproliferative Diseases," ed. J. G. Van Den Tweel, pp. 373–385 (1980). Leiden University Press, The Hague-Boston-London.
11. Sézary, A. and Bouvrain, Y. Erythrodermie avec presence de cellules monstreuses dans le derme et dans le sang circulant. *Bull. Soc. Fr. Dermatol. Syphiligr.*, **45**, 254–260 (1938).
12. Uchiyama, T., Sagawa, K., Takatsuki, K., and Uchino, H. Effect of adult T-cell leukemia cells on pokeweed mitogen induced normal B-cell differentiation. *Clin. Immunol. Immunopathol.*, **10**, 24–34 (1978).

EXPLANATION OF PHOTOS

PHOTO 1. Dermatopathic lymphadenitis with scattered tumor cells in an enlarged paracortex. Atypical cerebriform nuclei and mitotic cells in higher magnification are shown in the inset. H-E, ×64 and ×400.

PHOTO 2. Malignant histiocytosis-like infiltration. Atypical cells are seen scattered in single cell and small clumps in sinuses and parenchyma. H-E, ×200.

PHOTO 3.   T-zone distribution. ¡Tumor cells are distributed in paracortical or inferfollicular areas, sparing follicles with rather hyperplastic germinal centers. H-E, ×64.

PHOTO 4.   Angioimmunoblastic pattern. Tumor cells are proliferating along with conspicuous venules which are often arborizing. H-E, ×400.

PHOTO 5.   Generalized papular type. Solid erythematous papules disseminated on the arms and chest. Confluent papules in places. Case of leukemic medium-sized cell type.

PHOTO 6.   Generalized papular type. Tiny papules admixed with erythemas, reminiscent of measles. Case of leukemic medium-sized cell type.

PHOTO 7.   Generalized papulo-nodular type. Scattered solid nodules among papules. Some nodules showing ulcerations. Case of non-leukemic large cell type.

PHOTO 8.   Infiltrative plaque type. Confluent erythematous plaques on the abdomen. Absence of scaling and residual normal skin exclude erythrodermia. Case of leukemic medium-sized cell type.

PHOTO 9.   Ulcerative type. Large ulcers on the leg. Case of non-leukemic large cell type.

PHOTO 10.   Localized tumor type. Solitary flesh-colored tumor with satelite nodules on the buttock. Case of pleomorphic type with leukemic changes.

PHOTO 11.   Tumor in infiltrative plaque type. Soft mushroom-like tumors in scaly, brown-colored plaques with some neighboring scaly patches. Case of classical mycosis fungoides.

PHOTO 12.   Erythrodermic type. Exfoliative, erythematous rashes covering the whole body with no residual normal skin. Case of SS.

PHOTO 13.   Apparent Pautrier's microabscesses in medium-sized cell type with leukemic picture of ATL. Superficial, diffuse infiltration of highly convoluted lymphoid cells. H-E, ×460.

PHOTO 14.   Pleomorphic type. a) Histology of biopsied lymph node. Pleomorphic infiltrates with cerebriform giant cells. H-E, ×390. b) Cutaneous infiltration of same cases. Bizarre nucleated giant cells predominate. H-E, ×390.

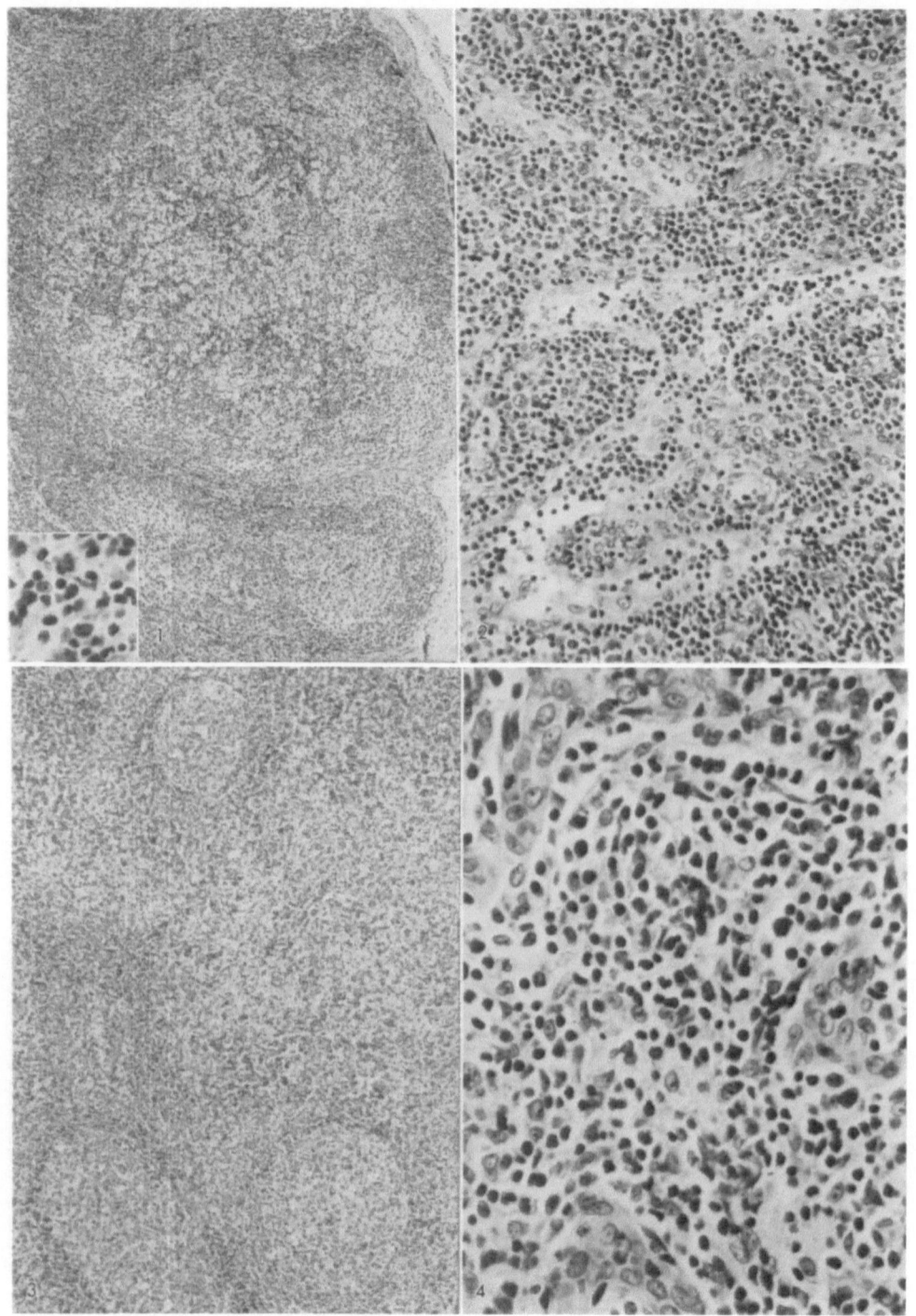

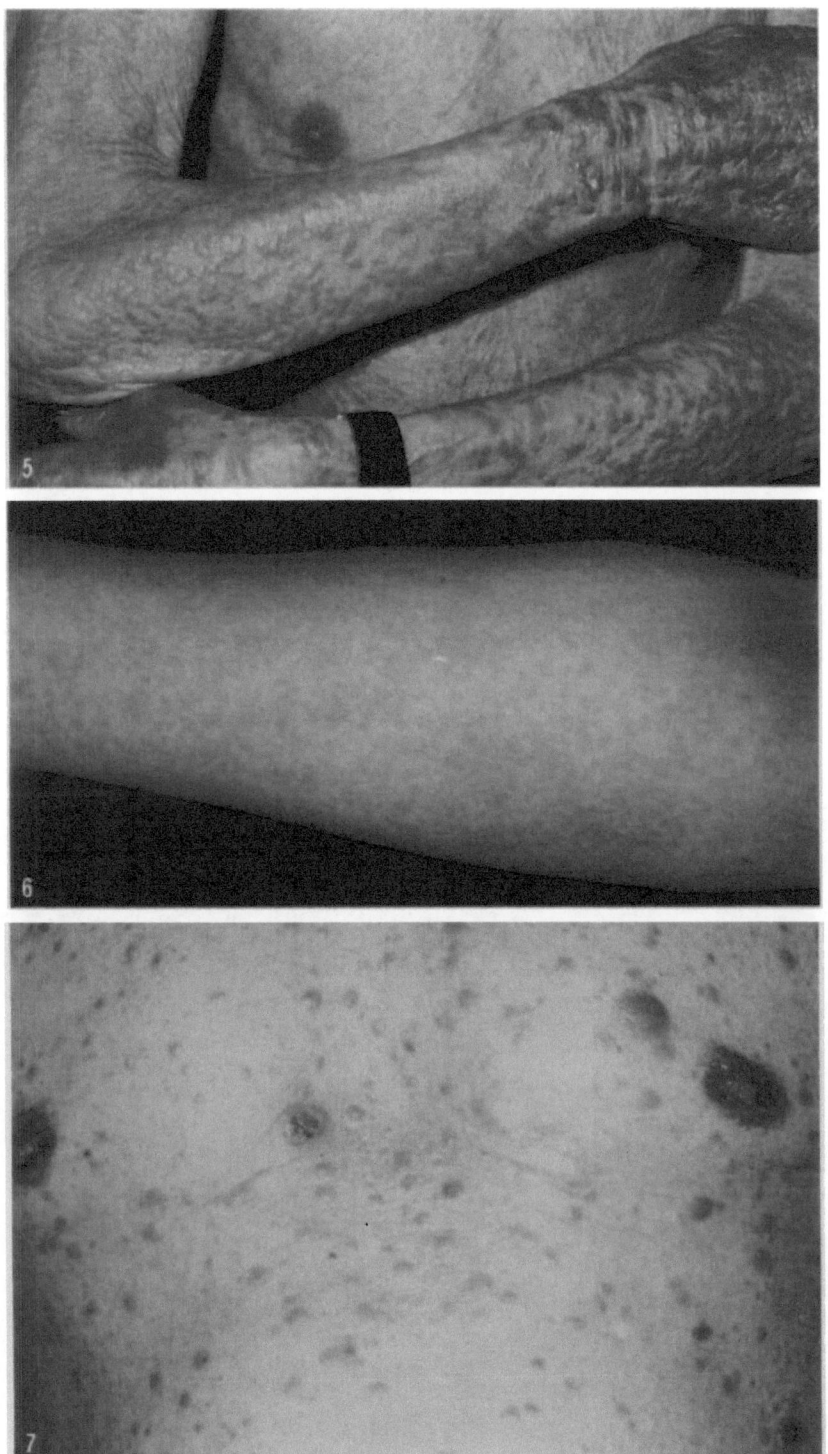

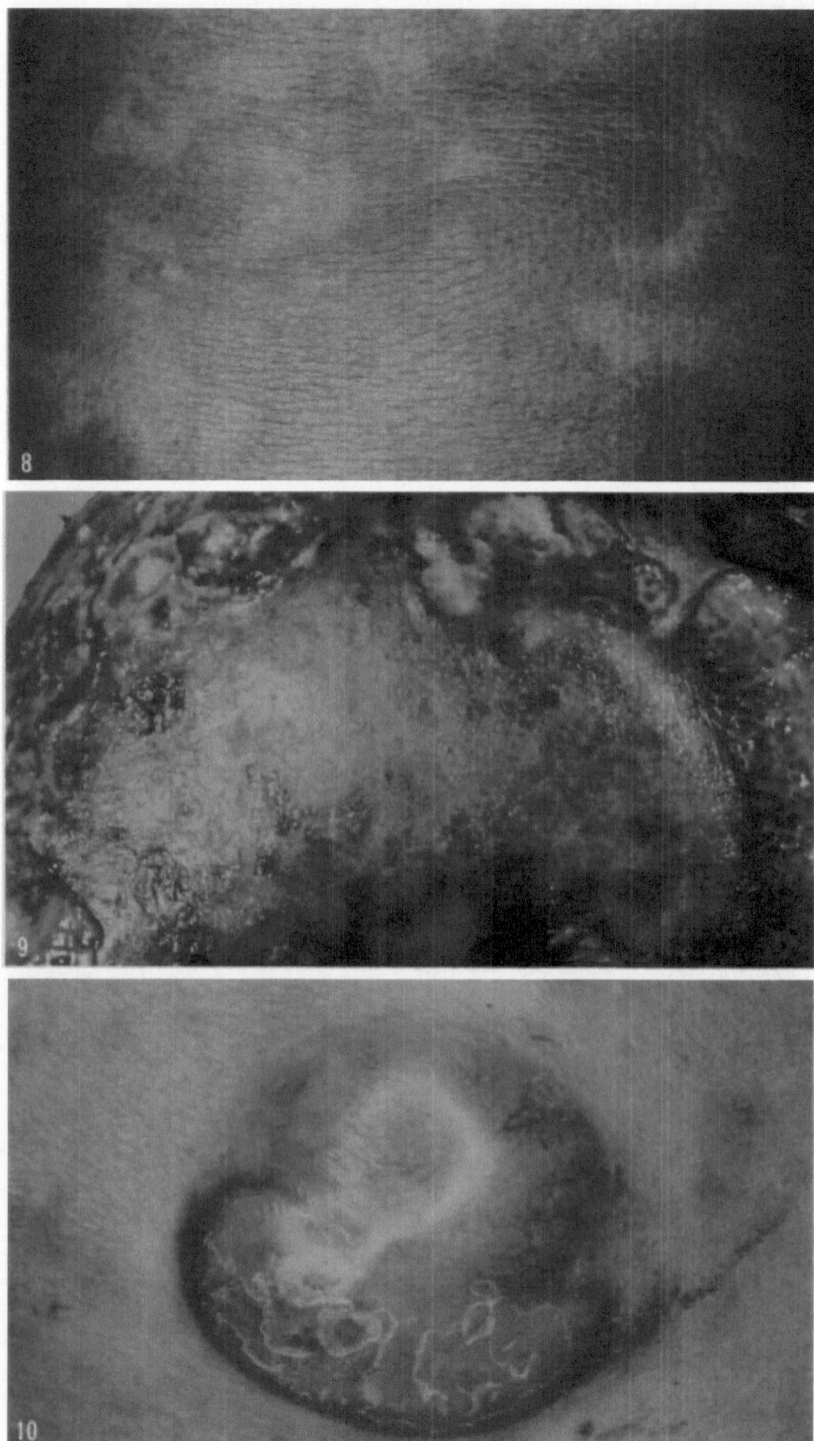

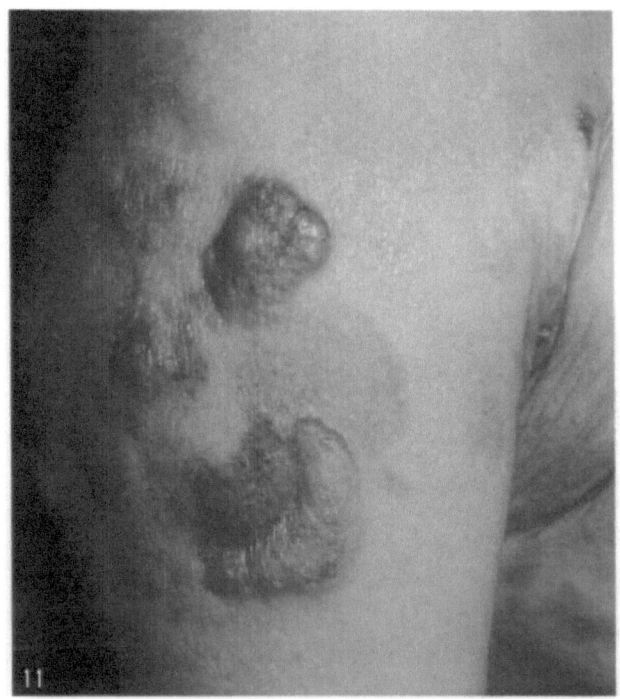

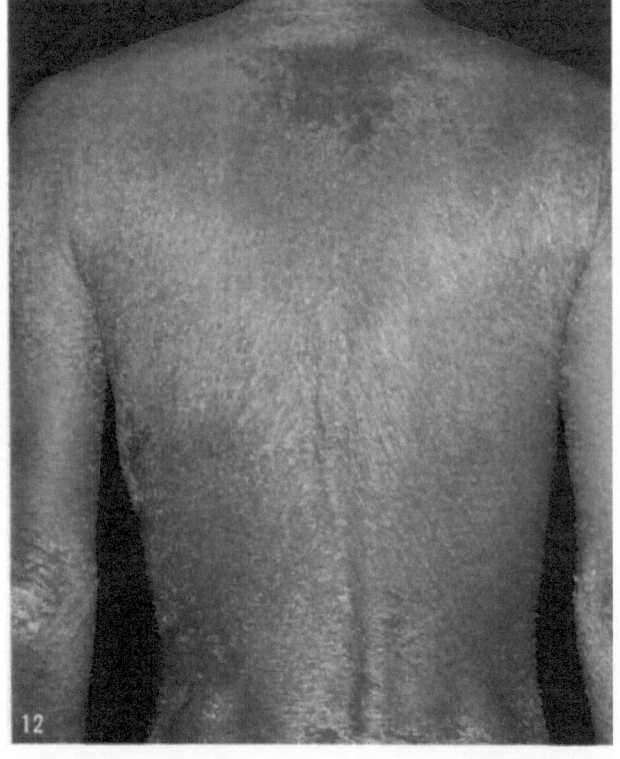

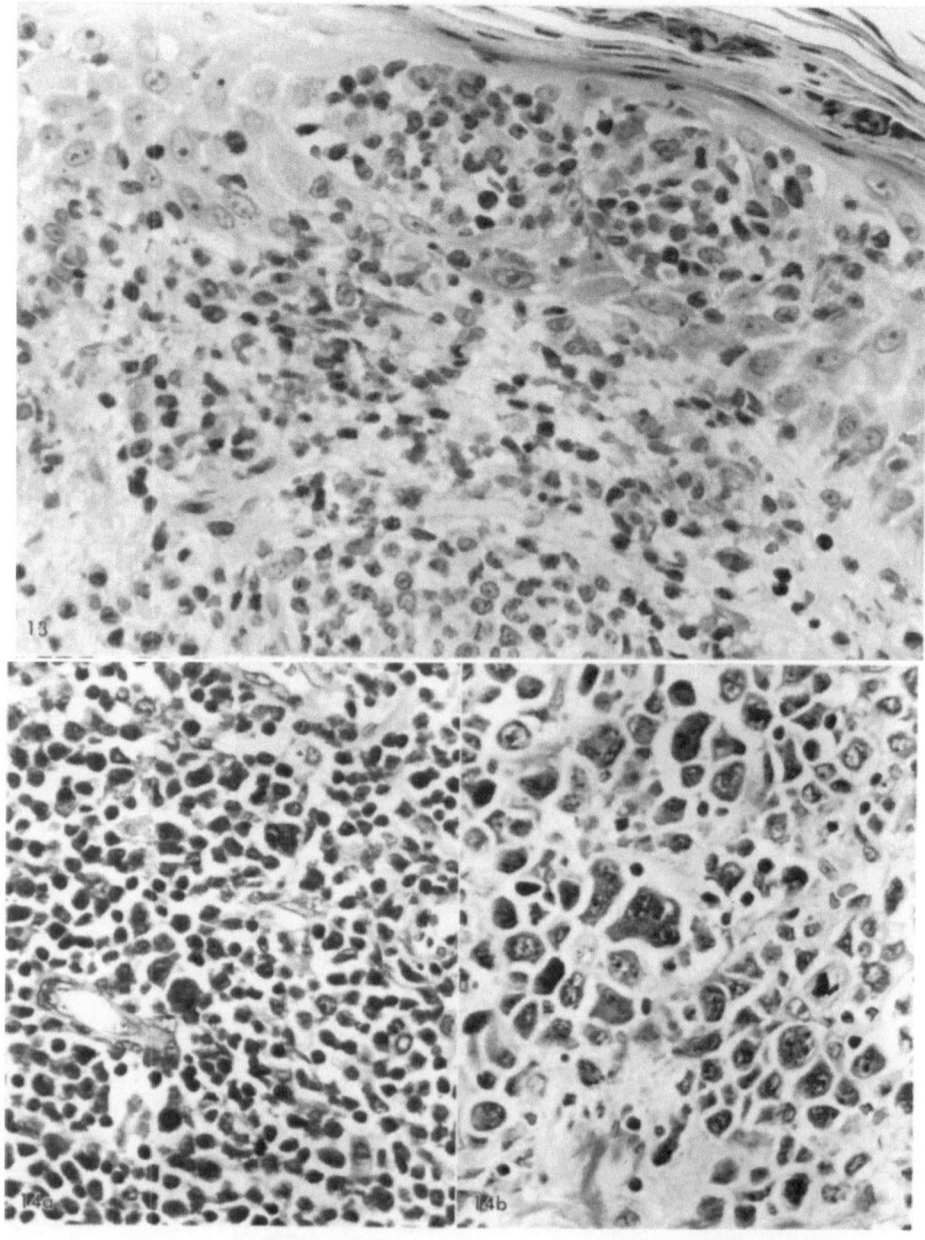

ADULT T CELL LEUKEMIA IN KAGOSHIMA: ITS CLINICAL FEATURES AND SKIN LESIONS

Kazuo Yunoki,*[1] Makoto Matsumoto,*[1] Tadashi Matsumoto,*[1] Hiroshi Kikuchi,*[1] Kouichiro Nomura,*[2] Hironori Furusho,*[2] Kouichiro Nishioka,*[2] and Shuichi Hanada*[2]

Institute of Cancer Research[1] *and The Second Department of Internal Medicine,*[2] *Faculty of Medicine, Kagoshima University*

Adult T-cell leukemia (ATL) and most of T-cell non-Hodgkin's malignant lymphoma (T-ML) in Kagoshima are presently considered different clinical manifestations of the same disease. Clinical features of ATL, therefore, are discussed in the same category with T-ML.

Of 187 lymphoproliferative malignant diseases recently studied 138 cases (73.8%) were T-cell malignancies, including 56 ATL and 68 T-ML. Malignant lymphomas in the Kagoshima district are characterized by a high incidence of T-cell malignancy. According to Lymphoma Study Group (LSG)-classification, all ATL and T-ML were diffuse lymphoma and about half of them were of the pleomorphic cell type. Leukemic cells in ATL were also characterized by the pleomorphism having a markedly deformed nucleus, and most cases of T-ML became leukemic in the course of disease. Hepatosplenomegaly was a common manifestation followed by liver function disorders and marked elevation of lactate dehydrogenase (LDH). Hypercalcemia was also an important manifestation and often attributable to unconsiousness. Clinical complications of pulmonary and skin lesions were found in about half of the cases of ATL and T-ML and the former was often lethal. Skin lesions were of neoplastic cell infiltration and many cases showed epidermal infiltration, similar to cutaneous lymphoma. Skin lesions were recognized to be one of the most characteristic manifestations in malignancies of peripheral T-cell origin, but the prognosis of ATL and T-ML was very poor, in contrast to the relatively good prognosis of cutaneous lymphoma.

Concerning the pathogenesis of ATL, antibodies to adult T-cell leukemia virus associated antigen (ATLA) were detected in all ATL and almost all T-ML. Anti-ATLA antibodies were also positive in about 15% of the healthy adults living in Kagoshima.

The concept of adult T-cell leukemia (ATL) proposed by Takatsuki *et al.* (*22–24, 27*) has presented important problems for the study of non-Hodgkin's lymphoma in Japan. On account of the peculiarity of this disease, such as its clinical, pathological, and geographical features, ATL occupies the attention of the investigators of lymphoid

---

[1],[2] Usuki-cho 1208-1, Kagoshima 890, Japan (柚木一雄, 松元　実, 松元　正, 菊池　博, 野村紘一郎, 古庄弘典, 西岡紘一郎, 花田修一).

neoplasias. We have already reported on the clinical features of ATL in the Kagoshima district of southwestern Japan, which is an endemic area of this disease (11, 12, 14).

A considerable amount of information accumulated on ATL and T-cell non-Hodgkin's malignant lymphoma (T-ML) has led us to believe that the two diseases are actually different clinical manifestations of the same disease, ATL being predominantly leukemic, in contrast to the predominant lymph node involvement in the leukemic state of T-ML. Based on our present knowledge, both ATL and T-ML are malignancies of peripheral T-cell origin. It is reasonable, therefore, to recognize these two diseases under the clinical concept of adult T-cell leukemia-lymphoma (ATLL).

About half of the ATLL patients experience various types of widespread cutaneous involvements, some of which resemble the skin lesion of cutaneous T-cell lymphoma (CTCL). The term cutaneous T-cell lymphoma, however, has been proposed by Lutzner et al. (9) for lymphoproliferative diseases, in which the disease is primarily confined to the skin and secondarily involves other organs. Therefore, a skin lesion of ATLL should be recognized as a different clinical manifestation than that of CTCL.

Patients and Diagnosis of ATL and T-ML

Fifty-five patients with ATL and 61 patients with T-ML, treated in our institution since 1976, were the subject of this study. Other types of lymphoid neoplasia were excluded.

A surface marker of neoplastic cells, obtained from peripheral blood or from lymph nodes by aspiration or biopsy, was determined by the spontaneous rosette-forming capacity with sheep erythrocytes for T-cell nature and by the direct detection of surface immunoglobulin for B-cell nature.

Our definition of ATL was as follows:
1) Neoplastic lymphoid cells are detected in both peripheral blood and bone marrow.
2) Neoplastic lymphocytes have relatively mature nuclei and the nucleus shows marked irregularity, such as convolution, lobulation, indentation, *etc.*
3) Cells having irregular nuclei, expressed with the pleomorphic cell, make up more than 30% of the peripheral lymphoid cells.

The residual cases of ATLL, excluding ATL, were determined to be T-ML. Patients with T-ML were further subdivided into a leukemic and a non-leukemic group. The leukemic state was defined by the existence of neoplastic cells in a quantity greater than 5% of the peripheral leukocyte count. Such cells in the non-leukemic group accounted for less than 5%.

Incidence

Incidences of lymphoid neoplasias based on the functional classification are shown in Table I. Out of 187 cases of lymphoproliferative malignant diseases, the numbers of T-cell, B-cell, and non-T, non-B-cell type were 138 (73.8%), 15 (8.0%), and 34 (18.2%), respectively. A high incidence of T-cell malignancy was noticeable in the Kagoshima district.

TABLE I. Incidence of Non-Hodgkin's Lymphomas Classified with Cell Surface Markers

	No. of cases		Total (%)
T-cell malignancy			138 (73.8)
ATLL			
ATL	56		
T-lymphoma	68		
Leukemic		35	
Non-leukemic		27	
T-chronic lymphocytic leukemia (T-CLL)	3		
Acute lymphoblastic leukemia (ALL)	3		
Mycosis fungoides	3		
Waldeyer's ring lymphoma	3		
Extranodal lymphoma	2		
B-cell malignancy	15		15 (8.0)
Non-T, non-B-cell malignancy	34		34 (18.2)
Total	187		187 (100)
Undetermined	21		

1. ATL and T-lymphoma

Out of 138 patients with T-cell malignancies, 124 cases (89.9%) were diagnosed as ATLL. The differentiation between ATL and T-cell lymphoma (T-ML) has been made on the basis of the above mentioned definition. This definition, however, was attended with some difficulties. Though all of the cases in which the peripheral lymphoid cell count was more than 30,000/mm^3 could be diagnosed as ATL, several cases were hardly classifiable as either ATL or T-ML. According to our definition, of the 124 cases of ATLL 56 (45.2%) were classified as ATL, and 68 (54.8%) as T-ML, including leukemic T-ML 35 and non-leukemic T-ML 27. These included several cases which could not be followed up.

2. Age and sex distribution

The mean age of patients with ATL and T-ML was 58.5 (25–76) and 56.3 (33–79), respectively. The male to female ratio was 1.4:1 in ATL and 2.8:1 in T-ML (Table III).

3. Seasonal distribution

The seasonal peak of the clinical onset of both ATL and T-ML was from May to August, and the lowest was from December to February. ATLL seems to have high incidence in summertime.

Histopathological Findings of Lymph Nodes

The histopathological findings of lymph node involvements in ATL and T-ML are summarized in Table II. The findings were classified as proposed by the Lymphoma Study Group (LSG) using the category best suited for lymphomas in Japan (20). All cases examined in this study were of the diffuse lymphoma type. Both in ATL and T-ML, the histologically predominant finding was the pleomorphic type which was

TABLE II. Histopathological Findings of Lymph Node Involvement in ATL and
T-lymphoma According to LSG-classification

	ATL No. of cases (%)	T-lymphoma No. of cases (%)	ATLL (total) No. of cases (%)
Follicular lymphoma			
Medium-sized cell type	0	0	0
Mixed type	0	0	0
Large cell type	0	0	0
Diffuse lymphoma			
Small cell type	0	1 (1.4)	1 (1.3)
Medium-sized cell type	6 (25.0)	13 (24.5)	19 (24.2)
Mixed type	7 (29.2)	9 (17.0)	16 (20.8)
Large cell type	1 (4.2)	6 (11.3)	7 (9.1)
Pleomorphic type	10 (41.7)	24 (45.3)	34 (44.2)
Lymphoblastic type	0	0	0
Burkitt type	0	0	0
Total	24	53	77

morphologically defined as lymphomas composed of neoplastic cells of various sizes, mixed in variable proportions, and showing convoluted and hyperconvoluted nuclei. The frequency of the pleomorphic type was 41.7% in 24 cases of ATL and 45.3% in 53 cases of T-ML.

The cytological findings in aspirated or touch smear of lymph nodes showed marked varieties in size, differentiation and maturation of neoplastic cells, even in cases of ATL which showed only mature-looking leukemic cells in peripheral blood. These neoplastic cells obtained from peripheral blood, bone marrow or lymph nodes had spontaneous rosette-forming activity with sheep erythrocytes.

Clinical Signs and Symptoms

Almost all of the cases were examined in a rather late stage and had a variety of clinical symptoms. All cases of ATL were at stage IV of the disease and most T-ML were at stage III or IV. Clinical signs and symptoms at the onset and during the course of the disease are summarized in Table III.

1. Lymphadenopathy

The enlargement of superficial lymph nodes was generally minimal in ATL and was hardly detectable in about one-fourth of the cases, as compared with the marked enlargement of these nodes in T-ML.

2. Hepatomegaly and splenomegaly

A majority of the ATL patients experienced hepatomegaly and splenomegaly in the course of disease. The frequency of hepto-splenomegaly was higher in ATL than in T-ML and marked enlargements were often observed in the former.

TABLE III. Clinical Signs and Symptoms at Presentation and in Cours of Disease

	ATL		T-lymphoma	
No. of patients	55		61	
Sex : male : female	32 : 23		45 : 16	
	(1.4 : 1)		(2.8 : 1)	
Age : mean	58.5		56.3	
(range)	(25–76)		(33–79)	
	At present. (%)	In course (%)	At present. (%)	In course (%)
Symptoms				
Fever	45.5	67.4	48.3	63.0
Upper abdominal pain and distension	23.6	34.8	18.0	20.0
Cough, dyspnea, shortness of breath	10.9	17.4	1.6	4.0
Diarrhea	5.5	10.9	1.6	1.7
Unconsiousness	3.6	12.7	0	8.6
Signs				
Lymphadenopathy	74.6	75.6	93.4	96.0
Hepatomegaly	50.9	60.0	37.9	42.0
Splenomegaly	36.4	51.1	12.0	17.2
Jaundice	1.8	9.8	0	2.2
Pulmonary lesion (chest X-ray)	29.1	60.8	5.2	44.0
Skin lesion				
Cutaneous infiltration	23.6	47.3	6.6	47.5
Various infection	23.1	23.6	13.2	21.3
Anemia (RBC$<3\times10^6$)	10.9	16.4	2.0	17.2
Mediastinal mass (chest X-ray)	0	0	0	0

RBC, red blood cells.

3. Skin lesions

Skin lesions are found in two manifestations, a cutaneous infiltration of neoplastic cells and an infectious lesion.

Non-infectious lesions of the skin are recognized to be one of the most characteristic manifestations in malignancies of peripheral T-cell origin. Various types of skin lesions, such as papule, nodule, erythroderma, node and tumor, were found in disseminated form even in the initial stage of ATLL, and more frequently in ATL. In the course of the diseases, about half of the cases of ATL and T-ML were accompanied by these non-infectious skin lesions. The detailed findings follow.

Infectious skin lesions were mostly fungal infections such as trichophytosis and candidiasis; herpes zoster was also found in both ATL and T-ML. These lesions all had a tendency to spread widely.

4. Pulmonary lesions

Pulmonary lesions were the most frequent, difficult to treat and lethal complications in ATL and T-ML. Some cases were already accompanied by pulmonary lesions even when first observed; pulmonary complications increased in the course of the diseases and over half of the patients suffered from this lethal complication. Pulmonary lesions revealed by autopsy were bacterial or fungal pneumonia, interstitial pneumonitis and a marked infiltration of neoplastic cells. *Pneumocystis carinii* and a cytomegalic inclusion body in pulmonary tissue was frequently found.

Laboratory Findings

1. Hematological findings
The diagnosis of ATL was based on the hematological definition which we proposed to differentiate it from the leukemic state of T-ML. Leukemic cells in ATL were characterized by pleomorphism, in which nuclei having dense chromatin showed marked deformity, such as convolution, lobulation, indentation, or clubbing. The cytoplasm of a leukemic cell sometimes had vague or distinct vacuolei and showed positive results for periodic acid-Schiff (PAS) reaction, acid phosphatase, β-glucuronidase, and non-specific esterase staining.

2. Blood chemistry
The abnormal elevation of glutamic oxalo-acetic transaminase (GOT) and alkaline phosphatase (ALP) was observed in about half the cases of ATL, and lactate

TABLE IV. Laboratory Findings of ATL

	Mean (range)	No. of examined cases
Peripheral blood		
RBC ($\times 10^4$/mm^3)	412 (109–667)	54
Platelet ($\times 10^4$/mm^3)	15.7 (1.1–50.5)	49
WBC ($\times 10^3$/mm^3)	86.9 (17.4–46.3)	55
Abnormal lymphocyte (%)	70.5 (16–97)	53
Bone marrow		
Nucleated cell count ($\times 10^4$/mm^3)	25.4 (1.3–174.0)	39
Dry tap		6
Abnormal lymphocyte (%)	48.2 (1.2–98.8)	50
Surface markers of abnormal lymphocyte		
E-RFC (%)	84.0 (20.6–98.8)	55
S-Ig (%)	1.7 (0–9.3)	55

	No. of examined cases
Blood chemistry	
GOT (elevation) (%)	26/51 (51.0)
GPT (elevation) (%)	17/51 (33.3)
LDH (elevation) (%)	48/51 (94.1)
ALP (elevation) (%)	26/51 (51.0)
Hypercalcemia ($>$6.0 mEq/l)	12/34 (35.3)
Hypoproteinemia ($<$6.0 g/dl) (%)	28/51 (54.9)

	No. of cases
PPD skin test	
−	24/30 (80.0)
±	5/30 (16.7)
+	1/30 (3.3)

WBC, white blood cells; E-RFC, sheep erythrocyte-rosette forming capacity; S-Ig, sulfate immunoglobulin; GOT, glutamic oxalo-acetic transaminase; GPT, glutamic pyruvate transaminase; PPD, purified protein derivative.

dehydrogenase (LDH) was abnormally elevated in almost all of the cases. Hypoproteinemia, under 6.0 g/dl, was frequently observed but was not accompanied by abnormalities of immunoglobulins. Hypercalcemia, over 6.0 mEq/1, was an important manifestation observed frequently in the course of the disease and was often attributable to the unconsiousness of a patient (6).

Skin Lesions

In the course of the disease, various types of skin lesions, other than infectious lesions, appeared in about half of the ATL and T-ML. Clinical appearance of an eruption was mostly nodular, and then erythrodermic and papular. Nodus-like or tumorlike eruptions were also observed in a few cases.

1. Histopathological examination

The histopathological findings of lymph nodes biopsied before anticancer chemotherapy were classified using the new classification proposed by the LSG of Japan (20). The enlargement of peripheral lymph nodes generally minimal in ATL and in some cases of ATL were irrelevant to the histopathological examination of these lymph nodes.

In cases with skin lesions, dermato-histopathological examinations were performed on specimens obtained by punched biopsy.

Relationships between histopathological findings of biopsied lymph nodes and skin lesions are shown in Table V. According to LSG classification, skin lesions were observed in about half of each histological type and no particular type showed high or low susceptibility to skin.

Histopathological examinations of skin lesions were performed on specimens obtained from 18 cases of ATL and 23 cases of T-ML. The histopathological findings were divided into two groups, according to the presence or absence of epidermal infiltration of neoplastic cells. Epidermal and dermal infiltration of neoplastic cells was found in 3 cases of ATL and 6 cases of T-ML. In other cases, the infiltration of neoplastic cells was limited to dermis. If many specimens from the same case were examined, the number of epidermal infiltrations would probably be increased. It is possible that the cutaneous lesions of ATLL are characterized by the epidermotropic nature of neoplastic cells.

Histopathological findings of skin lesions are shown in Photos 1–7.

TABLE V. Relationship between Histopathological Findings of Biopsied
Lymph Nodes and Skin Lesions

Histological findings of lymph node	ATL (24 cases) No. of cases with skin lesions / No. of cases with lymph node biopsy (%)	T-ML (53 cases)
Diffuse lymphoma		
Small cell type (%)	0	0/1
Medium-sized cell type	3/6 (50.0)	8/13 (61.5)
Mixed type	5/7 (71.0)	4/9 (44.4)
Large type	1/1	2/6 (33.3)
Pleomorphic type	5/10 (50.0)	13/24 (54.2)

Chemotherapy and Prognosis

1. Chemotherapy

Results of chemotherapy in the early stage of the research have been reported (*12*, *14*). Recent cases were treated with VEMP (vincristine, cyclophosphamide, 6-MP, prednisolone), VEPA (vincristine, cyclophosphamide, prednisolone, adriamycin) pro-posed by the Lymphoma Studp Group (*10*), and MEPA (methotrexate, cyclophosphamide, prednisolone, adriamycin). Remission rates in T-ML were 56.2% in 16 cases receiving VEMP, 58.3% in 12 cases receiving VEPA and 88.9% in 9 cases receiving MEPA. On the contrary, partial remission was obtained in only 2 cases of 9 ATL treated with VEMP and VEPA did not result in any remission in 4 cases of ATL. Mean survival from the beginning of chemotherapy in these 13 cases of ATL and 37 of T-ML was 5.1 and 4.8 months, respectively. Even these newly designed chemotherapy protocols did not contribute to survival.

2. Prognosis

Mean survival in 46 cases of ATL was 6.7 months from clinical onset and 3.4 months from the beginning of chemotherapy, while that in 50 cases of T-ML was 7.0 months from clinical onset and 3.8 months from the beginning of chemotherapy. There was no significant difference in survival between ATL and T-ML, nor could, any difference be observed between histological types based on the LSG classification.

Serological Examination

Sera obtained from patients with ATLL, other leukemias, lymphomas or other malignant diseases, were subjected to the serological examination of antibodies to ATL virus associated antigen (ATLA). The titer of anti-ATLA antibodies was determined in Dr. Y. Hinuma's laboratory (*7*). Titration was also performed on sera obtained from healthy adult residents in the Kagoshima district.

Antibodies to ATLA were estimated in sera obtained from patients with ATL and T-ML, and in control, including healthy adults living in the ATL-endemic area, Kagoshima and Okinawa. The results are summarized in Table VI.

All of the 33 ATL patients and 43 of 47 T-ML patients were anti-ATLA antibodies positive. In addition to this, all of the 5 mycosis fungoides and 4 of 7 Hodgkin's disease also showed positive results. On the other hand, the positive rate of anti-ATLA antibodies in healthy adults was 15.6% in Kagoshima and 10.4% in Okinawa. Except for the diseases mentioned above, the control group was the same as healthy and normal persons.

DISCUSSION

Hanaoka *et al.* (*5*) divided adult T cell leukemia into two types, monomorphic and pleomorphic, according to its histological and cytological features. Monomorphic T-cell leukemia was one of the ordinary types of lymphocytic leukemia composed of neoplastic cells derived from prothymocytes or immature thymocytes, as opposed to

TABLE VI. Frequency of Anti-ATLA Antibody in Lymphoproliferative
Diseases, Other Diseases, and Healthy

	Total cases	Anti-ATLA antibody	
		Positive cases (%)	Negative cases
Malignant lymphoma			
ATL	33	33 (100)	0
T-cell lymphoma	47	43 (91.5)	4
Mycosis fungoides	5	5 (100)	0
Non-T-cell lymphoma	15	1 (6.7)	14
Malignant lymphoma (Marker undetermined)	16	7 (43.8)	9
Hodgkin's disease	7	4 (57.1)	3
Other malignant diseases			
ALL (T and null cell)	10	0	10
CLL (T and B cell)	3	1 (33.3)	2
AML	18	3 (16.7)	15
Multiple myeloma and macroglobulinemia	7	1 (14.3)	6
Other malignancies	5	0	5
Benign disease			
Lymphocytosis			
Infectious mononucleosis	3	0	3
Tsutsugamushi disease	3	0	3
Unknown	4	2 (50.0)	2
Lymphadenitis (non-specific)	8	1 (12.5)	7
Collagen disease	15	5 (33.3)	10
Other diseases	23	3 (13.0)	20
Healthy adults			
Residents in Kagoshima	122	19 (15.6)	103
Residents in Okinawa	125	13 (10.4)	112

AML, acute myeloid leukemia.

pleomorphic T-cell leukemia which was composed of neoplastic cells derived from peripheral mature T-lymphocytes. The pleomorphic T-cell type should be applicable to the clinical entity of ATL proposed by Takatsuki. On the other hand, Shimoyama et al. (19) reported that the T-cell type of non-Hodgkin's lymphoma in Japan was divided into two types, thymus (+) T-cell type and thymus (−) T-cell type. The latter developed usually in adult and had no evidence of thymus involvement but a high leukemic manifestation. It was also found that both the pleomorphic T-cell leukemia and the thymus (−) T-cell lymphoma accompanied multiple skin lesions and showed geographically characteristic distribution in Japan. Moreover, information accumulated on both diseases has led us to understand that these two diseases are different clinical manifestations of the same disease. In this study, therefore, ATL and T-ML were recognized under the clinical concept of ATLL.

Though ATL and T-ML are substantially interpreted as ATLL in a broad sense, the clinical features could actually be divided into ATL and T-ML according to the definition mentioned above. In this study, to make clear the characteristics of ATLL the clinical features in 55 cases of ATL were compared with that in 61 cases of T-ML. As shown in our previous reports (11, 12, 14), both ATL and T-ML were characterized by the following clinical features: onset in adulthood, usually poor prognosis with rapid progression and various lethal complications due to immunological deficiencies, frequently severe pulmonary lesions, appearance of pleomorphic neoplastic cells with markedly deformed nuclei, neoplastic cells having peripheral T-cell nature, lymphadenopathy (in most cases), absence of mediastinal mass, high incidence of hepatosplenomegaly, frequent skin involvement, and frequent leukemic manifestation in T-ML. Lymph node enlargement was usually smaller in ATL than in T-ML and some cases of ATL lacked superficial lymph node enlargement. ATL, also in the leukemic stage of T-ML, was accompanied by bone marrow involvement.

On the basis of LSG-classification, histopathological findings showed lymph nodes to be predominantly of the pleomorphic type, postulated to be the typical one of adult T-cell malignancies in Japan (20). The pleomorphic type was found in 41.7 % of 24 cases with ATL and 45.3% of 53 cases with T-ML. These results were almost equal to data obtained by other investigators (8, 20, 21, 25, 26) who reported a high incidence of the pleomorphic type in Kyushu.

One of the clinical features peculiar to ATLL was skin involvement and varied skin lesions were found in 47.3% of 55 cases with ATL and 47.5% of 61 cases with T-ML. Brouet et al. (1, 2) observed skin involvement in nine of 23 cases with T-derived chronic lymphocytic leukemia and Hanaoka et al. (5) found skin affected in 66% of 59 cases with pleomorphic T-cell leukemia, probably correspondig to ATL. On the other hand, it is well known that neoplastic cells in the skin of CTCL, including mycosis fungoides and Sézary syndrome, have a T-cell nature (1, 3, 9). Schechter et al. (17) reported that abnormal lymphocytes appearing in circulating blood and lymph nodes had convoluted nuclei and T-cell nature, perhaps corresponding to neoplastic cells of ATL. It is very interesting that ATL and T-ML accompany skin involvement in about half the cases and that leukemic cells appearing in the late stage of CTCL have a morphological and immunological resemblance to neoplastic cells in ATL. The term cutaneous T-cell lymphoma has been proposed by Lutzner et al. (9) for lymphoproliferative diseases having the following characteristics: (1) The disease is primarily confined to the skin and secondarily involves other organs; (2) the neoplastic cell is a morphologically characteristic lymphoid cell of thymus-derived nature, involving preferentially T-cell dependent areas of lymphoid tissues; (3) the neoplastic cells infiltrate into the epidermis (13). The clinical features of ATLL differ from CTCL in the following respect: (1) about half of the patients with ATLL have no skin involvement; (2) the disease is primarily confined to blood or lymph nodes and secondarily involves the skin; (3) prognosis of ATLL is very poor, in contrast to the usually good prognosis of CTCL. It is also well known that neoplastic cells can be derived from a mature thymocyte or peripheral T-cell in both ATLL (28) and CTCL (17). The most characteristic histologic finding in CTCL is an epitheliotropism of the atypical cells, forming either intradermal clusters (Pautrier's microabscesses) or single cell pockets (4, 9). In our cases, epidermal infiltrations of neoplastic cells were found in 3 of 18 cases with ATL and in 6 of 23 cases with T-ML. The skin lesion of ATLL is characterized by epidermotropism of neoplastic cells, the same as that of CTCL.

Hinuma et al. (7) found antigens in cytoplasm of the MT-1 cell, a T-cell line established from the peripheral blood of a patient with ATL by Miyoshi et al. (15), and named them ATLA. The anti-ATLA antibodies were detectable in sera from patients with ATL. Soon after this, type C virus particles were found in the cytoplasm of ATLA positive ATL cells. In our cases, anti-ATLA antibodies were positive in all of 33 patients with ATL (100%), 43 of 47 patients with T-ML (91.5%), and all of 5 patients with mycosis fungoides. In ATL endemic areas the positive rate of anti-ATLA antibodies in healthy adults was 15.6% in Kagoshima (19 out of 122) and 10.4% in Okinawa (13 out of 125). Recently, Poiesz *et al.* (*16*) also found type C virus particles in lymphocytes of a patient with CTCL (mycosis fungoides) and named it HTLV. It is very interesting that all of our cases with mycosis fungoides showed anti-ATLA antibodies positive.

Acknowledgments
   We thank Prof. Y. Hinuma, Institute for Virus Research, Kyoto University, for measurement of anti-ALTA antibodies.
   This work was supported by a Grant-in-Aid for Cancer Research from the Ministry of Health and Welfare (Grant Number 53S-1).

REFERENCES

1. Brouet, J. C., Flandrin, G., and Seligmann, M. Indication of the thymus-derived nature of the proliferating cells in six patients with Sézary's syndrome. *N. Engl. J. Med.*, **289**, 314–344 (1973).
2. Brouet, J. C., Preud'homme, J. L., Flandrin, G., and Seligmann, M. Human T-derived lymphoproliferative diseases. *Recent Results Cancer Res.*, **64**, 131–137 (1978).
3. Ding, J. C., Adams, P. B., Patison, M., and Cooper, I. A. Thymic origin of abnormal lymphoid cells in Sézary syndrome. *Cancer*, **35**, 1325–1332 (1975).
4. Edelson, R. L. Cutaneous T cell lymphoma: Mycosis fungoides, Sézary syndrome and other variants. *J. Am. Acad. Dermatol.*, **2**, 89–106 (1980).
5. Hanaoka, M., Sasaki, M., Matsumoto, H., Tasaka, C., Fujiwara, H., Uchiyama, T., and Takatsuki, K. Adult T-cell leukemia; Histological classification and characteristics. *Acta Pathol. Jpn.*, **29**, 723–738 (1979).
6. Hanada, S., Kodama, M., Uematsu, T., Kato, Y., Nomura, K., Hashimoto, S., Matsumoto, T., Matsumoto, M., and Yunoki, K. Adult T-cell lymphoma-leukemia with hypercalcemia. *Acta Haematol. Jpn.*, **44**, 459 (1981) (in Japanese).
7. Hinuma, Y., Nagata, K., Hanaoka, M., Nakai, M., Matsumoto, T., Kinoshita, K., Shirakawa, S., and Miyoshi, I. Adult T-cell leukemia: Antigen in an ATL cell line and detection of antibodies to the antigen in human sera. *Proc. Natl. Acad. Sci. U.S.*, **78**, 6476–6480 (1981).
8. Kikuchi, M., Mitsui, T., Matsui, N., Sato, E., Tokunaga, M., Hasui, K., Ichimaru, M., Kinoshita, K., and Kamihira, S. T-cell malignancies in adults: Histopathological studies of lymph nodes in 110 patients. *Jpn. J. Clin. Oncol.*, **9** (Suppl.), 407–422 (1979).
9. Lutzner, M., Edelson, R., Schein, P., Green, I., Kirkpatrick, C., and Ahmed, A. Cutaneous T-cell lymphomas: The Sézary syndrome, mycosis fungoides, and related disorders. *Ann. Intern. Med.*, **83**, 534–552 (1975).
10. Lymphoma Study Group: Combination chemotherapy with vincristine, cyclophosphamide (endoxan), prednisolone and adriamycin (VEPA) in advanced adult non-Hodgkin's lymphoid malignancies: Relation between T-cell or non-T-cell phenotype and response. *Jpn. J. Clin. Oncol.*, **9** (Suppl.), 397–406 (1979).
11. Matsumoto, M. and Nomura, K. Clinical and hematological features of adult T-cell

leukemia in southern part of Kyushu, Japan. *Jpn. J. Clin. Hematol.*, **20**, 1040–1047 (1978) (in Japanese).

12. Matsumoto, M., Nomura, K., Matsumoto, T., Nishioka, K., Hanada, S., Furusho, H., Kikuchi, H., Kato, Y., Utsunomiya, A., Iwahashi, S., and Yunoki, K. Adult T-cell leukemia-lymphoma in Kagoshima district, southwestern Japan. Clinical and hematological characteristics. *Jpn. J. Clin. Oncol.*, **9** (Suppl.), 325–336 (1979).

13. Meijer, C.J.L.M., Van Der Loo, E. M., Van Vloten, W. A., Cornelisse, C. J., and Scheffer, E. Cutaneous T-cell lymphoma: morphological and immunological aspects. *In* "Malignant Lymphoproliferative Diseases," ed. J. G. van den Tweel, pp. 341–353 (1980). Leiden University Press, The Hague-Boston-London.

14. Nomura, K. and Matsumoto, M. Clinical features of adult T-cell leukemia in Kagoshima, the southernmost district in Japan—comparison with T-cell lymphoma—. *Acta Haematol. Jpn.*, **44**, 200–213 (1981).

15. Miyoshi, I., Kubonishi, I., Sumida, M., Yoshimoto, S., Hiraki, S., Tubota, T., Kobashi, H., Lai, M., Tanaka, T., Kimura, I., Miyamoto, K., and Sato, J. Characteristics of a leukemic T-cell line derived from adult T-cell leukemia. *Jpn. J. Clin. Oncol.*, **9** (Suppl.), 485–494 (1979).

16. Poiesz, B. J., Ruscetti, F. W., Gazdar, A. F., Bunn, P. A., Minna, J. D., and Gallo, R. C. Detection and isolation of type C retrovirus particles from fresh and cultured lymphocytes of a patient with cutaneous T-cell lymphoma. *Proc. Natl. Acad. Sci. U.S.* **77**, 7415–7419 (1980).

17. Reinherz, E. L. and Schlossmann, S. F. Derivation of human T-cell leukemias. *Cancer Res.*, **41**, 4767–4770 (1981).

18. Schechter, G. P., Bunn, P. A., Betty Fischmann, A., Matthews, M. J., Guccion, J., Soehnlen, F., Munson, D., and Minna, J .D. Blood and lymph node T lymphocytes in cutaneous T cell lymphoma: Evaluation by light microscopy. *Cancer Treat. Rep.*, **63**, 571–574 (1979).

19. Shimoyama, M. and Minato, K. Importance of immunological and functional classification of non-Hodgkin's lymphomas to establish their clinicopathological characteristics. *Recent Adv. RES Res.*, **16**, 119–130 (1976).

20. Suchi, T., Tajima, K., Nanba, K., Wakasa, H., Mikata, A., Kikuchi, M., Mori, S., Watanabe, S., Mohri, N., Shamoto, M., Harigaya, K., Itagaki, T., Matsuda, M., Kirino, Y., Takagi, K., and Fukunaga, S. Some problems on the histopathological diagnosis of non-Hodgkin's malignant lymphoma. A proposal of a new type. *Acta Pathol. Jpn.*, **29**, 755–776 (1979).

21. Suchi, T. and Tajima, K. Peripheral T-cell malignancy as a problem in lymphoma classification. *Jpn. J. Clin. Oncol.*, **9** (Suppl.), 443–450 (1979).

22. Takatsuki, K., Uchiyama, T., Sagawa, K., and Yodoi, J. Surface markers of malignant lymphoid cells in the classification of lymphoproliferative disorders, with special reference to adult T cell leukemia. *Jpn. J. Clin. Hematol.*, **17**, 416–421 (1976) (in Japanese).

23. Takatsuki, K. Adult T-cell leukemia: Concept and problems. *Jpn. J. Clin. Hematol.*, **20**, 1036–1039 (1979) (in Japanese).

24. Takatsuki, K., Uchiyama, T., Ueshima, Y., and Hattori, T. Adult T-cell leukemia: Further clinical observations and cytogenetic and functional studies of leukemic cells. *Jpn. J. Clin. Oncol.*, **9** (Suppl.), 317–324 (1979).

25. Tajima, K., Tominaga, S., Kuroishi, T., Shimizu, H., and Suchi, T. Geographical features and epidemiological approach to endemic T-cell leukemia/lymphoma in Japan. *Jpn. J. Clin. Oncol.*, **9** (Suppl.), 495–504 (1979).

26. The T- and B-cell Malignancy Study Group. Statistical analysis of immunologic, clinical and histopathologic data on lymphoid malignancies in Japan. *Jpn. J. Clin. Oncol.*, **11**, 15–32 (1981).
27. Uchiyama, T., Yodoi, J., Sagawa, K., Takatsuki, K., and Uchino, H. Adult T cell leukemia. Clinical and hematologic features of 16 cases. *Blood*, **50**, 481–492 (1977).
28. Yamanaka, N., Ishii, Y., Koshiba, H., Mikuni, C., Ogasawara, M., and Kikuchi, K. A study of surface markers in non-Hodgkin's lymphoma by using anti-T and anti-B lymphocyte sera. *Cancer*, **47**, 311–318 (1981).

EXPLANATION OF PHOTOS

Histopathological findings of skin lesions in ATL and T-ML (Photos 1–7)

PHOTO 1. ATL (M.K.; 47, male). Histopathological finding of lymph node: diffuse lymphoma, medium-sized cell type. Skin: diffuse infiltration of rather uniform medium-sized lymphoid cells with irregular nuclei, containing several giant cells similar to Reed-Sternberg cell. Epidermis is free from infiltration of neoplastic cells. ×200.

PHOTO 2. ATL (I.S.; 76, male). Histopathological finding of lymph node: diffuse lymphoma, pleomorphic type. Skin: intradermal proliferation of pleomorphic lymphoid cells containing ginat cells. Epidermis contains several Pautrier's microabscesses. ×200.

PHOTO 3. T-ML (K.K.; 35, male). Histopathological finding of lymph node: diffuse lymphoma, mixed type. Skin: dermal and epidermal proliferation of atypical lymphoid cells, mixed medium and large-sized cells. Lymphoid cells in epidermis form single cell pockets. ×200.

PHOTO 4. T-ML (S.S.; 55, male). Histopathological finding of lymph mode: diffuse lymphoma, pleomorphic type. Skin: sporadic infiltration of lymphoid cells in dermis and epidermis. Epidermis contains Pautrier's microabcess. ×200.

PHOTO 5. ATL (S.U.; 56, male). Histopathological finding of lymph node: diffuse lymphoma, pleomorphic type. Skin: perivascular infiltration of atypical lymphoid cells. Epidermis is free from infiltration of lymphoid cells. ×100.

PHOTO 6. T-ML (M.O.; 34, female). Histopathological finding of lymph node: diffuse lymphoma, pleomorphic type. Skin: dermal infiltration of pleomorphic lymphoid cells. Epidermis contains Pautrier's microabscess. ×100.

PHOTO 7. T-ML, leukemic (A.A.; 63, female). Histopathological finding of lymph node: diffuse lymphoma, medium sized cell type. Skin: intradermal proliferation of atypical lymphoid cells. Neoplastic cells have no affinity for epidermis. ×40.

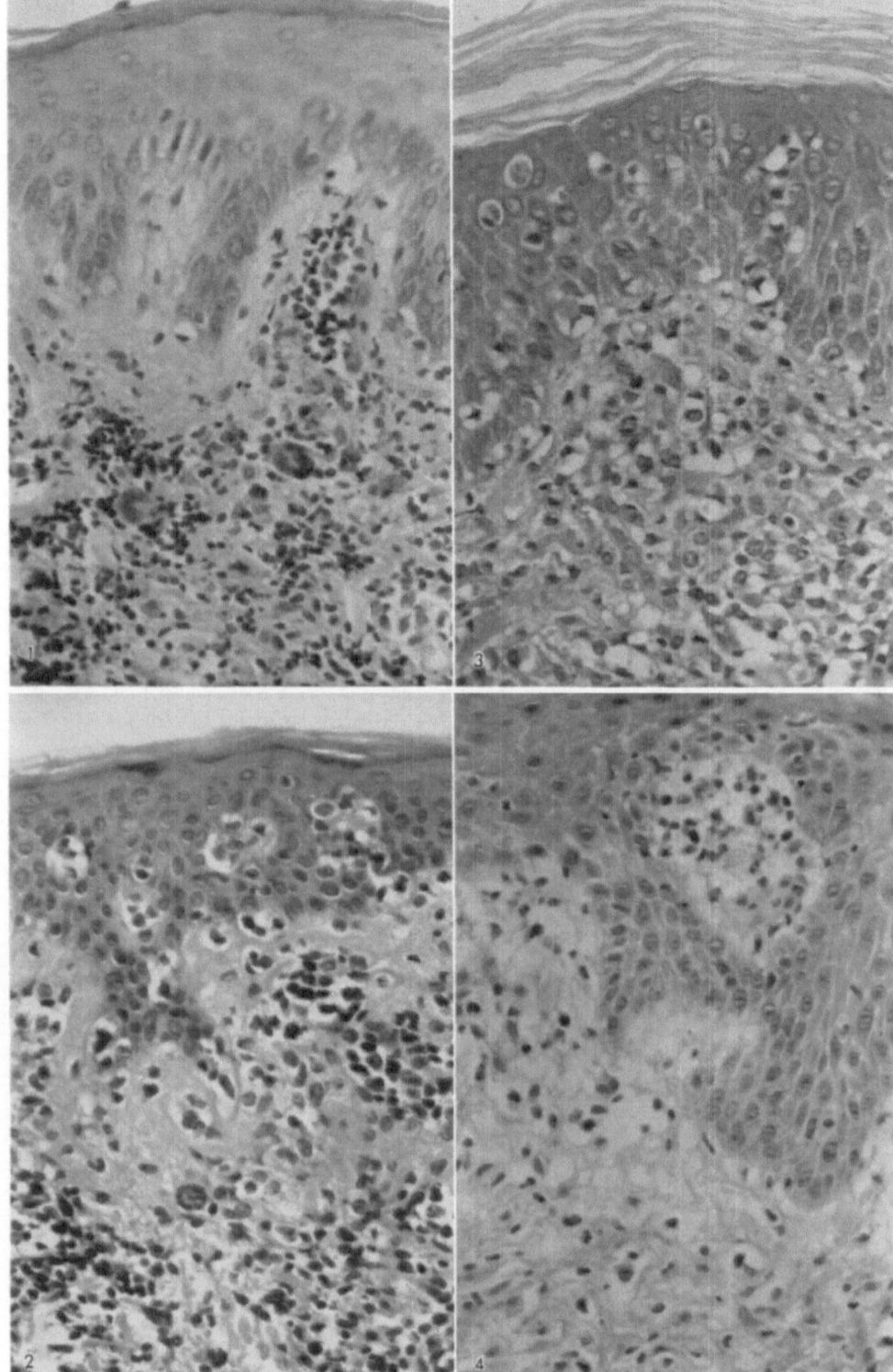

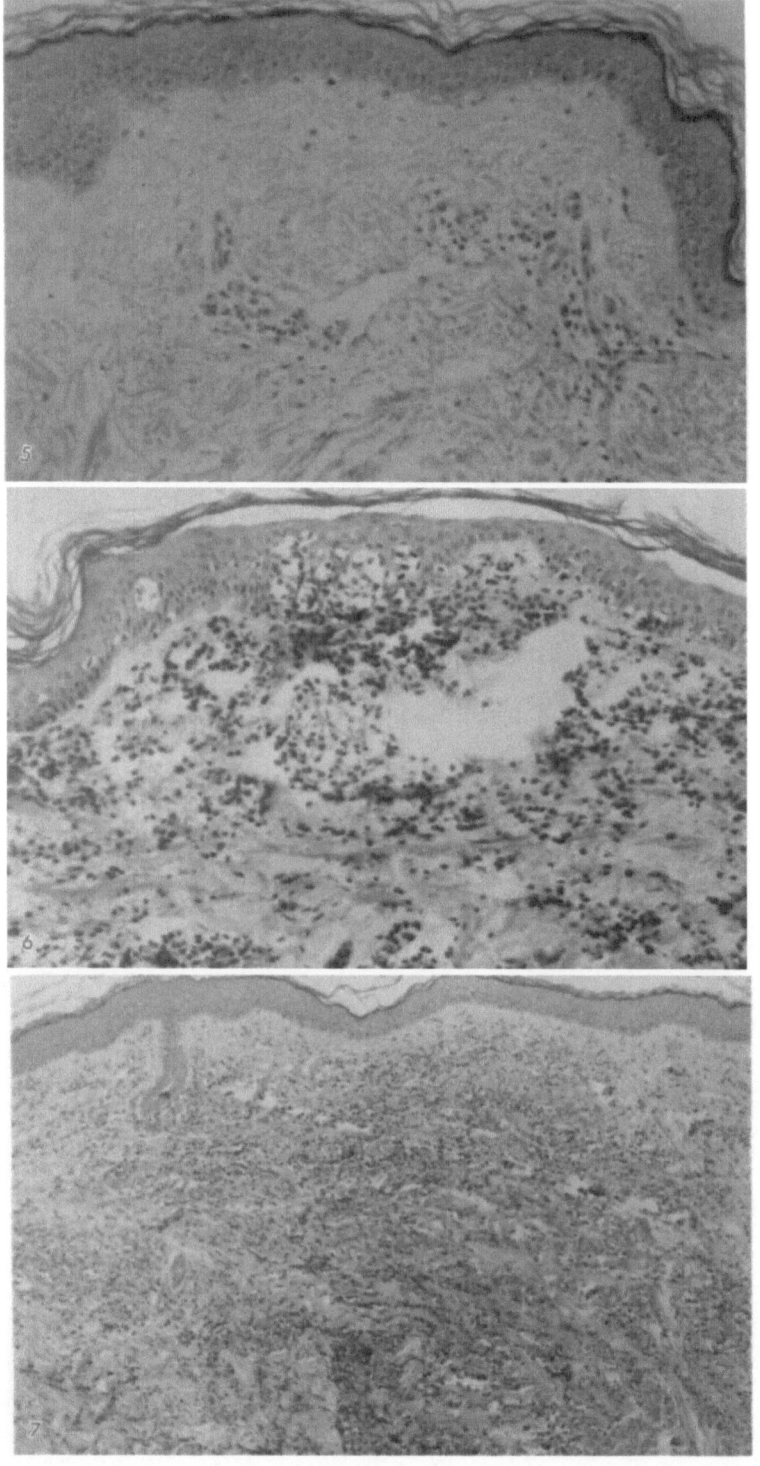

ADULT T CELL LEUKEMIA-LYMPHOMA IN THE NAGASAKI DISTRICT

Kenichiro KINOSHITA, Shimeru KAMIHIRA, Yasuaki YAMADA,
Tatsuhiko AMAGASAKI, Shūichi IKEDA, Saburo MOMITA,
and Michito ICHIMARU

*Department of Hematology, Atomic Disease Institute,
Nagasaki University School of Medicine**

Clinical, hematological and pathological findings of 84 cases with adult T-cell leukemia (ATL) were compared with those of 54 cases with T-cell malignant lymphoma (T-ML) in the Nagasaki district. ATL was characterized by pleomorphism in the peripheral blood cell size and histological appearance. However, most of the leukemic T-cell showed obvious lymphocytic differentiation, with condensed nuclear chromatin and scant cytoplasm, although in many cases lymphomatous infiltrate was dominated by either pleomorphic lymphoid cells or mediumsized cells, accompanied by occasional large multinucleated lymphoid cells. Clinically, they primarily involved middle-aged and elderly subjects, and were characterized by widespread organ invasion (particularly of the liver, spleen, and skin), susceptibility to various infections, complication of hypercalcemia and a poor prognosis. No mediastinal mass was observed in any of the case. The patients had a median survival of only 7.5 months. On the other hand, non-leukemic T-cell lymphomas, half of which histologically showed the monotonous infiltrations of large lymphoid cells, were not different in any way from the usual manifestation of malignant lymphoma with massive lymphadenopathy. These patients were generally resistant to chemotherapy and many of them died of the progression of the lymphoma within less than one year. On the basis of DNA synthesis of the malignant pleomorphic T-cells, it was suggested that large lymphoid cells, namely, T-immunoblast differentiated to mature lymphocytes, resulting in a pleomorphism of the lymphoid infiltrates and leukemic manifestation. We could detect adult T-cell leukemia associated antigen (ATLA) in a short-term culture of the malignant T-cells from 7 patients with ATL, 3 patients with T-ML, one patient with T-chronic lymphocytic leukemia (T-CLL) and one patient with mycosis fungoides (MF).

In recent years an unusual T-cell leukemia of adulthood has been reported in Japan. A new entity, adult T-cell leukemia (ATL) was proposed for this disease by Takatsuki *et al.* (*35*) in 1977. The most striking finding of this leukemia is the geographic clustering of the patients' birthplaces in the Kyushu district in Japan. So far, there have been

---

* Sakamoto-machi 12-4, Nagasaki 852, Japan (木下研一郎, 上平　憲, 山田恭暉, 尼ケ崎辰彦, 池田柊一, 樅田三郎, 市丸道人).

many more cases of adult T-cell leukemia-lymphoma (ATLL) in the Nagasaki district than in other parts of Japan (except in the Kagoshima district). Therefore, the purpose of this paper is to report clinical, hematological, and pathological features of ATLL in the Nagasaki district.

Patient Population and Diagnosis of ATLL

In the current study a detailed analysis of 199 lymphoid malignancies admitted to our institute or referred to us from 1974 to 1982 was performed, including the determination of T- or B-lymphocyte surface markers and the examination of clinical and pathological characteristics of the ATLL. The tumor was histologically classified using the criteria of the Lymphoma Study Group (31) in Japan.

ATL was determined as follows. In the initial examination, neoplastic cells appeared in the peripheral blood and leukemia was defined as the presence of more than 10% neoplastic T-cells in the leukocyte differential count of the peripheral blood.

Preparation of Specimens

Mononuclear cell suspensions were prepared from lymph nodes, peripheral blood and pleural fluids. Lymph nodes were obtained immediately following excision and teased apart in TC 199. The resulting cell suspension was filtered through gauze and centrifuged through a Ficoll-Conray gradient to obtain viable mononuclear cells. Isolation of lymphocytes from heparinized peripheral blood or pleural fluid was accomplished by dilution with two volumes of physiological saline and centrifugation through a Ficoll-Conray gradient for 30 min at 1,000 g. The mononuclear cells at the interphase were collected, washed three times with phosphate buffered saline (PBS), and examined for viability by the exclusion of trypan blue dye. Cells of more than 98% viability were used.

Distribution of T- and B-cells in 199 Lymphoid Malignancies

The ratio of lymphoid malignancies classified by morphologic and functional classification is shown in Table I. The majority of the cases were classified as T-cell lymphoproliferative disease (145 cases (72.9%)), while 44 cases (22.1%) were of B-cell and 9 cases (4.5%) were of non T-, non B-cell. Many of the T-cell malignancies were classified as ATLL which comprised 69.3% of all the lymphoid malignancies. In this report we summarize the characteristics of 138 cases with ATLL.

Clinical, Hematological, and Pathological Features of ATLL

1. Clinical features

The clinical features of ATLL are summarized in Table II. The T-cell form primarily involved middle-aged and elderly subjects. The mean age at onset of the leukemic form (ATL) was 54 years with a range of 16 to 82 years and that of the non-leukemic form (T-cell malignant lymphoma (T-ML)) was 57 years with a range of 18 to 85 years. The male/female ratio was 1.5:1 in the ATL and 1:1 in the T-ML.

TABLE I. Distribution of T- and B-cells in 199 Lymphoid Malignancies

	No. of cases	Total (%)
T-cell malignancy		145 (72.9)
ATLL		
ATL	84	
T-ML	54	
T-CLL	2	
Sézary syndrome	2	
MF	1	
IBL-like T-ML	2	
B-cell malignancy		44 (22.1)
B-malignant lymphoma	19	
Burkitt type	2	
B-CLL	21	
Macroglobulinemia W	2	
Non T-, non B-cell malignancy	9	9 (4.5)
True histiocytic malignancy	1	1 (0.5)
Total		199
Undetermined	3	

TABLE II. Clinical Features of ATLL in the Nagasaki District

	ATL (84 cases)	T-ML (49 cases)
Age	Mean 54.8 years (16–82 years)	Mean 57.0 years (18–85 years)
Sex	Male : Female=1.5 : 1 (%)	Male : Female=1 : 1 (%)
Initial symptom		
Lymphadenopathy	22 (26.2)	36 (73.5)
Skin eruption	20 (23.8)	1 (2.0)
Constitutional symptoms (fever, malaise, anorexia, etc.)	20 (23.8)	4 (8.2)
Routine blood examination	9 (10.7)	0 (0)
Hypercalcemia	4 (4.8)	0 (0)
Jaundice	2 (2.4)	0 (0)
Others	7 (8.3)	4 (8.2)
Signs		
Lymphadenopathy	74 (88.1)	43 (87.7)
Hepatomegaly	56 (66.7)	18 (36.7)
Skin eruption	43 (51.2)	6 (12.2)
Splenomegaly	24 (28.6)	6 (12.2)
Hepatosplenomegaly	19 (22.6)	5 (10.2)
Mediastinal mass	0 (0)	1 (2.0)

Lymphadenopathy (26.2%), constitutional symptoms (23.8%) including general malaise, anorexia and low grade fever, and skin eruption (23.8%) was the usual triad in the ATL cases. On the other hand, the most common and usually the earliest symptom in the T-ML was characterized by enlargement of the lymph nodes or obstructed symptoms due to the sarcomatous process. Sometimes the patients with ATL were asymptomatic and diagnosed through blood examinations. Some complained of thirst, fatigue or consciousness disturbance from onset, because of hypercalcemia. On physical examination, inconspicuous but systemic lymphadenopahty, hepatomegaly and/or splenomegaly and skin rash were predominant findings in the ATL, while only lymph node enlargement was predominant and the other findings were less frequent in the T-ML. Skin rash, one of the distinctive manifestations in the ATL, appeared in various forms including papules, erythematous plaque, nodules, and erythroderma. Histologically, the skin lesions demonstrated dermal and subcutaneous perivascular infiltration by lymphoid cells. Pautrier's microabscess-like infiltrates extending to the epidermis were occasionally found. A mediastinal mass was present in only one of the T-ML subjects.

2. Hematological findings

The blood picture of the patients is shown in Table III. In the blood picture of ATL, anemia was absent or not remarkable. Generally, the leukocyte count was markedly elevated with a high percentage of neoplastic T-cells. The leukocyte count ranged from 4,400 to 486,000/mm³ (mean value 56,300/mm³) and was distributed most frequently between 10,000/mm³ and 50,000/mm³. The mean percentage of leukemic cells in the peripheral blood was 52.8% (range 10.0–99.5%). Most of the neoplastic T-cells in the peripheral blood were pleomorphic, but the majority of them were

TABLE III. Hematological Findings of ATLL

	ATL (84 cases)	T-ML (48 cases)
Anemia (Hb≦10 g)	7 (8.3%)	2 (4.2%)
Thrombocytopenia (≦10×10⁴)	14 (16.6%)	2 (4.2%)
WBC count (per mm³)	Mean 56,320 (4,400–486,000)	Leukemic change (7 cases) at the terminal stage
<10,000	8 (9.5%)	
10,000–50,000	48 (57.1%)	
50,000–100,000	15 (17.8%)	
100,000≦	13 (15.5%)	
Abnormal cell	Mean 52.8% (10.0–99.5%)	
BM involvement (+)	60/65 (92.3%)	7/40 (17.5%)
BM abnormal cell	Mean 30.1% (0–100%)	

WBC, white blood cells; Hb, hemoglobin.

TABLE IV. Histological Subtype of ATLL and Leukemic Manifestation of Each Subtype

	No. of cases	ATL	T-ML	Leukemic manifestation (%)
Small cell	4	4	0	4/4 (100)
Mixed type	8	5	3	5/8 (62.5)
Pleomorphic type	37	30	7	30/37 (81)
Medium-sized cell	40	24	16	24/40 (60)
Large cell	36	9	27	9/36 (25)
IBL-like	3	1	2	1/3 (33)
Lennert's lymphoma	1	0	1	0/1 (0)
Dermatopathic, etc.	4	4	0	4/4 (100)
Total	133	77	56	77/133 (58)

9-13 μm in size with indented, convoluted or lobulated nuclei, and exhibited obvious lymphocytic differentiation with coarsely clumped nuclear chromatin and scanty cytoplasm (Photo 1a, 2a, 3a). In contrast to overt leukemic changes, infiltration of the bone marrow (BM) with these leukemic T-lymphocytes was less striking. Three patients had no bone marrow involvement, although a marked leukocytosis with a high percent of leukemic cells was present in the peripheral blood. On the other hand, leukemic manifestation was observed in only 7 cases at the terminal stage of the T-ML, and at the same time bone marrow involvement was less frequent.

3. Histology

Table IV shows the histological distribution of lymph node specimens according to the criteria of the Lymphoma Study Group (LSG) in Japan. Most of them showed variable histology of diffuse lymphoma (small cell, mixed, pleomorphic, medium-sized, and large cell type) and few exhibited specific lymphomatous lesion (immunoblastic lymphadenopathy (IBL)-like, Lennert's lymphoma, and dermatopathic type). However, the medium-sized cell type (40 cases), pleomorphic type (37 cases), and large cell type (36 cases) were the major histological subtypes. These three subtypes included 85% of all the T-cell leukemia-lymphomas. As compared to the histological subtypes between the leukemic and non-leukemic forms, the small cell and pleomorphic types were more predominant in the former, whereas the large cell type was more common in the latter. Medium-sized cell type was equally distributed in both forms. In many cases of the leukemic forms the lymphoid infiltrate exhibited striking pleomorphism in cell size and nuclear transformation. In some lymph nodes, occasional large multi-nucleated lymphoid cells indistinguishable from Reed-Sternberg's giant cells were seen, mimicking Hodgkin's disease. In the current study, these were classified as the pleomorphic or mixed type. An increase of post-capillary venules (PCV) in a variable degree was found in many cases of ATL. Thirteen out of 20 cases examined showed apparent migration of numerous abnormal lymphocytes through the PCV wall (Photo 4a, 4b). PCV with excessive lymphocyte migration were most conspicuous in 3 cases which showed the chronic lymphocytic leukemia (CLL)-like blood picture, but also present in 10 cases with leukemic T-cells showing lymphocytic differentiation in their peripheral blood.

4. Blood chemistry

Liver function studies frequently revealed slight to moderate elevation of transaminase, alkaline phosphatase, and total bilirubin, suggesting liver involvement. Hypoproteinemia was common and serum immunoglobulin values tended to be low.

The Properties of Neoplastic T-cells (Table V)

1. Surface marker

The presence of T-lymphocyte was determined by non-immune rosette formation with sheep red blood cells (SRBC). A rosette containing three or more SRBCs was defined as a positive E-rosette. The neoplastic cells were confirmed to form an E-rosette by staining with May-Grünwalds-Giemsa dye. The presence of surface membrane immunoglobulins (S-Ig) as a B-cell marker was evaluated in a direct immuno-

TABLE V. Properties of the Malignant T-cell

	ATL	T-ML
Surface marker		
E-RFC	PB: 13.0–99.0%	
	LN: 30.0–88.5%	LN: 5.0–86.5%
S-Ig	PB: 0–16%	LN: 0–10%
Leu 1 (+), Leu 2a (−), Leu 3a (+)	23/25 cases	6/7 cases

	ATL (22 cases)	T-ML (7 cases)	
DNA synthesis			
Labeling indices	PB: mean 2.4% (0.1–13.7%)		
	LN: mean 4.4% (0.8–20.8%)	LN: mean 9.0% (3.3–12.5%)	

	ATL (20 cases)	T-CLL (one cases)	Sézary syndrome (one cases)
Cytochemistry			
β-GL	(+)–(卌)	(卄)	(卄)
Acid phosphatase	(+)–(卌)	(+)	(+)
PAS	(−)–(卌)	(−)	(卌)

	ATL (20 cases)	T-CLL (one case)	Healthy persons (20 cases)
Function			
PHA response	Mean		
(Blast transformation %)	12.3% (0–50.5%)	67.5%	82.0% (72.0–90.0%)
Effect on B-cell	Suppressive effect (+) 14/20	1/1	
Differentiation	Helper activity 1/20		
	No effect 5/20		

PB, peripheral blood; LN, lymph node; E-RFC, E-rosette cell forming.

fluorescent procedure, using FITC-conjugated rabbit anti-human antiserum (Behring diagnostics).

The results of the surface marker studies are shown in Table V. The range of E-rosette positive cells was 5–99% of the lymphoid cells in suspensions prepared from the peripheral blood and lymph node. Many of the cases showed 50–80% E-rosette formation.

E-rosette forming cells were identified in each smear preparation stained by May-Grünwalds-Giemsa dye (Photo 5). Two cases which had E-rosette positive cells of only 5% and 12% were confirmed as of T-cell origin with monoclonal antibodies of the Leu series. Twenty-three of 25 cases with ATL, 6 of 7 cases with T-ML, and one case with T-CLL showed phenotypically inducer/helper T-cell properties using monoclonal antibody [Leu 1 (+), Leu 2a (−), Leu 3a (+)].

2. DNA synthesis of neoplastic T-cells

Cell suspensions from lymph nodes or peripheral blood were incubated for 1 hr at 37°C with ³H-thymidine. After fixation in absolute methyl alcohol for 15 min, the smears were dipped into Fuji NR-M2 emulsion, exposed for 7 days at 4°C, developed, fixed and stained with May-Grünwalds-Giemsa dye.

The labeling index (LI) of neoplastic T-cells was similar to that of acute myelogenous leukemia. LI of leukemic cells in the peripheral blood was generally lower than that of the node cells. LI was extremely high (25–50%) in the large lymphoid cells, while it was less than 1% in the small malignant T-cells (Photo 6). The results obtained by the analysis of DNA labeling of the pleomorphic neoplastic T-cells indicated that the large lymphoid cells are dividing cells and small lymphocyte-like T-cells are not capable of DNA synthesis.

3. Cytochemistry

Cytochemically, β-glucuronidase and acid phosphatase activity in the cytoplasm of the neoplastic T-cells can be seen as a red deposit in the area of the Golgi apparatus and considerable numbers of the cases showed coarse granular PAS positivity in the leukemic T-cells (Photo 7a, 7b, 7c).

4. Function of neoplastic T-cells

The majority of the leukemic T-cells in cluture failed to respond to PHA stimulation. However, there appeared to be a proportion of abnormal T-cells responding to phytohemagglutinin (PHA), since those cases showed a moderate degree of blastoid transformation and almost all of the peripheral blood cells were neoplastic T-cells. The percentage of blastoid transformation from one case with T-CLL was 67.5%. The leukemic T-cells in 14 out of 20 cases with ATL showed marked suppressive effect on the capacity of normal B-lymphocyte to produce immunoglobulin examined by the method of Gronowicz et al. (13). The dissociation between antigenic phenotype (inducer/helper T-cells) and functional properties (suppressor T-cells) of the same leukemic cells remains unsolved.

5. Adult T-cell leukemia associated antigen (ATLA) and anti-ATLA antibody

Mononuclear cells of peripheral blood, thoracic duct lymph and pleural effusion derived from 7 patients with ATL, 3 patients with T-ML, one patient with mycosis fungoides and one patient with T-CLL were cultured in RPMI 1640 medium con-

TABLE VI. ATLA and Anti-ATLA Antibody in the ATLL

Case	Age/Sex	Diagnosis	Materials	Anti-ATLA (titer)	ATLA positive cells (culture day)	(%)
1	49/F	ATL	PB	20	2	8.3
2	73/M	ATL	PB	40	16	9.3
3	75/M	ATL	PB	160	3	15.3
4	51/M	ATL	PB	1,240	4	8.2
5	32/M	ATL	PB	160	4	73.2
6	51/M	ATL	PB	160	5	14.4
7	64/F	ATL	Thoracic duct lymph	320	3	16.5
8	47/M	T-CLL	PB	160	3	7.7
9	70/M	T-ML (leukemic stage)	PB	640	8	17.8
10	49/F	MF (leukemic stage)	PB	160	2	3.2
11	57/M	T-ML (leukemic stage)	PB	160	2	55.5
12	49/F	T-ML	Pleural effusion	40	9	16.3

taining 10% heat-inactivated fetal calf serum and T-cell growth factor and examined for ATLA using anti-ATLA positive sera from ATL patients. Sera from ATL patients in the Nagasaki district was sent to the Hinuma Laboratory in Kyoto University and antibodies against the antigens in MT-1 cells (anti-ATLA antibodies) were examined (16).

Antibodies against the ATLA in MT-1 cells (anti-ATLA antibodies) (13, 16) were found in all 23 examined ATL patients and in 9 of 12 patients with T-ML in the Nagasaki district. Anti-ATLA antibodies were also demonstrated in a patient with T-CLL and in 2 patients with mycosis fungoides. We also detected ATLA in the cytoplasm of short-term cultured neoplastic T-cells from 7 patients with ATL, 3 patients with T-ML, and one patient with T-CLL. All of these patients were ATLA antibody positive (Table VI).

Drainage of Thoracic Duct Lymph and Appearance of Neoplastic T-cells in the Thoracic Duct Lymph

ATL is the leukemic form of T-ML. But the major pathway through which neoplastic T-cells enter the circulating blood is unclear. The thoracic duct is generally accepted as the major pathway of normal lymphocytes into the circulating blood. Hence, thoracic duct lymph from 2 patients with ATL was obtained by cannulation of the duct and examined for the appearance of neoplastic T-cells. Following is a report of a patient with ATL who received thoracic duct drainage.

Case Report

A 49-year old female complained of blurred vision and it was found that her leukocyte count was markedly elevated. The peripheral blood contained 200,000/mm³ leukocytes with 99% of the cells being abnormal lymphocytes (Photo 8a). The majority of these cells, as well as abnormal lymphocytes from a lymph node, formed rosettes with SRBC and were identified as T-cells. A biopsied lymph node had the features of a pleomorphic lymphoma using LSG criteria (Photo 8b). Thoracic duct lymph of this patient was obtained over a continuous period of 19 days. Unexpectedly, the leukocyte count in the thoracic duct lymph was low at 15,000/mm³. However, unlike the peripheral blood, approximately 20–30% of the cells in the lymph were transformed large lymphocytes and the others were small lymphocytes similar to the peripheral blood cells (Photo 8c). The abnormal lymphocytes from the thoracic duct lymph formed E-rosettes with SRBC and showed an inducer/helper T-cell phenotype using monoclonal antibody. Therefore, the abnormal lymphocytes in the thoracic duct as well as in the peripheral blood were identified to be of the same T-cell origin and it was ascertained that the major pathway for abnormal lymphocytes into the blood is through the thoracic duct *via* efferent lymphatic vessels.

Complications

Major complications in ATLL are shown in Table VII. They can be divided into 3 groups: infections, hypercalcemia and infiltrations to various organs (predominantly

TABLE VII. Major Complications of ATLL

	ATL	T-ML
Infection	47/76 (61.8%)	18/48 (20.8%)
Pneumonia	29	6
Bacterial	24	3
Pneumocystis carinii	5	3
Fungus	8	5
Sepsis	3	3
Generalized varicella	4	3
Tuberculosis	2	1
Isospora belli	1	0
Hypercalcemia	44/81 (54.3%)	14/48 (29.2%)
	6 cases with osseous destruction	5 cases with osseous destruction
Extranodal involvement	More than half of the cases	20/40 (50.0%)
Skin, liver, lung, bone, meninges, pleura, *etc.*		

to skin, liver, bone, lung, meninges, and pleura). More than 60% of the ATL were complicated with various infections, especially bacterial pneumonia (31.6%), whereas the infections complicated with T-ML were less frequent. The other infections included *Pneumocystis carinii* penumonia, fungus, sepsis, generalized varicella, tuberculosis, and isospora belli. The majority of these infections did not improve in spite of intensive supportive therapy and finally became the cause of death. Hypercalcemia was observed in 58 cases (45%) out of 129 ATLL during their course, with 11 cases showing osseous destruction on X-ray. More than half of the ATL were hypercalcemic. The incidence of hypercalcemia was compared between ATL and T-ML and was found more frequently demonstrated in ATL. Many of the hypercalcemic patients, even though transiently improved by chemotherapy, relapsed as the disease progressed in the terminal stage. One of the other important complications is extranodal involvement, especially of skin, liver, bone, lung, meninges, and pleura. The infiltration of these organs was observed in more than 57% of the ATL and in 50.0% of the T-ML.

Course, Cause of Death, and Survival

The clinical course of T-cell form was variable, but a poor prognosis was apparent. About 40% of the leukemic form died of various infections as mentioned above or progression of the disease 2 to 3 months after admission. Such fatal infections developed from the onset of the disease in some cases. Leukemic T-cells in the peripheral blood were gradually reduced by chemotherapy 3 or 4 months to one year after treatment, but also during this period many of them (40% of the cases) died of opportunistic infections (Table VIII). A few cases in this group, who were fortunately free from complications, achieved a partial remission. About 20% of all the leukemic cases under partial remission owing to chemotherapy, terminally deteriorated and died of leukemic progression to various organs 6 months to 2 years after admission, even in the longest survivors. On the other hand, the non-leukemic cases were generally resistant to chemotherapy. Many of them died of the progression of lymphomas 3 to 4 months after admission and a few died of complicating infections. The remaining cases, even though

TABLE VIII.   Causes of Death in ATLL

	ATL (58 cases)	T-ML (30 cases)
Infection	26 (44.8%)	11 (36.7%)
Pneumonia (bacterial)	12 (20.7)	1 (3.3)
(*Pneumocystis carinii*)	6 (10.3)	2 (6.6)
Sepsis	4 (6.9)	3 (10.0)
Generalized varicella	2 (3.4)	1 (3.3)
Fungus	2 (3.4)	4 (13.3)
Progression of leukemia-lymphoma	26 (44.8%)	19 (63.3%)
Emaciation	22 (37.9)	
Renal failure due to hypercalcemia	4 (6.9)	
Others	6 (10.3%)	0 (0 %)

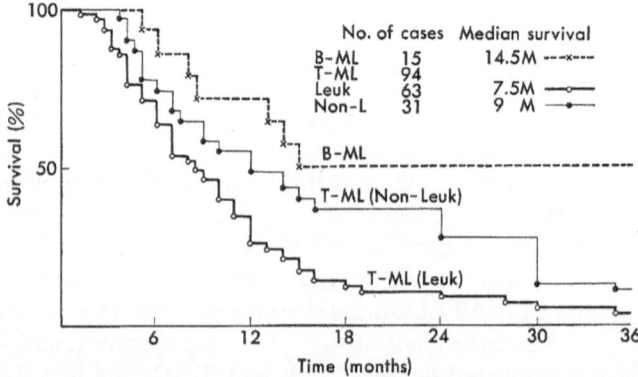

FIG. 1.   Survival rate of ATLL and B-cell lymphoma. B-ML, B-cell lymphoma; T-ML, T-cell lymphoma; Leuk, leukemic group; Non-Leuk, non-leukemic group.

transient remission was obtained, relapsed rapidly and died within less than one year after admission. The median survival time from oneset of the leukmic form was only 7.5 months and 9 months with the non-leukemic form. As compared to B-cell lymphomas, they had a significantly worse prognosis (Fig. 1).

DISCUSSION

Immunological surface marker study of neoplastic cells of non-Hodgkin's lymphomas (NHL) has revealed that the majority of NHL with identifiable markers have been classified as B-cell disorders and few of them have been identified as T-cell neoplasias in the western countries (*2, 4, 7, 9, 10, 12, 14, 18, 20, 21, 23, 26*). On the other hand, the proportion of T-cell lymphoma has been much more frequent in Japan, especially in the Kyūshu district located in southwestern Japan (*15, 17, 19, 25, 30, 33, 34*). Approximately 70% of the NHL in our series were of T-cell origin and many of them first appeared with a leukemic manifestation in the Nagasaki district. Clinically, this peculiar T-cell leukemic variety of NHL was characterized by widespread organ invasion, increased susceptibility to infection and poor prognosis. A mediastinal mass was present in only one case. Morphologically, the leukemic T-cell exhibited a wide spectrum of morphological variations. However, the majority of the cells showed obvious lymphocytic differentiations, with condensed nuclear chromatin and scant cytoplasm and were characterized by multiple nuclear abnormalities such as notching, indentation, lobulation, and convolution. This peculiar T-cell leukemic variety of NHL was identical to the disease concept of "adult T-cell leukemia (ATL)" proposed by Takatsuki, et al. (34, 35). This disease, as described in this report, is clinically, morphologically, and histologically clearly different from previously reported malignancies of the T-cell type (6, 22, 24, 27, 32, 37), including Sézary syndrome, the leukemic form of lymphoblastic lymphoma with mediastinal mass and rare cases of chronic lymphocytic leukemia. Histologically, employing the criteria of LSG, T-cell leukemic variety was of a diffuse type with pleomorphic, medium-sized cells, large cell, mixed, and small cell types present in decreasing order of frequency. Many of them exhibited a histology composed of a mixture of large and small lymphoid cells with occasional Reed-Sternberg-like giant cells. Such cases were difficult to classify by Rappaport's criteria and have been classified as pleomorphic T-cell lymphoma in this report. Sometimes they were mistaken as Hodgin's lymphoma because of pleomorphic lymphoid infiltrates. However, the atypism of the surrounding lymphocytes distinguishes this lesion from Hodgkin's disease. The pathology observed in our cases was partly consistent with the histological descriptions reported by Berard (3), Waldron (36), Pinkus (29), Palutke (28), and Gaeke (11). Unlike their reports, the most striking finding in our series was the presence of the peripheral blood involvement, which was not apparent in any of the other investigations. Another striking feature, recognized in some of the leukemic varieties, was the morphological discrepancy between the peripheral blood cells and node cells. A large number of small lymphocyte-like malignant T-cells were noted in the peripheral blood, whereas lymph nodes of the same patient showed an histology of large lymphoid cells or pleomorphic lymphoid infiltrates. On the basis of DNA synthesis of pleomorphic T-cells in the peripheral blood and lymph node with ATL, it was suggested that large lymphoid cells, namely T-immunoblasts, differentiated to mature lymphocytes, resulting in a pleomorphism of the lymphoid infiltrates and leukemic manifestation; this was because neoplastic cells often retain the properties of their normal counterparts, and are presumably capable of differentiation to smaller effector T-cells. Therefore, the pleomorphic cell component of the node cells from ATL patients may be considered the same as that of malignant lymphoma with plasmacytic differentiation which reflects a broad spectrum of cells at different stages of B-cell differentiation into plasma cells. Lennert has pointed out that an increase of PCV with many migrating lymphocytes is the most prominent feature in the histology of T-CLL. Migrating lymphocytes were also evident in many cases with ATL and in addition leukemic T-cells in the thoracic duct lymph were observed in 2 patients with ATL. From these observations, it seems possible that malignant T-cells appear through the thoracic duct in the peripheral blood after differentiation, and recirculate into the lymph node via the PCV. On the other hand, non-leukemic T-ML showed the monotonous proliferation of large lymphoid cells and was not different in any way from the usual manifestation of malignant lymphoma with massive lymphadenopathy. ATL in the Nagasaki district included a wide spectrum of T-cell proliferative diseases which ranged from subacute to prolonged T-cell proliferation. T-CLL could be classified into the latter group of ATL, because ATLA was demonstrated in the cytoplasm of short-term cultured T-cells from one T-CLL patient. The leukemic T-cells from 14 out of 20 patients with ATL acted as suppressor T-cells. So, ATL appeared to be different from Sézary syndrome which shows helper activity on B-cell differentiation (5). This leukemic, T-cell form was characterized by complications of various infections and hypercalcemia. Many cases died of complicating pulmonary infection, most frequently caused by gram-negative bacteria. Increased susceptibility to infection was presumably due to decreased immunity, since the PPD reaction and PHA-induced blastogenesis were diminished. Hypercalcemia was one of the characteristic complications found in half of the leukemic cases. Osseous destruction was seen in 11 patients and in those cases it was suggested that hypercalcemia was induced by the release of Ca^{2+} from destroyed bone by tumor cell infiltration. However, the remaining cases did not exhibit bone destruction on X-ray and the concentration of parathyroid hormone (PTH), examined in a few of the patients was within normal limits. It has been reported that T- and B-cell distribution of NHL differs considerably in various areas of Japan (33). As a rule, B-cell type is more predominant in northern Japan and the proportion of T-cell variety tends to increase toward southwestern Japan. Moreover, the birthplaces of the patients with leukemic T-cell variety cluster markedly in the Kyūshu district located in southwestern Japan. On considering the etiology of this disease with such peculiar geographic distribution, it was of interest that in this population this disease frequently occurred in the same family. We have encountered 13 families, with two or more patients in the same family having lymphoproliferative disorders, of which this leukemic T-cell form was observed in 9 (shown in another chapter by Ichimaru). Many of these patients came from Goto Island, located west of Nagasaki City. We mapped the birthplaces of the patients with ATL and B-cell lymphomas in the Nagasaki district (Fig. 2). The ATL patients were clustered with relatively high frequency on Goto Island in spite of its small population, rather than in Nagasaki City. On the other hand, the birthplaces

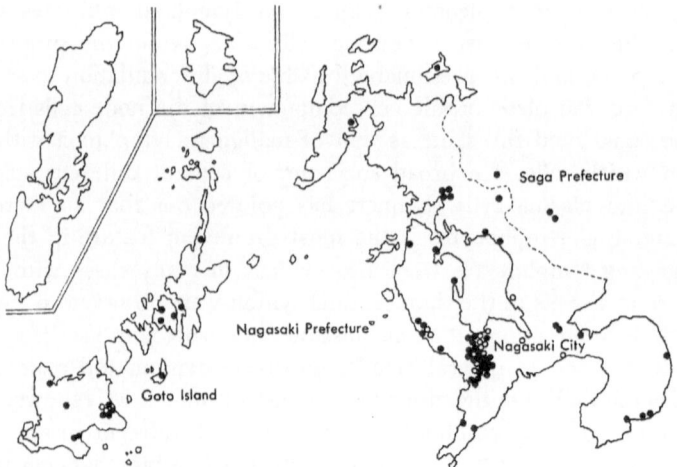

FIG. 2. Distribution of ATL and B-malignant lymphoma in the Nagasaki district. ○ B-ML; ● ATL.

of the patients with B-cell lymphomas center in Nagasaki City which comprises one-third of the population of Nagasaki Prefecture.

Retroviruses are involved in the etiology of naturally occurring leukemia and lymphoma of animals (*1, 8*). However, whether or not they are involved in human leukemia-lymphoma has yet to be revealed. Type C retrovirus particles were found in the leukemic T-cells from ATL patients as well as in the T-cell line by Hinuma *et al.* Moreover, they have reported that proviral DNA from retrovirus is integrated into the DNA of peripheral leukemic cells of ATL patients (*38*). We also could detect ATLA in the short term culture of the malignant T-cells from 7 patients with ATL, 3 patients with T-ML, one patient with T-CLL and one patient with mycosis fungoides (MF). In the near future it is expected that a mechanism of leukemogenesis by the type C retrovirus will be clarified.

Acknowledgment

This work was supported in part by a Research Grant from the Ministry of Public Welfare for Japanese Adult T-cell Leukemia.

REFERENCES

1. Aaronson, S. A., Tronick, S. R., and Stephenson, J. R. Endogenous type-C RNA viruses of mammalian cells. *Biochim. Biophys. Acta*, **458**, 323–354 (1976).
2. Aisenberg, A. C. and Long, J. C. Lymphocyte surface characteristics in malignant lymphoma. *Am. J. Med.*, **58**, 300–306 (1975).
3. Berard, C. W. An overview of neoplasia. *In* "The Reticuloendothelial System," ed. J. W. Rebuck, C. W. Berard, and M. R. Abell, pp. 301–317 (1975). Williams and Wilkins Co., Baltimore.
4. Berard, C. W., Jaffe, E. S., Braylan, R. C., and Nanba, K. Immunologic aspects and pathology of the malignant lymphomas. *Cancer*, **42**, 911–921 (1978).
5. Broder, S., Edelson, R. L., Lutzner, M. A., Nelson, D. L., MacDermott, R. P., Durm, M. E., Goldman, C. K., Meade, B. O., and Waldmann, T. A. The Sézary syndrome: A malignant proliferation of helper T cells. *J. Clin. Invest.*, **58**, 1297–1306 (1976).
6. Brouet, J. C., Flandrin, G., Sasportes, M., Preud'-Homme, J. L., and Seligmann, M. Chronic lymphocytic leukemia of T-cell origin. Immunological and clinical evaluation in eleven patients. *Cancer*, **2**, 890–893 (1975).
7. Brouet, J. C., Labeume, S., and Seligmann, M. Evaluation of T and B lymphocyte membrane markers in human non-Hodgkin's malignant lymphoma. *Br. J. Cancer*, **31** (Suppl. II), 121–127 (1975).
8. Callahan, R., Lieber, M. M., Todaro, G. J., Garves, D. C., and Ferrer, J. F. Bovine leukemia virus genes in the DNA of leukemic cattle. *Science*, **192**, 1005–1007 (1976).
9. Cooper, D. A., Petts, V., Luckhurst, E., Biggs, J. C., and Penny, R. T and B cell populations in blood and lymphnode in lymphoproliferative disease. *Br. J. Cancer.*, **31**, 550–558 (1975).
10. Davey, F. R., Goldberg, J., Stockman, J., and Gottlieb, A. J. Immunologic and cyto-chemical cell markers in non-Hodgkin's lymphomas. *Lab. Invest.*, **35**, 430–438 (1976).
11. Gaeke, M. E., Vardiman, J. W., Miller, W., Medenica, M., Hopper, J. E., and Rowley, J. D. Human T-cell lymphoma with suppressor effects on the mixed lymphocyte reaction (MLR). I. Morphological and cytogenetic analysis. *Blood*, **57**, 634–641 (1981).
12. Gajl-peczalska, K. J., Bloomfield, C. D., Coccia, P. F., Sosin, P. F., Sosin, H., Brunning,

180   K. KINOSHITA ET AL.

R. D., and Kersey, J. H. B and T cell lymphomas. Analysis of blood and lymphnodes in 87 patients. *Am. J. Med.*, **59**, 674–675 (1975).

13. Gronowicz, E., Coutinho, A., and Melchers, F. A plaque assay for all cells secreting Ig of a given type or class. *Eur. J. Immunol.*, **6**, 588 (1976).

14. Habeshaw, J. A., Macaulay, R.R.A., and Stuart, A. E. Correlation of surface receptors with histological appearance in 29 cases of non-Hodgkin lymphoma. *Br. J. Cancer*, **35**, 858–867 (1977).

15. Hanaoka, M., Sasaki, M., Matsumoto, H., Tankawa, H., Yamabe, H., Tomimoto, K., Tasaka, C., Fujiwara, H., Uchiyama, T., and Takatsuki, K. Adult T cell leukemia— Histological classification and characteristics—. *Acta Pathol. Jpn.*, **29** (5), 727–738 (1979).

16. Hinuma, Y., Nagata, K., Hanaoka, M., Nakai, M., Matsumoto, T., Kinoshita, K., Shirakawa, S., and Miyoshi, I. Adult T-cell leukemia: Antigen in an ATL cell line and detection of antibodies to the antigen in human sera. *Proc. Natl. Acad. Sci. U.S.*, **78**, 6476–6480 (1981).

17. Ichimaru, M., Kinoshita, K., Kamihira, S., Ikeda, S., Yamada, Y., and Amagasaki, T. T-cell malignant lymphoma in Nagasaki district and its problems. *Jpn. J. Clin. Oncol.*, **9** (Suppl. 1), 337–347 (1979).

18. Jaffe, E. S., Shevach, E. M., Sussmann, E. H., Frank, M., Green, I., and Berard, C. W. Membrane receptor sites for the identification of lymphoreticular cells in benign and malignant conditions. *Br. J. Cancer*, **31** (Suppl. II), 107–120 (1975).

19. Kikuchi, M., Mitsui, T., Matsui, N., Sato, E., Tokunaga, M., Hasui, K., Ichimaru, M., Kinoshita, K., and Kamihira, S. T-cell malignancies in adults: Histopathological studies of lymph nodes in 110 patients. *Jpn. J. Clin. Oncol.*, **9** (Suppl. 1), 407–421 (1979).

20. Koziner, B., Filippa, D. A., Mertelsmann, R., Gupta, S., Clarkion, B., Good, R. A., and Siegel, F. P. Characterization of malignant lymphomas in leukemic phase by multiple differentiation markers of mononuclear cells. *Am. J. Med.*, **63**, 556–567 (1977).

21. Lennert, K. "Malignant Lymphomas Other Than Hodgkin's Disease." pp. 83–469 (1978). Springer-Verlag, New York-Heidelberg-Berlin.

22. Lille, I., Desplaces, A., Meeus, L., Saracino, R. T., and Brouet, J. Thymus derived proliferating lymphocytes in chronic lymphocytic leukemia. *Lancet*, **ii**, 263–264 (1972).

23. Lukes, R. J., Parker, J. W., Taylor, C. R., Tindle, B. H., Cramer, A. D., and Lincoln, T. L. Immunologic approach to non-Hodgkin lymphomas and related leukemia, analysis of the results of multiparameter studies of 425 cases. *In* "Seminars in Hematology," pp. 322–351 (1978). Grune and Stratton, New York.

24. Lutzner, M., Edelson, R., Shein, P., Green, I., Kirkpatrick, C., and Ahmed, A. Cutaneous T-cell lymphomas: The Sézary syndrome, mycosis fungoides, and related disorders. *Ann. Intern. Med.*, **83**, 534–552 (1975).

25. Matsumoto, M., Nomura, K., Matsumoto, T., Nishioka, K., Hanada, S., Furusho, H., Kikuchi, H., Kato, Y., Utsunomiya, A., Uematsu, T., Iwahashi, M., Hashimoto, S., and Yunoki, K. Adult T-cell leukemia-lymphoma in Kagoshima district, southwestern Japan: Clinical and hematological characteristics. *Jpn. J. Clin. Oncol.*, **9** (Suppl. 1), 325–336 (1979).

26. Morris, M. W. and Davey, F. R. Immunologic and cytochemical properties of histiocytic and mixed histiocytic-lymphocytic lymphomas. *Am. J. Clin. Pathol.*, **63**, 403–414 (1975).

27. Palutke, M., Patt, D. J., Weise, R., Varadachari, C., Wylin, R. F., Bishop, C. R., and Tabaczka, P. M. T cell leukemia-lymphoma in young adults. *Am. J. Clin. Pathol.*, **68**, 429–439 (1977).

28. Palutke, M., Tabaczks P. M., Weise, R. W., Axelrod, A., Palacas, C., Margolis, H.,

Khilanai, P., Ratanatharathorn, V., Piligian, J., Pollard, R., and Husain, M. T-cell lymphomas of large cell type. *Cancer*, **46**, 87–101 (1980).

29. Pinkus, G. S., Said, J. W., and Hargreaves, H. Malignant lymphoma, T-cell type. *Am. J. Clin. Pathol.*, **72**, 540–550 (1979).

30. Shimoyama, M., Minato, K., Saito, H., Kitahara, T., Konda, M., Nakazawa, M., Watanabe, S., Inada, N., Nagatani, T., Deura, K., and Mikata, A. Comparisons of clinical, morphologic and immunologic characteristics of adult T-cell leukemia-lymphoma and cutaneous T-cell lymphoma. *Jpn. J. Clin. Oncol.*, **9** (Suppl. 1), 357–372 (1979).

31. Suchi, T., Tajima, K., Nanba, K., Wakasa, H., Mikata, A., Kikuchi, M., Mori, S., Watanabe, S., Mohri, N., Shamoto, S., Harigaya, K., Itagaki, T., Matsuda, M., Kirino, Y., Takaga, K., and Fukunaga, S. Some problems on the histopathological diagnosis of non-Hodgkin's malignant lymphoma—A proposal of a new type—. *Acta Pathol. Jpn.*, **29** (5), 755–776 (1979).

32. Sullivan, A. K., Vera, J. C., Jerry, L. M., Rowden, G., and Bain, B. Small lymphocyte T-cell leukemia in the adult. *Cancer*, **42**, 2920–2927 (1978).

33. Tajima, K., Tominaga, S., Kuroishi, T., Shimizu, H., and Suchi, T. Geographical features and epidemiological approach to endemic T-cell leukemia/lymphoma in Japan. *Jpn. J. Clin. Oncol.*, **9** (Suppl. 1), 495–504 (1979).

34. Takatsuki, K., Uchiyama, T., Ueshima, Y., and Hattori, T. Adult T-cell leukemia. Further clinical observations and cytogenetic and functional studies of leukemic cells. *Jpn. J. Clin. Oncol.*, **9** (Suppl. 1), 317–328 (1979).

35. Uchiyama, T., Yodoi, J. Sagawa, K., Takatsuki, K., and Uchino, H. Adult T-cell leukemia: Clinical and hematologic features of 16 cases. *Blood* **50**, 481–492 (1977).

36. Waldron, J. A., Leech, J. H., Glick, A. D., Flexner, J. M., and Collins, R. D. Malignant lymphoma of peripheral T-lymphocyte origin. *Cancer*, **40**, 1604–1617 (1977).

37. Williams, A. H., Taylor, C. R., Higgins, G. R., Quinn, J. J., Schneider, B. K., Swanson, V., Parker, J. W., Pattengale, P. K., Chandor, S. B., Powars, D., Lincoln, T. L., Tindle, B. H., and Lukes, R. J. Childhood lymphoma-leukemia: I. Correlation of morphology and immunological studies. *Cancer*, **42**, 171–181 (1978).

38. Yoshida, M., Miyoshi, I., and Hinuma, Y. *Proc. Natl. Acad. Sci. U.S.*, in press.

EXPLANATION OF PHOTOS

PHOTO 1a. Three leukemic T-cells have condensed nuclear chromatin with prominent lobulation and distortion. In the center there is a "lymphoblast"-like cell with nucleoli. May-Giemsa, ×1,000.

PHOTO 1b. Histology of the lymph node from same patient shows the pleomorphic lymphoid infiltration. Hematoxylin-eosin (H-E), ×400.

PHOTO 2a. On the right is a malignant T-cell with convoluted nucleus. May-Giemsa, ×1,000.

PHOTO 2b. A lymph node from same patient diffusely infiltrated with rounded lymphoid cells, showing slight variation in size. H-E, ×400.

PHOTO 3a. A transformed lymphocyte is seen in the center. Majority of leukemic cells are small and show obvious lymphocytic differentiation. May-Giemsa, ×1,000

PHOTO 3b. A biopsied lymph node from same patient shows the feature of a "histiocytic lymphoma" using the Rappaport classification or immunoblastic sarcoma employing the Lukes'criteria. H-E, ×400.

PHOTO 4a. Large numbers of PCV with many migrating lymphocytes in lymph node from ATL. H-E, ×200.

PHOTO 4b. A great increase of PCV with numerous recirculating small lymphoid cells in the wall. H-E, ×400.

PHOTO 5. Malignant T-cells forming sheep E-rosettes. Note that sheep erythrocytes rosette not only
with large lymphoid cells, but also with small abnormal lymphocytes. May-Giemsa, ×1,000.

PHOTO 6. DNA labeling with tritiated thymidine employing an autoradiographic technique. Note the
large lymphoid cells synthesizing DNA. The DNA labeling indices were high in the large lymphoid
cells, but extremely low in the small lymphoid cells.

PHOTO 7a. β-Glucuronidase reaction. β-Gucuronidase activity in the cytoplasm of pleomorphic T-cells
can be seen as a red deposit in the area of the Golgi apparatus. ×1,000.

PHOTO 7b. Acid phosphatase reaction in the leukemic T-cells from ATL. ×1,000.

PHOTO 7c. PAS reaction, positive in the vacuoles of cytoplasm, appears as granular deposit. ×1,000.

PHOTO 8a. The majority of the leukemic T-cells are small with cleft and convoluted nuclei. May-
Giemsa ×1,000.

PHOTO 8b. A biopsied lymph node from this patient diffusely infiltrated with pleomorphic lymphoid
cells. H-E ×400.

PHOTO 8c. Unlike the peripheral blood, T-immunoblasts are more frequently admixed with small lymphoid cells in the lymph of thoracic duct than in the peripheral blood. May-Giemsa ×1,000.

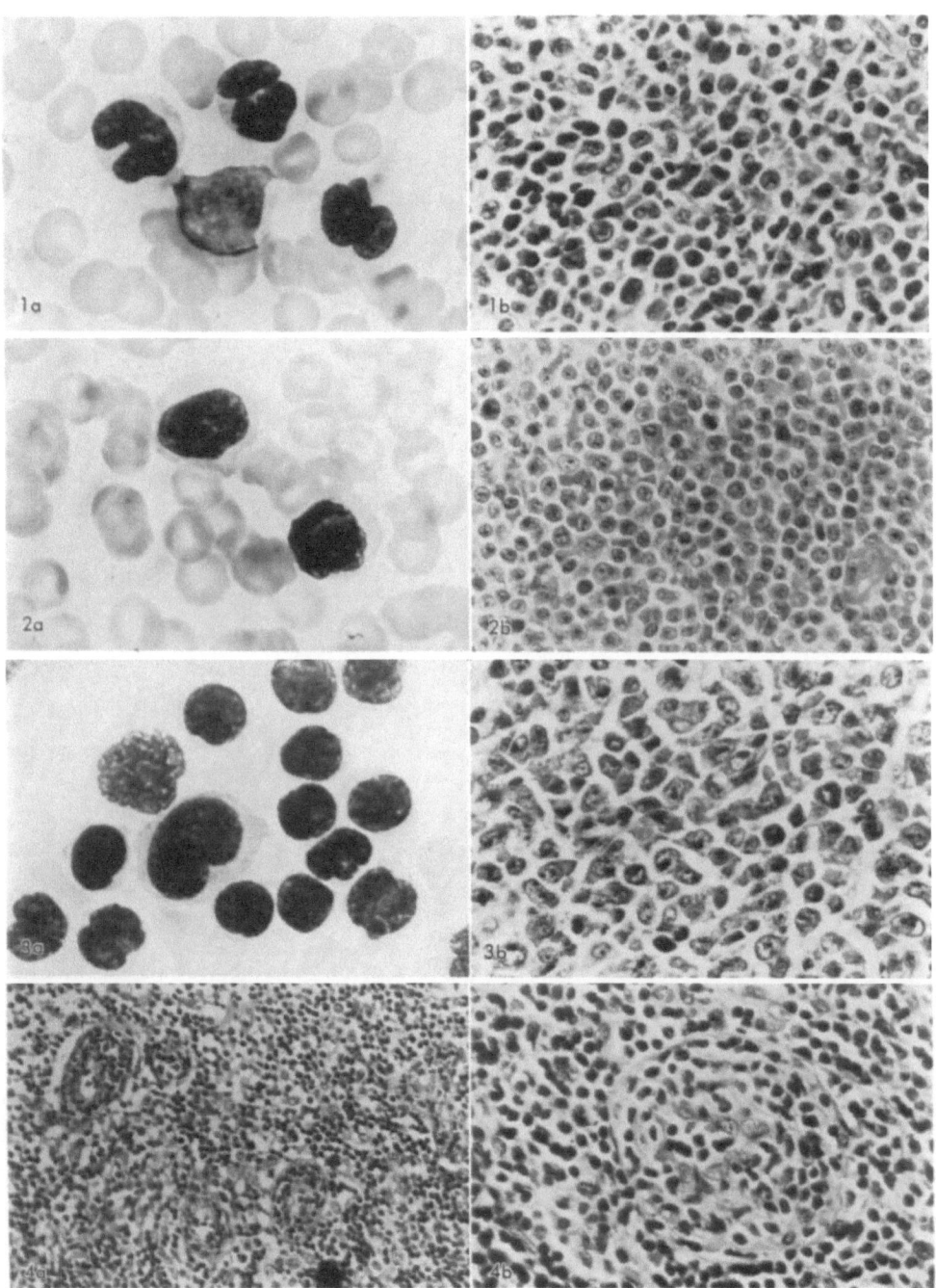

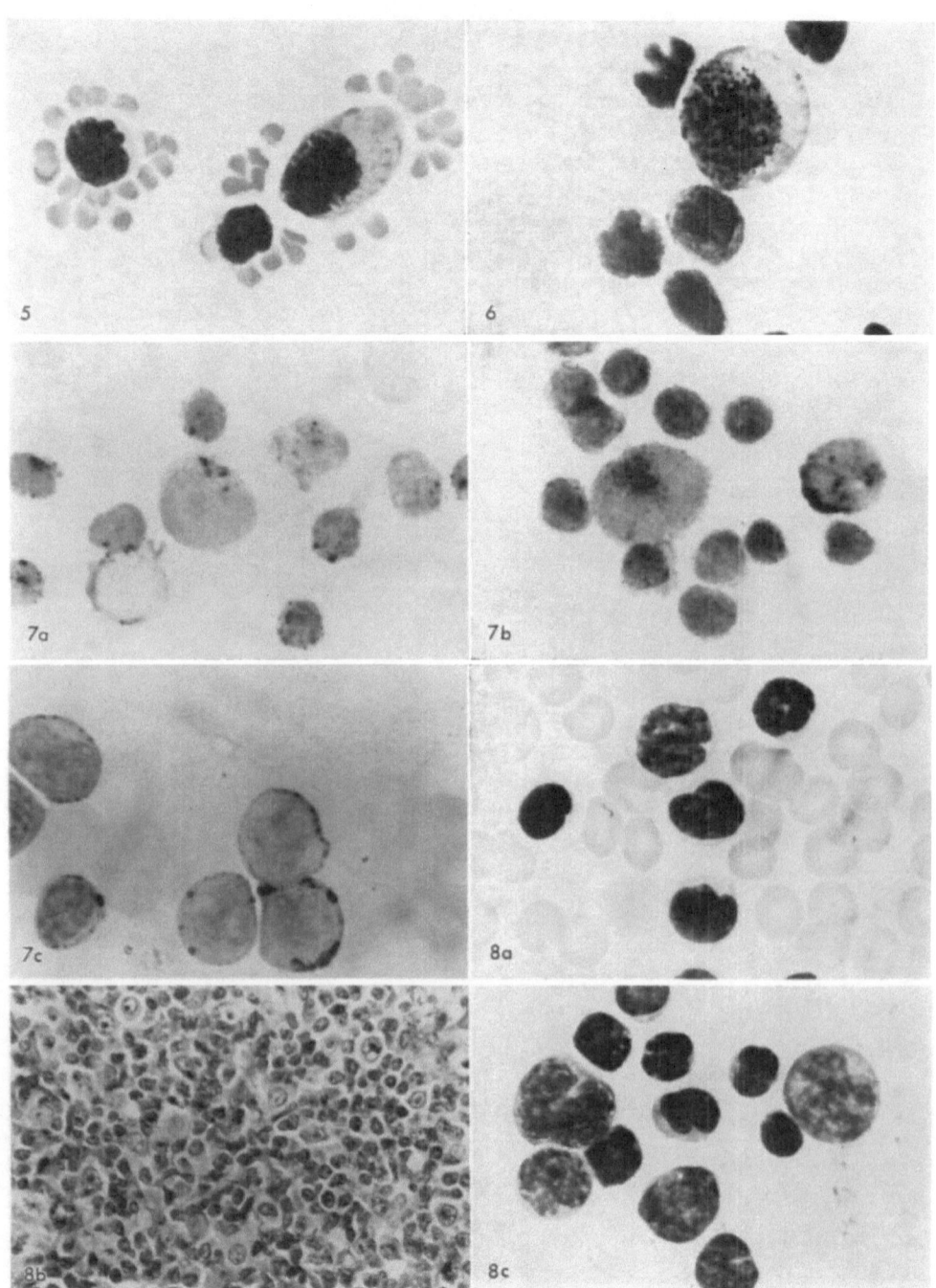

FAMILIAL DISPOSITION OF ADULT T CELL
LEUKEMIA AND LYMPHOMA

Michito Ichimaru, Kenichiro Kinoshita, Shimeru Kamihira,
Yasuaki Yamada, Yukinobu Oyakawa, Tatsuhiko Amagasaki,
and Miyuki Kusano

Department of Clinical Hematology, Atomic Disease Institute,
Nagasaki University School of Medicine*

Thirteen families with familial disposition among 137 cases of adult
T-cell leukemia and T-cell lymphoma (ATLL) were found. Seven of
these cases have a parent with lymphoma, 6 cases have other lymphoma
cases in siblings. Three families of sibling cases with clinicopathological
findings are presented; these sibling cases were all T-cell malignancies.

Adult T-cell leukemia associated antigen (ATLA) antibody in the
cases of ATL patients were all positive, and 57.1% of T-cell malignant lymphoma (T-ML) were positive. Positive rate of healthy spouses
and siblings of ATLL patients for ATLA-virus (ATLV) antibody was
high (71.4%, 50% respectively).

The meaning of high familial disposition of ATLL is discussed.

With the recent elucidation of geographical distribution of malignant lymphoma
by surface marker in Japan, a disease entity of adult T-cell leukemia (ATL) has been
established for a special T-cell type non-Hodgkin lymphoma with leukemic manifestation (*10*).

In this report, we refer to adult leukemic T-cell non-Hodgkin lymphoma as ATL,
non-leukemic T-cell non-Hodgkin lymphoma as T-ML (T-cell malignant lymphoma),
and ATL and T-ML together as ATLL. These reported cases were all observed by
the authors. Geographic specificity has been recognized in the occurrence of ATL in
Japan with higher prevalence in the southwestern part of the country (Kyushu and
southern Shikoku) (*9*). Many ATL cases have been personally observed in Nagasaki,
and many ATL and T-ML cases with familial disposition were found in that district
our study.

Hinuma (*2*) reported that C type retrovirus was found in the tumor cells of ATL
patients and that the sera of these patients had a specific antibody for an antigen in
the ATL cell line. This antigen is called ATLA. From this point of view, the existence
of many cases with familial disposition seems important, because there may be virus
infection in the family or some genetic factor may participate in the onset of this disease. Reported in this paper are 13 families having two or more lymphoma or leukemia
cases, with special reference to 3 families in which ATL or T-ML cases were observed
in siblings. The results of examinations for ATLA antibody in the serum of the cases

---

* Sakamoto-machi 12-4, Nagasaki 852, Japan (市丸道人, 木下研一郎, 上平　憲, 山田恭暉, 親川幸信, 尼
ケ崎辰彦, 草野みゆき).

with ATL, T-ML or some other related disorders, healthy persons having ATL or T-ML cases in their families, and control healthy persons are reported.

In this report, 171 cases of non-Hodgkin lymphoma were classified into T, B and non T, non B type by surface marker study. A family study was performed on all these non-Hodgkin lymphoma cases. Of the 13 families with familial disposition, 3 having sibling cases are presented since satisfactory data on their clinicopathological features is available.

Surface Marker Study

Tumor cells in the peripheral blood or lymph node cells in saline suspension were examined for the determination of surface markers. T-lymphocytes were determined by non-immune rosette formation with sheep red blood cells (SRBC) and B-lymphocytes by the presence of cell surface immunoglobulin (S-Ig) in the direct immunofluorescent procedure. Reaction for monoclonal antibody using Leu series monoclonal antibody was tested for the T-cells in several ATL and T-ML cases.

ATLA Antibody

The classification of non-Hodgkin lymphoma by surface marker study is shown in Table I. One hundred thirty-seven out of 171 cases of non-Hodgkin lymphoma (80%) were T-cell type, and 83 of these (60%) were leukemic. These leukemic non-Hodgkin T-cell lymphoma cases were compatible with ATL. Non-leukemic type T-cell non-Hodgkin lymphoma were T-ML.

TABLE I. Classification of Non-Hodgkin's Lymphomas by Surface Markers (Dec. 1981)

	No. of cases (%)	Non-leukemic	Leukemic
T-cell	137 (80.1)	54 (T-ML)	83 (ATL)
B-cell	21 (12.2)	19	2
Non T-, non B-cell	9 (5.2)	8	1
True histiocytic	1 (0.5)	0	1
Undetermined	3 (1.8)	3	0
Total	171	84	87

Familiar Study

Table II shows 13 cases of T-cell malignancy having two or more cases of malignant lymphoma or leukemia within their families. These 13 cases were confirmed as T-cell malignancy by the surface marker study; the diagnosis was ATL in 10 cases, T-acute lymphoblastic leukemia (ALL) in 1 case and T-ML in 2 cases. Seven of these cases have other cases in their parents, and 6 cases have other lymphoma cases in their siblings. Three families of sibling cases with satisfactory clinicopathological findings are presented below.

TABLE II.   Families with 2 or More Cases of T-cell Lymphoma or Leukemia

Case	Age	Sex	Diagnosis	Other cases in family	
1. H. F.	27	F	ATL	Father: RCS	Uncle: ML
2. S. S.	32	M	ATL	Mother: RCS	Aunt: RCS
3. H. N.	10	M	T-ALL	Father: ML	Gramdmother: ML
4. T. Y.	54	M	ATL	Mother: AL	
5. T. O.	41	M	ATL	Mother: ML	Uncle: AL
6. Y. F.	37	F	ATL	Father: AL	
7. M. K.	56	F	ATL	Sister: ATL	
8. S. Y.	37	F	ATL	Brother: ML	
9. M. H.	65	M	T-ML	Sister: T-ML	
10. Y. Y.	54	M	ATL	Sister: T-ML	Brother: T-ML
11. A. K.	65	M	T-ML	Brother: ML	
12. M. I.	58	M	ATL	Sister: B-ML	
13. K. S.	54	M	T-ML	Mother: Neck sarcoma	

AL, acute leukemia; ML, malignant lymphoma; RCS, reticulum cell sarcoma.

TABLE III.   Family 1

Hometown: Kishuku-cho, Minamimatsuura-gun (Goto), Nagasaki Prefecture

Case	1) Y. Y. age 54	2) K. Y. age 46	3) C. S. age 43
Onset	Nov., 1974	Sep., 1980	May, 1979
Onset to death (months)	18	12	4
Diagnosis	ATL	T-ML	T-ML
Histology (LSG-classification)	Large cell type	Pleomorphic type	Pleomorphic type
WBC (per μl)	27,600	7,900	4,400
Blood leukemia cells (%)	40	19	0
Liver function GOT	39(178)	16 (85)	18 (88)
GPT	46(86)	17 (62)	7 (16)
Ca in serum (mg/dl)	15	15.2	16.2
PPD skin test	—	—	—
Lymphadenopathy	+	+	Abdominal bulky mass

WBC, white blood cells; GOT, glutamic oxaloacetic transaminase; GPT, glutamic pyrvic transaminase; PPD, purified protein derivative tuberculin.

1. Family 1 (Table III)

These siblings were born in the Goto area of Nagasaki Prefecture which is known for a high incidence of malignant lymphoma. The elder brother who had a different father was ATL while his sister and younger brother were T-ML. Histological diagnosis by Lymphoma Study Group in Japan (LSG) classification (8) of their tumors was large cell type in the elder brother, and pleomorphic type in the sister and younger brother (Photo 1). In their clinical course, liver function disturbance and hypercalcemia, probably due to tumor cell infiltration, were observed.

2. Family 2

These sisters have already been reported on. (3). They showed clinical features of ATL. Lymph node swelling was minimal and not palpable. Tumor cells in their peri-

TABLE IV. Family 3
Hometown: Tokitsu-cho, Nishisonogi-gun, Nagasaki Prefecture

Case	H. A. age 39	S. Y. age 37
Onset	April, 1973	March, 1980
Onset to death (months)	5	10
Diagnosis	Malig. lymphoma (RCS)	ATL
Histology (LSG-classification)	Med-sized cell type ?	Pleomorphic type
Blood	Non-leukemic	WBC 14,700 (leuk. cell 37%)
Lymph node enlargement	‐‐‐	‐‐
Hypercalcemia	Unknown	+

RCS, reticulum cell sarcoma.

pheral blood showed typical ATL cells with lobulated nuclei and similar clinical features were observed. They were born in Fukuda, a seaside town in Nagasaki Prefecture.

3. Family 3 (Table IV)

This was a brother and a sister. The brother suffered from malignant lymphoma in 1973 at the age of 39; the sister's ATL occurred in 1980 at age 37. The pathological diagnosis for the brother's lymphoma was reticulum cell sarcoma and no surface marker study was made for the tumor cells. However, clear pleomorphism of tumor cells in the tissue which is characteristic of ATL cells could be observed, strongly suggesting his lymphoma to be the T-cell type. Their histological lymph node features are shown in Photo 2. Histological findings of the sister's lymph nodes were pleomorphic. Tumor cells in her peripheral blood were confirmed as T-cells. These siblings were born in Tokitsu, another seaside area in Nagasaki Prefecture.

Evaluation of Antibody

Determination of ATLA antibody was performed at Hinuma's laboratory in the Institute for Virus Research, Kyoto University. In brief, an using MT 1 cells established as a cultured cell line in the laboratory of Miyoshi (7). The positive rates of ATLA antibody in the sera of 34 cases of malignant lymphoma, 48 cases of miscellaneous blood diseases other than lymphoma, 40 persons (9 families) having ATL or T-ML patients in their families, and 40 healthy control persons are shown in Table V. ATL patients were all positive for the ATLA antibody (100%). Four of 7 T-ML patients (57.1%) were positive, 4 cases of non-T non-Hodgkin malignant lymphoma were all negative, and 3 cases of 4 Hodgkin lymphoma were positive (75%). As described above, 3 cases of T-ML were negative for ATLA antibody. However, 2 of these were immunoblastic lymphadenopathy (IBI)-like T-cell lymphoma and the other case was a somewhat different type of T-cell lymphoma as compared with common T-cell type non-Hodgkin lymphoma. Tumor cells in the latter case were in the bone marrow only, and these were large cells with big nuclei without T-cell specific nuclear lobulation but with many granulations and E rosette formation. The ATLA antibody was positive in 7 out of 18 acute leukemia cases. These acute leukemia cases were all myelogenous leukemia and they had received many blood transfusions over a long period. One positive case of

TABLE V. ATLA Antibody Reactivity of Sera from Adult Patients with Various Diseases and from Healthy Adults

	Positive cases/ subjects examined	Rate (%)
ATLL		
ATL	19/19	100
T-ML	4/7	57.1
Non T-ML (non-Hodgkin's lymphoma)	0/4	0
Hodgkin's lymphoma	3/4	75.0
Blood disorders		
Acute leukemia	7/18	38.9
Others	1/30	3.3
ATLL family	13/40	32.5
Normal control subjects	4/40	10.0

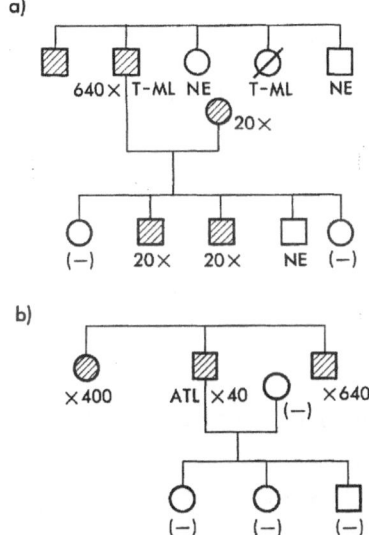

FIG. 1. Pedigree of ATLL cases examined for ATLA antibody. a) M. H. (T-ML). b) I. W. (ATL). □ male; ○ female; / dead; ▨ ● Anti-ATLA (+); □ ○ Anti-ATLA (−); NE not examined.

another blood disease was aplastic anemia and she had also received many blood transfusions. Thirteen out of 40 persons in 9 families having ATL or T-ML patients were positive for ATLA antibody (32.5%). Four out of 40 adult healthy controls in Nagasaki City were positive (10%). The pedigree of 2 families having ATL or T-ML patients examined for the ATLA antibody are shown in Fig. 1. Figure 1a shows a family having sibling cases of malignant lymphoma: a brother with T-ML was positive for antibody, a sister with malignant lymphoma was not examined. The wife and two sons of the T-ML case were positive, however, two daughters were negative. Figure 1b shows another family having an ATL patient. The two siblings were positive but the wife and three children were negative for ATLA antibody. The positive rate of antibody in 40

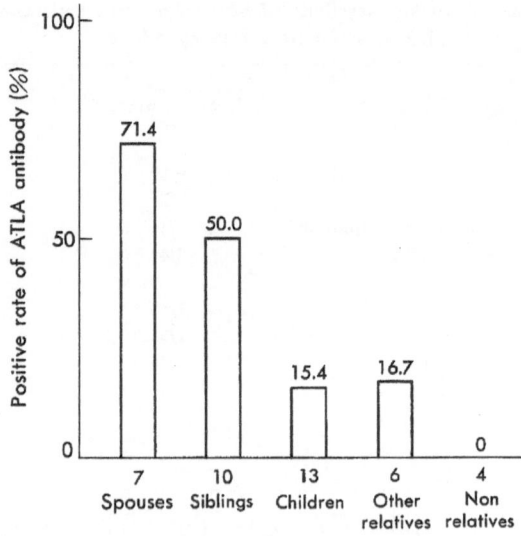

FIG. 2. Positive rate of ATLA antibody in 40 members of 9 families having ATLL patients.

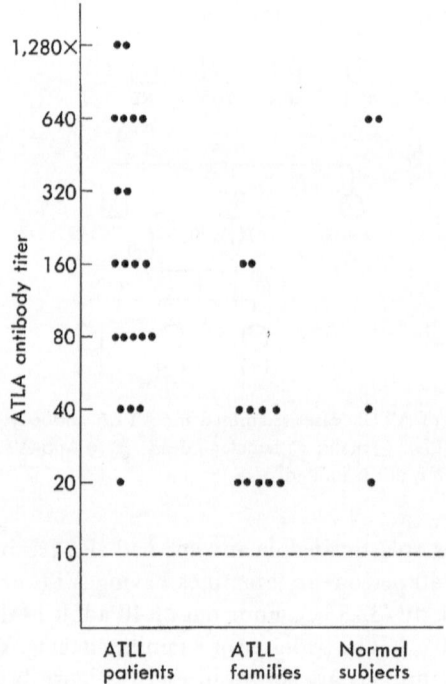

FIG. 3. ATLA antibody titer of ATLL patients and families.

subjects having ATL or T-ML patients in their family is shown in Fig. 2 (32.5%). The positive rate in spouses and sibilings was high (71.4% and 50%). On the other hand, the rate in children and other relatives was 15.4 and 16.7%, respectively. Non-relatives in the families all showed negative results for the antibody test. The ATLA antibody titer of ATL and T-ML patients was compared with that of their healthy family members and healthy controls as shown in Fig. 3. The patients titer appeared higher than that of positive family members without the disease.

DISCUSSION

It seems important to elucidate the relationship of human leukemia or malignant lymphoma with viral infection. A close relationship of Burkitt lymphoma with EB virus has been recognized in Central Africa, however, so far we have been unable to find any other virus having a direct relationship with human leukemia or malignant lymphoma. Therefore, Hinuma's report of C type retrovirus (ATLV) probably being related to ATLL has great meaning. Hinuma named this virus ATLA-virus (ATLV), and its nature and relationship with ATL and T-ML have been studied. If there is any relationship between ATLV infection and the occurrence of these diseases, the existence of many cases of ATL and TML with familial disposition seems very important to clarify the feature and the time of viral infection and to solve problems which may possibly exist during the period from viral infection to actual onset. The incidence of ATL and T-ML with familial disposition is much higher than that of other myelogenous leukemias. Guasch (1) reported the incidence of familial leukemia to be one case out of 220 (0.45%); Miyata (6) reported that Japanese familial leukemia is one case per 200 (0.5%) stating that its incidence is very rare.

Three families having sibling patients are presented in this report. It is noteworthy that all the cases in these three families examined for surface marker were T-cell malignancies. Although a brother case in Family 3 whose pathological diagnosis about 10 years ago was reticulum cell sarcoma was not examined for surface marker of tumor cells, it was strongly suggested that his disease was T-ML in view of the nuclear pleomorphism of tumor cells in the lymph node tissue as stated above. Since the development of the lymphocyte surface marker study, almost all the reticulum cell sarcomas morphologically diagnosed have been identified as T- or B-cell malignancy. In the Nagasaki district, we found such T-cell lymphoma in many cases. (5). Hodgkin's lymphoma also might possibly have been misdiagnosed in reference to its histological structure resembling the pleomorphic type of T-ML (4). The existence of many of the above incidents of ATL and T-ML having sibling cases suggests the possibility of a horizontal infection virus. So far, the number of cases examined for ATLA antibody has not been adequate, however, 100% of the ATL cases and 57.1% of the T-ML were positive for ATLA antibody. As previously stated, 3 ATLA antibody negative cases of T-ML were somehow different from the common type of non-Hodgkin lymphoma in clinicopathological features as well as in the pattern of reaction to monoclonal antibody, whereas common types of ATL and T-ML by Leu series monoclonal antibody showed Leu-1, Leu-3a positive and Leu-2a negative. Two cases of ATLA antibody negative T-ML were only Leu-3a positive, and the other case was Leu-1, Leu-2a positive and Leu-3a negative. (We will report the details of the reactions for monoclonal antibodies in another paper).

Among the other family members of ATL or T-ML patients, the positive rate of ATLA antibody showed high values in spouses and siblings. However, we have not experienced any occurrence in both spouses although many sibling cases of ATLL have been observed. ATL or T-ML of these sibling cases all occurred at an age beyond 35 years. Their lives and environments in their adulthood certainly differed from each other, therefore, ATLV infection, if any, is likely to have taken place in their childhood. The percentage of positive ATLA antibody in the husband or wife of the patient was high but there has been no occurrence of the disease in either spouse. These facts may suggest that there is participation of some genetic factor other than viral infection in the occurrence of this disease. It may be suggested also that a long latent period is necessary for the occurrence of the disease after the first viral infection. In our study, 10% of the healthy controls were positive for ATLA antibody. Hinuma et al. (2) reported a positive rate of ATLA antibody in healthy Japanese persons in endemic areas and non-endemic areas to be 26% and 1–2%, respectively. The Nagasaki district has been noted as one of the endemic areas, but there may be some difference in the positive rate of ATLA antibody among different areas within Nagasaki Prefecture; for example, it may be higher in seaside areas. In any event, if 10–25% of the healthy persons are positive, the total number of patients suffering from ATL or T-ML *versus* the total positvie persons seems to be very low. Almost all the sera of ATL patients, however, show positive reaction for ATLA antibody and there are many cases of ATL or T-ML with familial disposition. These facts may suggest that there is a strong correlation between ATLV and these diseases. Therefore, it seems important in the future to clarify which positive persons are likely to develop the diesase, what factors are involved during the latent period from viral infection to the onset, what the mechanism is whereby ATLV transforms T-cells into tumor cells, and what preventative measures are possible.

That the positive rate of ATLV antibody was high in the sera of those with blood diseases other than ATLL who received blood transfusions over long periods may suggest that the transfusions themselves may be one of the important routes of ATLV infection.

Acknowledgments

The authors wish to thank Prof. Y. Hinuma and his laboratory staff for their cooperation in the determination of ATLA antibody.

This study was supported by a Grant-in-Aid for Cancer Research from the Ministry of Health and Welfare.

REFERENCES

1. Guasch, J. Hérédité des leucémies. *Sang*, **25**, 384–421 (1954).
2. Hinuma, Y., Nagata, K., Hanaoka, M., Nagai, M., Matsumoto, T., Kinoshita, K., Shirakawa, S., and Miyoshi, I. Adult T-cell leukemia: Antigen in an ATL cell line and detection of antibodies to the antigen in human sera. *Proc. Natl. Acad. Sci. U.S.*, **78**, 6467–6480 (1981).
3. Ichimaru, M., Kinoshita, K., Kamihira, S., Ikeda, S., Yamada, Y., and Amagasaki, T. T-cell malignant lymphoma in Nagasaki district and its problems. *Jpn. J. Clin. Oncol.*, **9** (Suppl), 337–346 (1979).
4. Ichimaru, M. Clinical features of T-cell malignant lymphoma. *J. Jpn. Soc. Intern. Med.*, **70**, 511–524 (1981) (in Japanese).
5. Kinoshita, K., Nonaka, H., Amagasaki, T., Yamada, Y., Ikeda, S., Kamihira, S.,

Ichimaru, M., Matsuo, T., and Tsuda, N. T-cell derived non-Hodgkin's lymphoma showing Hodgkin's disease-like histology. *J. Kyushu Hematol. Soc.*, **28**, 61–66 (1981) (in Japanese).

6. Miyata, H. and Enomoto, H. Familial leukemia. *Jpn. J. Clin. Hematol.*, **5** (Suppl.), 15–25 (1964) (in Japanese).
7. Miyoshi, I., Kubonishi, M., Sumida, M., Yoshimoto, S., Hiraki, S., Tsubota, T., Kobashi, H., Lai, M., Tanaka, T., Kimura, I., Miyamoto, K., and Sato, J. Characteristics of a leukemic T-cell line derived from adult T-cell leukemia. *Jpn. J. Clin. Oncol.*, **9** (Suppl.), 485–494 (1979).
8. Suchi, T. and Tajima, K. Peripheral T-cell malignancy as a problem in lymphoma classification. *Jpn. J. Clin. Oncol.*, **9** (Suppl.), 443–450 (1979).
9. Tajima, K., Tominaga, S., Shimizu, H., and Suchi, S. A hypothesis on the etiology of adult T-cell leukemia/lymphoma. *Gann*, **72**, 684–691 (1981).
10. Takatsuki, K., Uchiyama, T., Ueshima, Y., and Hattori, T. Adult T cell leukemia: Farther clinical observations and cytogenetic and functional studies of leukemic cells. *Jpn. J. Clin. Oncol.*, **9** (Suppl.), 312–324 (1979).

EXPLANATION OF PHOTOS

PHOTO 1. Family 1 lymph nodes. a) Histology of elder brother's lymph node. Hematoxylin-eosin H-E. b) Histology of sister's lymph node. H-E. c) Histology of younger brother's lymph node. H-E.
PHOTO 2. Family 3 lymph nodes. a) Histology of brother's lymph node. H-E. b) Histology of sister's lymph node. H-E.

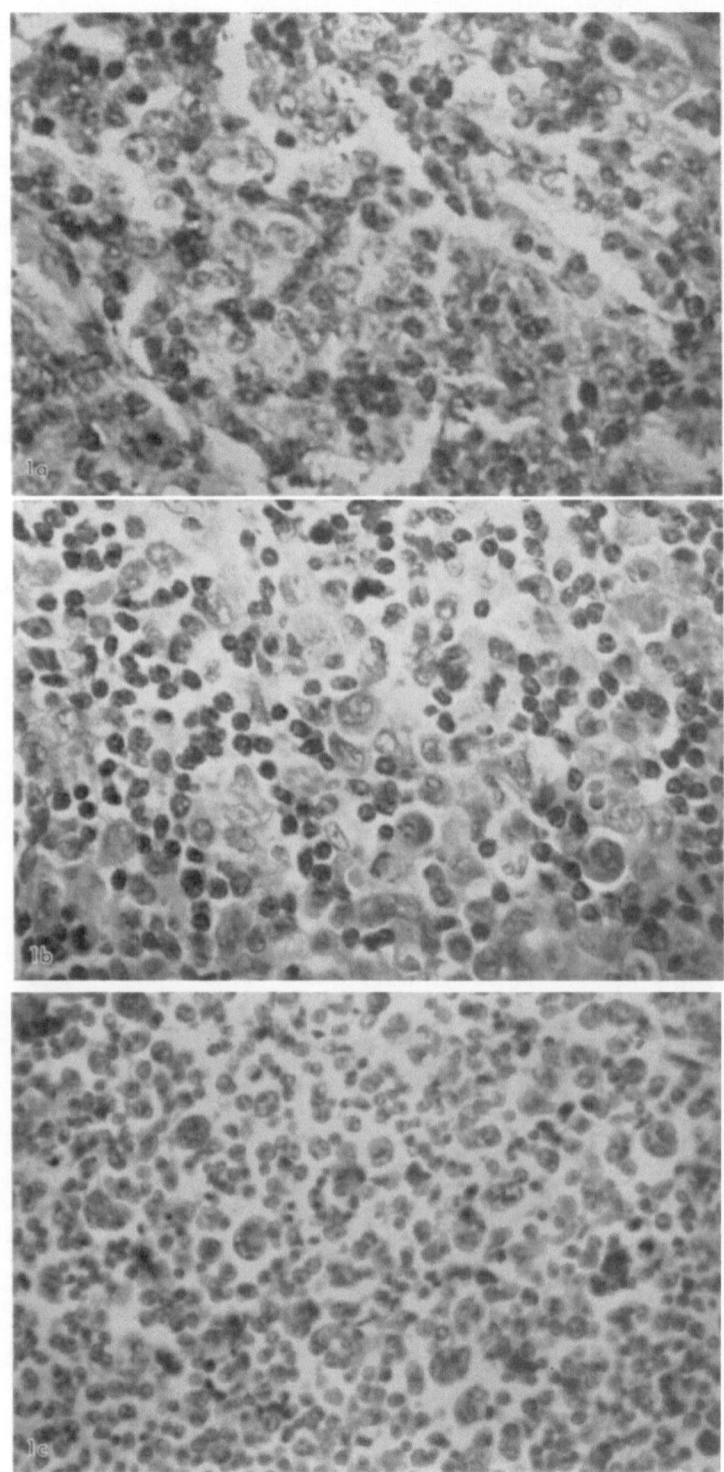

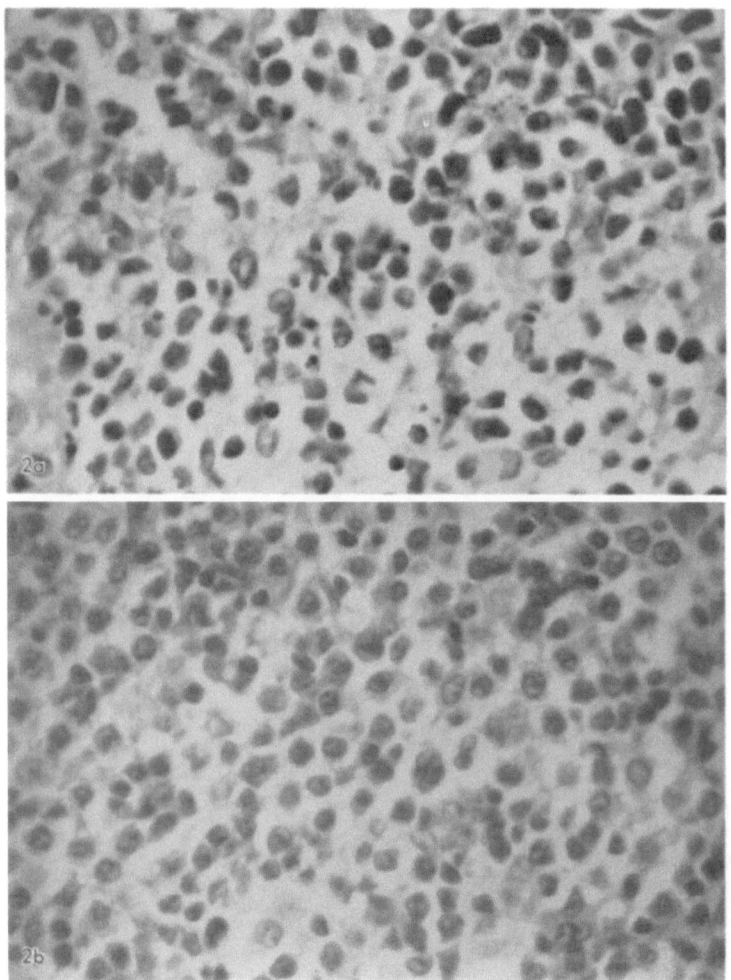

CLINICO-EPIDEMIOLOGICAL ANALYSIS
OF ADULT T CELL LEUKEMIA

Kazuo Tajima,*1 Suketami Tominaga,*1 and Taizan Suchi*2

*Division of Epidemiology, Aichi Cancer Center Research Institute*1 and*
Department of Pathology and Clinical Laboratory,
*Aichi Cancer Center Hospital*2

According to an analysis of the Vital Statistics, the mortality from malignant lymphomas in Japan is remarkably high in the Kyushu district. Evidence from a nationwide survey performed by the T and B-cell Malignancy Study Group revealed that the excessive rate in that area was mainly due to a high incidence of adult T-cell malignancy. This was characterized by clinico-epidemiological findings which contrasted with B-cell malignancy and other endemic malignant lymphomas such as Burkitt's lymphoma and Mediterranean intestinal lymphoma.

Furthermore, adult T-cell leukemia (ATL) was prevalent in limited zones in Kyushu, mainly in rural coastal areas which are warm in winter and humid in summer. It was found that the geographical distribution of filariasis was very similar to that of ATL. It is known that filariasis affects lymphatic vessels and results in several lymphoreticular ailments, and that microfilaria is transmitted by mosquitoes which may transfer not only tumor viruses, including adult T-cell leukemia virus (ATLV), but also tumor cells. Analyses of the time trends of the average weight and height of schoool children by perfecture suggested that the nutritional condition of inhabitants in Kyushu might have been poorer than that of inhabitants of other areas in Japan, especially in the past.

In order to elucidate the etiology of ATL, relevant geographic-pathological and other related information was accumulated. An etiological hypothesis was formulated that repeated exposure to filarial antigen and ATL virus might have played an important role in the etiology of ATL and that undernutrition had also contributed to its progression.

A marked geographical variation in the mortality due to malignant lymphoma has been observed within Japan. The evidence of high mortality from malignant lymphoma limited in Kyushu district suggests the existence of some special risk factors for this rare but characteristic malignancy.

On the other hand, some epidemiological studies on malignant lymphomas have shown time-space clusters and a characteristic age-distribution of several subtypes of malignant lymphomas in the world. However, except for the endemic Burkitt's lymphoma in Africa (4), only a few analytical epidemiological studies to identify risk

---

*1,*2 Kanokoden 81-1159, Tashiro-cho, Chikusa-ku, Nagoya 464, Japan (田島和雄, 富永祐民, 須知泰山).

factors of human malignant lymphomas, including Hodgkin's disease, have been conducted, because the disease is too rare for meaningful analysis on a statistical basis.

Since about 10 years ago, it has become possible to distinguish the two types of lymphocytes, T-lymphocytes, and B-lymphocytes, in terms of their immunological function. Human neoplastic lymphoid cells have been studied for their expression of cell surface markers of the two types. From these investigations, it has been revealed that the proportion of the patients with T-cell lymphoma is large in Japan, especially in Kyushu district, than in the Western countries (15).

Furthermore, the places of birth of patients with adult T-cell leukemia (ATL) clustered to the limited zones in Japan. The facts of the specific geographical distribution of ATL advanced to the next step investigation in the epidemiological field to elucidate the etiology of malignant lymphomas of Japan.

In order to determine the cause of this disease, much information concerning ATL and related diseases was accumulated and was analyzed from the viewpoint of epidemiology.

Time Trend and Geographical Distribution of Malignant Lymphoma in Japan

The age adjusted death rate from malignant lymphomas in Japan is much lower than those in western countries and the USA (13). The time trends in age adjusted death rates of malignant lymphoma from 1960–1978, however, have shown a marked increase in both sexes in recent years (Fig. 1). To examine these increasing trends, deaths were calculated by age groups and are graphed in Fig. 2 (14). The death rate of individuals over 40 years old is higher as age progresses. According to the Vital Staitstics of Japan Series, the age distribution of the Japanese population has changed gradually in such a way that the proportion of old age groups, generally a high risk group for malignant lymphomas, has become relatively larger year by year. Additionally, the recent improvements in diagnostic techniques may have resulted in fewer

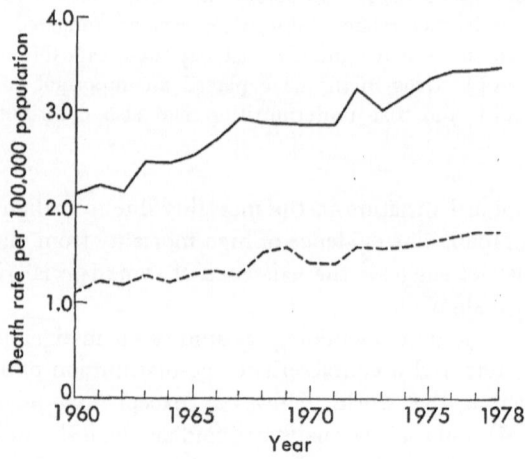

Fig. 1. Trends in the age-adjusted mortality rate* of malignant lymphomas (ICDs, 200–202) by sex (1960–1978) in Japan. —— male; - - - - female.
* Standardized on the age distribution of the Segi's world population.

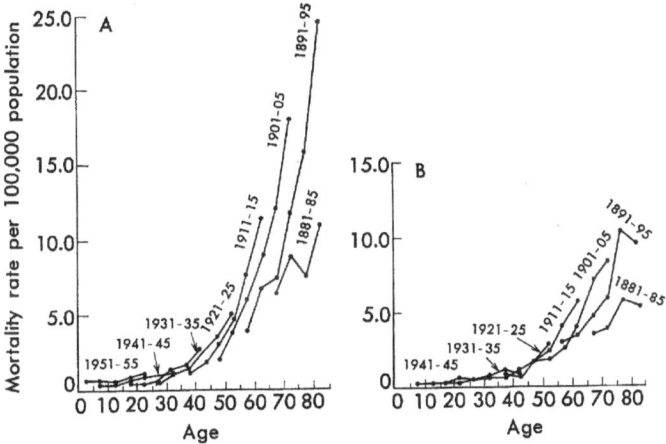

FIG. 2. Age specific mortality rates of malignant lymphomas (ICDs, 200–202) by birth-year grouping (1881–1955) in Japan. A) male. B) female (from Shimizu, et al., 1980).

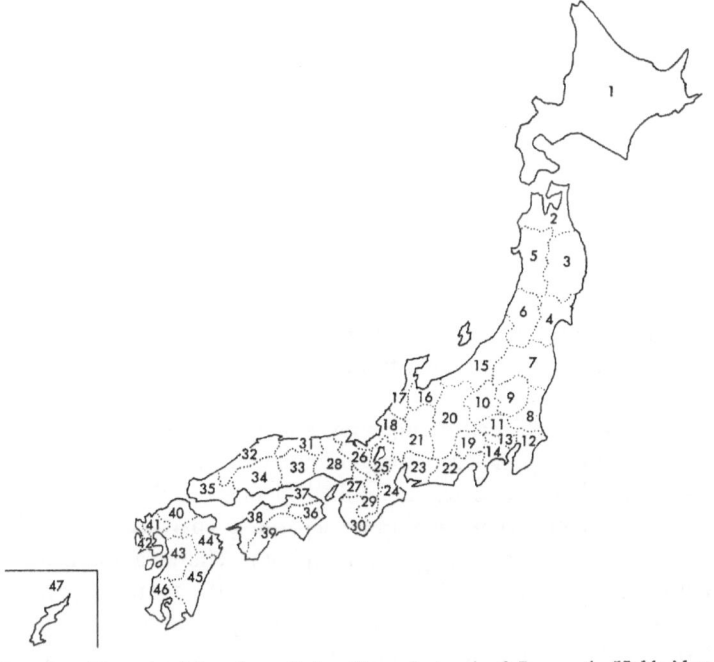

FIG. 3a. Name and location of the 47 prefectures of Japan. 1, Hokkaido; 2, Aomori; 3, Iwate; 4, Miyagi; 5, Akita; 6, Yamagata; 7, Fukushima; 8, Ibaraki; 9, Tochigi; 10, Gunma; 11, Saitama; 12, Chiba; 13, Tokyo; 14, Kanagawa; 15, Niigata; 16, Toyama; 17, Ishikawa; 18, Fukui; 19, Yamanashi; 20, Nagano; 21, Gifu; 22, Shizuoka; 23, Aichi; 24, Mie; 25, Shiga; 26, Kyoto; 27, Osaka; 28, Hyogo; 29, Nara; 30, Wakayama; 31, Tottori; 32, Shimane; 33, Okayama; 34, Hiroshima; 35, Yamaguchi; 36, Tokushima; 37, Kagawa; 38, Ehime; 39, Kochi; 40, Fukuoka; 41, Saga; 42, Nagasaki; 43, Kumamoto; 44, Oita; 45, Miyazaki; 46, Kagoshima; 47, Okinawa.

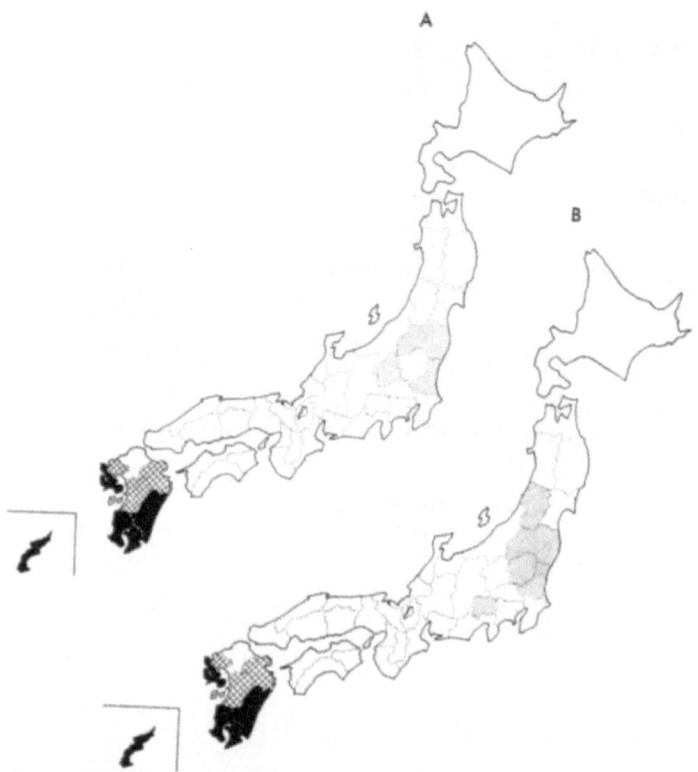

FIG. 3b. Geographical comparison of SMR of malignant lymphomas (ICDs, 200–202) in Japan (1973–1977). A) male. B) female. ■ ≧1.75; ※ 1.25–1.74; □ 0.75–1.24; ▦ ≦0.74.

underdiagnoses of malignant lymphomas. Without more detailed information it is impossible to know whether this increasing trend reflects a true increase in risk factors or merely artificial factors.

Because the proportion of T-cell malignancy among all lymphomas is relatively large in Japan (15, 21) and T-cell lymphoma originates from T-lymphocytes which are quite different from B-lymphocytes in biological characteristics, the etiological risk factors of the two lymphoma types should be separately analyzed.

A geographical comparison of malignant lymphoma shows a marked variation (Fig. 3a, 3b, Table I). In the four prefectures of Kyushu in the southern part of Japan, the standardized mortality ratio (SMR) for malignant lymphoma in adults (older than 24 years) from 1973 to 1977 was twice as high as for all Japan, but this disease was rarely seen in children (younger than 15 years) (15).

According to a nationwide survey performed by the T- and B-cell Malignancy Study Group in 1980 (21), the proportion of patients with T-cell malignancy is very large in Kyushu and southern Shikoku and there is an increasing gradient from north to south (Fig. 4). It was revealed that the excessive rate of adult malignant lymphomas in the Kyushu district was attributable to the very high incidence of adult T-cell malignancy.

TABLE I. Deaths, Standardized Mortality Rations (SMR) and Age-adjusted Mortality Rates (AAMR) of Malignant Lymphomas (ICDs 200–202) by Prefecture in Japan (1973–1977)

		Male			Female		
		Deaths	AAMR[a]	SMR[b]	Deaths	AAMR[a]	SMR[b]
1	Hokkaido	409	3.21	96.8	233	1.67	99.3
2	Aomori	118	3.29	103.0	60	1.42	85.5
3	Iwate	98	2.68	82.4	76	1.73	105.9
4	Miyagi	154	3.29	98.3	75	1.34	80.3
5	Akita	106	3.27	97.7	69	1.79	103.2
6	Yamagata	98	2.81	86.1	50	1.22	70.3*
7	Fukushima	122	2.27	70.6**	53	0.80	50.1**
8	Ibaraki	126	2.12	64.4**	80	1.14	68.9**
9	Tochigi	112	2.58	79.4*	62	1.25	73.4*
10	Gunma	95	2.10	62.9**	70	1.25	78.1*
11	Saitama	238	2.32	74.1**	140	1.26	77.7**
12	Chiba	259	2.80	87.2*	140	1.34	82.1*
13	Tokyo	723	2.77	85.2**	407	1.39	84.6**
14	Kanagawa	348	2.65	79.4**	219	1.50	91.5
15	Niigata	192	2.91	89.2	107	1.35	81.0*
16	Toyama	86	2.94	89.8	52	1.39	88.4
17	Ishikawa	74	2.59	80.3	57	1.65	100.4
18	Fukui	62	2.80	87.3	37	1.42	85.6
19	Yamanashi	60	2.86	82.9	29	1.10	66.0*
20	Nagano	187	3.21	96.4	135	1.76	114.7
21	Gifu	146	2.97	91.6	70	1.21	76.1*
22	Shizuoka	235	2.91	88.4	123	1.29	78.5**
23	Aichi	327	2.51	76.6**	183	1.24	75.6
24	Mie	151	3.36	104.1	81	1.53	91.6
25	Shiga	72	2.84	85.1	51	1.60	98.6
26	Kyoto	227	3.75	113.6	113	1.54	92.6
27	Osaka	612	3.49	107.6	358	1.79	107.9
28	Hyogo	380	3.20	95.7	221	1.54	93.7
29	Nara	94	3.43	106.9	48	1.38	89.4
30	Wakayama	105	3.52	106.1	63	1.68	103.4
31	Tottori	65	3.80	116.7	34	1.45	95.8
32	Shimane	76	3.20	94.5	50	1.58	100.9
33	Okayama	165	3.12	97.0	92	1.40	89.9
34	Hiroshima	225	3.28	99.5	136	1.67	100.8
35	Yamaguchi	152	3.57	106.2	100	1.76	113.9
36	Tokushima	60	2.61	78.3	52	1.84	110.8
37	Kagawa	87	3.19	96.2	58	1.77	104.6
38	Ehime	121	2.92	89.3	74	1.45	89.1
39	Kochi	90	3.58	110.5	56	1.90	108.7
40	Fukuoka	418	3.88	120.2**	238	1.83	111.1
41	Saga	119	5.20	155.1**	68	2.37	138.4**
42	Nagasaki	364	8.82	269.5**	234	4.44	275.3**
43	Kumamoto	226	4.70	142.7**	149	2.39	148.3**
44	Oita	158	4.66	142.1**	101	2.49	146.4**
45	Miyazaki	183	6.31	192.2**	114	3.12	192.2**
46	Kagoshima	325	6.51	197.7**	226	3.41	207.7**
47	Okinawa	130	6.49	190.7**	98	3.64	213.1**
	All	8,980	3.27	100.0	5,342	1.64	100.0

[a] Rate per 100,000 population.   [b] All Japan=100.
Standardized on the age distribution of the Segi's world population.
* $p < 0.05$; ** $p < 0.01$ . . . compared to the SMR of all Japan.

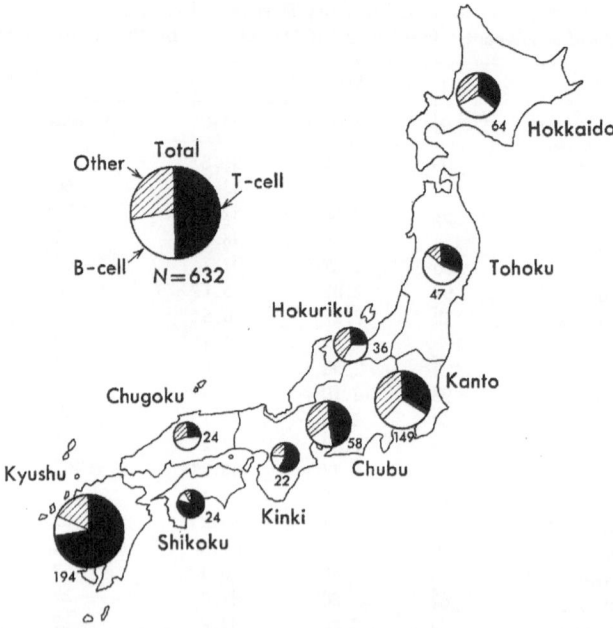

FIG. 4. Geographical distribution of the immunological cell types of 632 patients with lymphoid malignancy (from report of the T- and B-cell Malignancy Study Group, 1981).

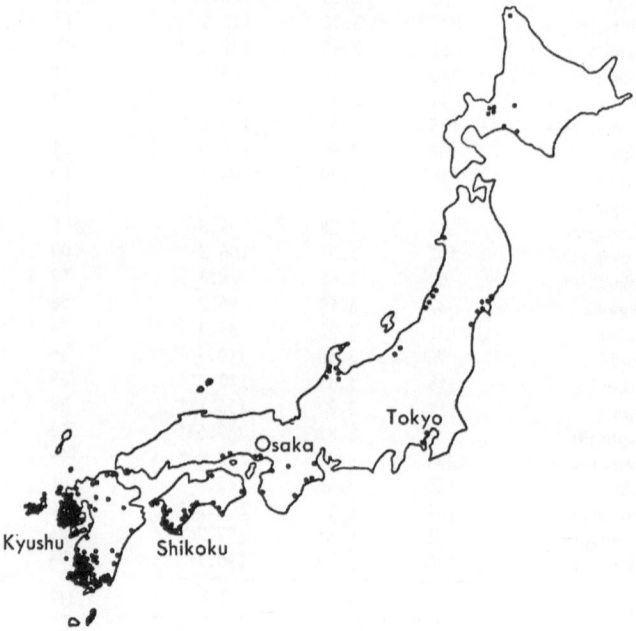

FIG. 5. Distribution of birthplaces of patients with ATL (from report of the T- and B-cell Malignancy Study Group, 1981).

Moreover, the geographical distribution of the birthplaces of patients with "adult T-cell leukemia (ATL)" which was first reported by Takatsuki et al. (20) showed clusters in the coastal areas of Kyushu and southern Shikoku (Fig. 5). It is noted that the birthplaces of ATL patients are localized, mainly in coastal areas, in this southern part of Japan, where it is warm in winter and humid in summer, and it is speculated (15) that some environmental risk factors may therefore exist in these areas.

Clinico-epidemiological Features of ATL and B-cell Malignancy

According to the analyses of the 102 cases of ATL and 162 cases of B-cell malignancy which were collected from 27 institutes throughout Japan by the T- and B-cell Malignancy Study Group (21), marked differences in clinico-epidemiological features were observed between those two types of lymphoid malignancies.

The age distribution of patients with ATL and B-cell malignancy is shown in Figs. 6 and 7 (21). The main age distribution in males was in the 50–59 year group for B cell malignancy and ATL. However, in females it shifted to the 60–69 age group

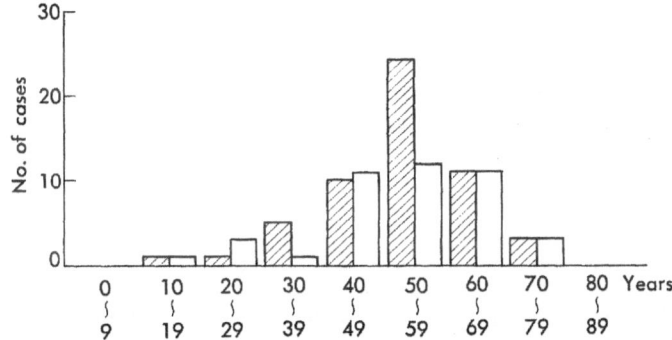

FIG. 6. Age distribution and mean age of 97 patients with ATL (from report of the T- and B-cell Malignancy Study Group, 1981). ▨ males; □ females. Mean age±2S.E.; male 52.9 years±3.0; female 52.4 years±4.1.

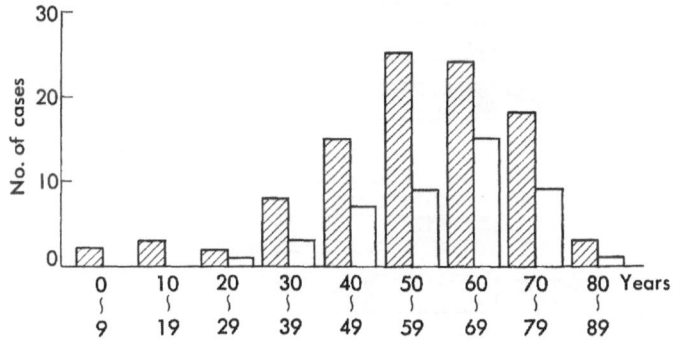

FIG. 7. Age distribution and mean age of 145 patients with B-cell malignancy (from report of the T- and B-cell Malignancy Study Group, 1981). ▨ males; □ females. Mean age±2S.E.; males 55.7 years±3.3; females 58.2 years±4.3.

TABLE II. Mean Age and Male/Female Ratios in Patients with ATL and B-cell Malignancy

Clinical diagnosis	No. of cases	Range	Age (years) (mean±2 S.E.)	Sex ratio (male/female)
ATL	102 (5)	16–78	52.7±2.5	1.3
B-cell malignancy	162 (17)	4–82	59.5±2.6	2.2

Figures in parenthesis indicate the numbers of patients whose ages were unknown.

for B-cell malignancy. The mean age of male patients with ATL was 52.9 years and for B-cell malignancy was 55.7 years. The mean age of female patients with ATL was 52.4, and for B-cell malignancy was 58.2. The age distribution of patients with ATL was younger than that of the patients with B-cell malignancy.

The sex ratio of patients with B-cell malignancy in this series is almost the same (2. 2) as that calculated from the Vital Statistics Japan series for the period 1950–1978 (17). However, the male/female ratio of patients with ATL was 1: 3, the proportion of female patients being larger than that in B-cell malignancy (Table II) (21).

Initial clinical manifestations of patients with ATL are markedly different from those with B-cell malignancy; in the former leukemic manifestation, skin lesion and hepatosplenomegaly appear in larger numbers. (21).

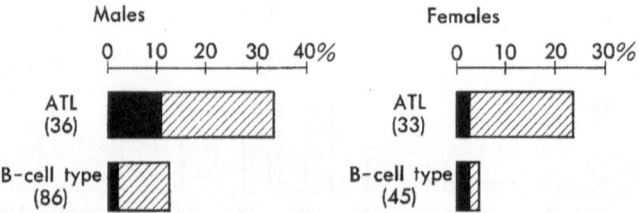

FIG. 8. Proportion of patients with abnormal serum GPT in cases of ATL and B-cell malignancy. Figures in parenthesis indicate the numbers of cases available for analysis (from report of the T- and B-cell Malignancy Study Group, 1981). ■ ≥100IU of GPT; ▨ 41–99 IU of GPT.

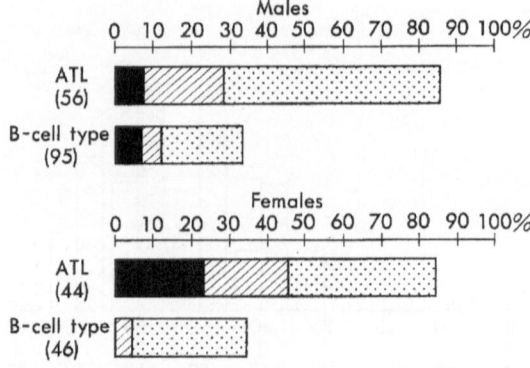

FIG. 9. Proportion of patients with abnormal serum LDH in cases of ATL and B-cell malignancy. Figures in parenthesis indicate the numbers of cases available for analysis (from report of the T- and B-cell Malignancy Study Group, 1981). ■ ≥2,000 IU of LDH; ▨ 1,010–2,000 IU; ▦ 400–1,000IU.

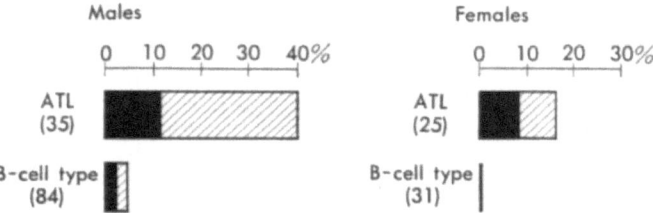

FIG. 10. Proportion of patients with hypercalcemia in cases of ATL and B-cell malignancy. Figures in parenthesis indicate the numbers of cases available for analysis (from report of the T- and B-cell Malignancy Study Group, 1981). ■ ≥ 8.0 mEq of Ca^{2+}/ml; ▨ 5.6–7.9 mEq of Ca^{2+}/ml.

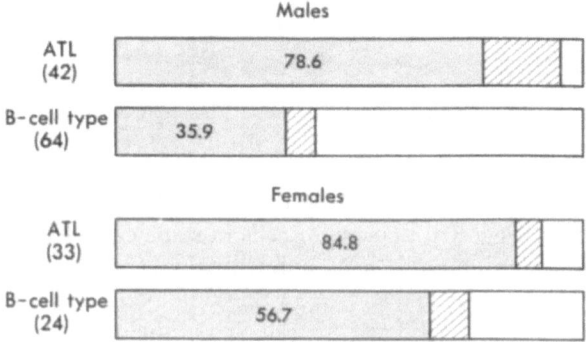

FIG. 11. Distribution of reactions to the PPD skin test in cases of ATL and B-cell malignancy by sex. Figures in parenthesis indicate the numbers of cases available for analysis (from report of the T- and B-cell malignancy Study Group, 1981). ▒ negative; ▨ weakly positive; □ positive.

Results of laboratory data on patients with ATL and B-cell malignancy are shown in Figs. 8–10 (27). Abnormal values of glutamic pyruvic transaminase (GPT) and lactate dehydrogenase (LDH) were detected in few patients with B-cell malignancy but were seen in most patients with ATL and in both sexes because of the frequent line involvement and the advanced clinical stage. Hypercalcemia was observed in 40% of the male patients with ATL and in only 5% with B-cell malignancy. In female patients, hypercalcemia was observed in 16% with ATL and in none with B-cell malignancy. It was suggested that the hypercalcemia was due not only to the release of Ca^{2+} from the bone destroyed by tumor infiltration but also, possibly, to the secretion of some humoral factor from the tumor cells. Such a humoral factor could be a parathyroid hormonelike substance, or some other substance that induces bone reabsorption (12).

As an indication of the activity of cell-mediated immunity, the results of the purified protein derivatives (PPD) skin test were analyzed and are shown in Fig. 11 (27). Because of the impairment of cellular immune function in patients with ATL, the proportion of positive tests was much smaller than those with B-cell malignancy, especially in male patients. However, it is yet to be clarified whether these immunological disorders were a cause of the disease, or whether the function of cellular immunity was disturbed by

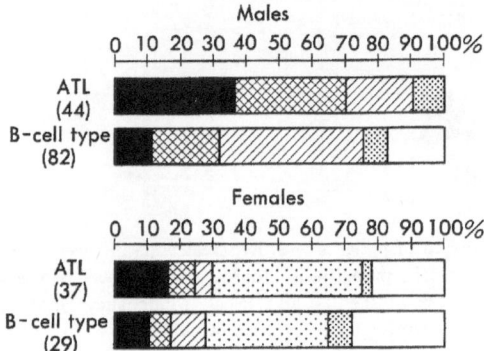

FIG. 12.   Distribution of the occupation of patients with ATL and B-cell malignancy by sex. Figures in parenthesis indicate the numbers of cases available for
analysis (from report of the T- and B-cell malignancy Study Group, 1981).
■ agriculture, fishery and forestry workers; ▨ merchant and operative workers;
▨ clerical professional and technical workers; ▨ houseworkers; ▨ other workers;
☐ without occupation.

tumor cells as a result of the disease. Based on research on tumor cell function in cases
of ATL, it has been suggested that tumor cells in some cases have a suppressive effect
on pokeweed mitogen-induced B-cell differentiation (22). In the case of Sézary
syndrome caused by neoplastic disorders of the same peripheral T-lymphocytes, some
researchers suggested that these leukemic cells have a helper effect on immunoglobulin
synthesis by bone marrow-derived lymphocytes (B-cells) (3).

The 3 year survival rate of patients with ATL was only 1%, but of patients with
B-cell malignancy it was 42% in males and 29% in females.

The distribution of the occupations of male patients with ATL is markedly
different from those with B-cell malignancy (Fig. 12) (21). A larger proportion of the
former whose birthplaces were in rural or coastal areas were engaged in primary in-
dustry.

In addition to this geographical clustering of ATL, a seasonal grouping of the times
of clinical onset, with a peak in the summer, was observed (21). This may provide a
clue in elucidating the etiology of ATL in Japan.

Epidemiological Analysis of the Risk Factors for ATL

Some epidemiological studies on malignant lymphomas have shown time-space
clusters and a characteristic age distribution of several subtypes in the world. Among
them, two endemic lymphomas, Burkitt's lymphoma in Africa and Mediterranean
intestinal lymphoma (5), which show important epidemiological features have been
reported in the world during the last two decades (Table III). It has been revealed
(9) that Epstein-Barr virus may play an important role in the etiology of Burkitt's
lymphoma accompanied by an immunological disturbance with serious malarial
manifestation.

In eastern parts of the Mediterranean coastal area, a particular intestinal lymphoma
with malabsorption and a higher IgA level in the serum is prevalent, mainly in young

TABLE III. Endemic Lymphomas in the World

	Adult T-cell leukemia/lymphoma	Burkitt's lymphoma	Mediterranean intestinal lymphoma
Place	Kyushu, South Shikoku South Kii Peninsula	Tropical Africa New Guinea	Eastern coast of the Mediterranean sea
Geographical features	Coastal areas, warm in winter and humid in summer	Hot and moist area	Moist sea coast area
Age	Adult (40–70 years)	Child (3–12 years)	Young adult
Sex ratio (male/female)	1.3	2.8	1.2
Locality	General lymph nodes and peripheral blood	Jaw and orbita	Small intestine
Familial aggregation	+	+	− ?
Target cell	Peripheral T-cell	B-cell	B-cell
Possible causal agents	ATL virus Filariasis?	Epstein-Barr virus Malaria	Chronic infestation with some antigen
Chromosome abnormality	14q	14q	?
Other features	Helper T-cell	Surface immuno-globulin (IGM)	IgA production

adults. It seems likely that immunological stimulation of the gut by chronic intestinal infestation leads to the development of this intestinal lymphoma (11).

In view of the specific geographical distribution of ATL cases and characteristic climate, the geographical distribution of some kinds of tropical diseases caused by viruses, parasites, and other agents was reviewed to check for vectors which might be related to the cause of ATL. From these analyses it was found (18) that the distribution of filariasis, which is transmitted by several kinds of mosquitoes (Culex pipens pallens, C. tritaeniorhynchus, and Anopheles hyrcanus sinensis), resembled that of ATL. The distribution of Culex pipens pallens is especially similar (10).

Furthermore, the filarial worm which is parasitic in the human body affects the lymphatic vessels, and causes several lymphoreticular ailments, for example, lymph-angitis, lymphadenitis, and high fever. A mass screening test showed that most adult inhabitants in affected areas had a positive intradermal reaction to filarial antigen (1). Therefore, it is possible that people in areas with high rates of microfilaria carriers have frequently been bitten by mosquitoes which transmit microfilaria. It has been reported (23) that some mosquitoes transferred circulating tumor cells of hamster reticulum cell sarcoma from tumor-bearing to tumor-free hamsters. It was also suggested (18) from analyses of the chronological changes of average weight and height of school children by prefecture in Japan that the nutritional condition of inhabitants in Kyushu might have been poorer than that of other districts, especially in the past.

Generally, T-cells in humans are divided, differentiated and maturated in the thymus which appears in the fetus before the fourth month of pregnancy and reaches its maximum development in a child of school (2). It was reported that the progression of the thymic gland and the function of cell mediated immunity are rather related to the nutritional condition. It is noteworthy that the thymic organ markedly involuted after 40 years of age when most patients had contracted ATL.

Recently, a type of RNA virus known as adult T-cell leukemia virus (ATLV) which may be the main agent of the abnormal transformation of T-cells, was identified by Hinuma et al. (6) from cultivated ATL tumor cells (MT1) (8). The sera of all cases

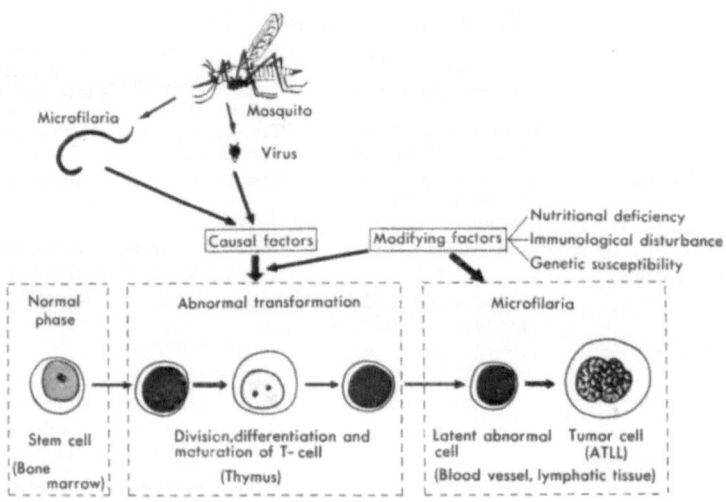

Fig. 13.   Flowchart of our epidemiological hypothesis on the etiology of ATL.

of ATL tested have been shown to be ATLV associated antigen (ATLA) reactive. Also of note is the fact that one-third of the healthy persons older than 40 years in the endemic areas also have positive reactivity to ATLA (*19*).

The role of the genetic factors should not be ignored in the etiology of ATL because of the presence of familial clusters of ATL (*7, 21*), but environmental factors may actually be playing a more important role. Some epidemiological evidence concerning familial infectivity of ATLV (*19*) suggests a route of transmission of this virus among family members from parents to children and between a married couple, especially husband to wife. There is one possibility of the horizontal transmission of not only virus particles but also of T-cells infected with ATLV from repeated biting by mosquitoes.

It was hypothesized from information obtained to date that normal T-cells may be activated by the oncogenic virus (ATLV) in company with repeated stimulation of non-specific antigens such as filarial worm antigens, and then transformed to abnormal T-cell by chance. Malignant transformed T-cells could be carried in the host for a long time and could suddenly begin to divide and multiply due to some disturbance of the immunological regulation depending on the thymus of the host who had so far experienced no adult illness. Nutritional deficiency may be a modifying factor and genetic susceptibility of the host may also be an underlying factor in the etiology of ATL (Fig. 13).

In order to confirm this hypothesis, further studies are planned. Moreover, a nationwide case-control study of ATL is being carried on by the T- and B-cell Malignancy Study Group. Surveys on patients with ATL and the infestation of ATLV in some Southeast Asian countries and in China are also being carried on to clarify the frequency of this disease in the world.

Acknowledgment
   This study was carried out in cooperation with the T- and B-cell Malignancy Study

Group and was supported by Grants-in-Aid for Cancer Research from the Ministry of Health and Welfare (Grant Number 53S-1, 54–29)

REFERENCES

1. Ando, M. Studies on epidemiology and mass-treatment of filariasis. *Kagoshima Igaku Zasshi*, **23**, 133–168 (1971) (in Japanese).
2. Boyd, E. The weight of the thymus gland in health and in disease *Am. J. Child.*, **43**, 1162–1214 (1932).
3. Broder, S., Edelson, R. L., Lutzner, M. A., Nelson, D. L., MacDermott, R. P., Durm, M. E., Goldman, D. K., Meade, B. D., and Waldmann, T. A. The Sézary syndrome. A malignant proliferation of helper T-cells. *J. Clin. Invest.*, **58**, 1297–1306 (1976).
4. Burkitt, D. A sarcoma involving the Jaws in African children. *Br. J. Surg.*, **46**, 218–223 (1958).
5. Fairley, N. T. and Mackie, F. P. The clinical and biochemical syndrome in lymphadenoma and allied diseases involving the mesenteric lymph glands. *Br. Med. J.*, **1**, 375–380 (1937).
6. Hinuma, T., Nagata, K., Hanaoka, M., Nakai, M., Matsumoto, T., Kinoshita, K., Shirakawa, S., and Miyoshi, I. Adult T-cell leukemia: Antigen in an ATL cell line and detection of antibodies to the antigen in human sera. *Proc. Natl. Acad. Sci. U.S.*, **78**, 6478–6480 (1981).
7. Ichimaru, M., Kinoshita, K., Kamihira, S., Ikeda, S., Yamada, Y., and Amagasaki, Y., T-cell malignant lymphoma in Nagasaki district and its problems. *Jpn. J. Clin. Oncol.*, **9** (Suppl. 1), 337–346 (1979).
8. Miyoshi, I., Kubonishi, I., Sumida, M., Yoshimoto, S., Hiraki, S., Tsubota, T., Kobashi, H., Lai, M., Tanaka, T., Kimura, I., Miyamoto, K., and Sato, J. Characteristics of a leukemic T-cell line derived from adult T-cell leukemia. *Jpn. J. Clin. Oncol.*, **9** (Suppl. 1), 485–494 (1979).
9. O'Conor, G. T. Persistent Immunologic stimulation as factor in oncogenesis to a vector virus. *Am. J. Med.*, **48**, 279–285 (1970).
10. Oda, T. Personal communication.
11. Ramot, B. and Many, A. Primary intestinal lymphoma: Clinical manifestations and possible effect of environmental factors. *In* "Recent Results in Cancer Research Current Problems in the Epidemiology of Cancer and Lymphomas," ed. E. Grundmann, pp. 193–199 (1972). Springer-Verlag, Berlin-Heiderberg-New York.
12. Richard, S. N. Hypercalcemia in undifferentiated leukemia. *Cancer*, **30**, 942–944 (1972).
13. Segi, M. "Age-adjusted Death Rates for Cancer for Selected Sites (A-classification) in 46 Countries in 1975" (1980). Segi Institutes of Cancer Epidemiology, Nagoya.
14. Shimizu, H., Tajima, K., Kuroishi, T., Tominaga, S., and Aoki, K. An epidemiological study on mortality from malignant lymphomas in Japan. *J. Jpn. Soc. RES*, **20**, 1–12 (1980) (in Japanese).
15. Tajima, K., Tominaga, S., Kuroishi, T., Shimizu, H., and Suchi, T. Geographical features and epidemiological approach to endemic T-cell leukemia/lymphoma in Japan. *Jpn. J. Clin. Oncol.*, **9** (Suppl. 1), 495–504 (1979).
16. Tajima, K. Epidemiology of malignant lymphoma. *Biomed. Ther.*, **7**, 495–502 (1981) (in Japanese).
17. Tajima, K., Shimizu, H., and Tominaga, S. Epidemiology of malignant lymphoma. *In* "MOOK", ed. M. Ogawa, Vol. 18, pp. 1–13 (1981). Kanehara, Tokyo (in Japanese).

18. Tajima, K., Tominaga, S., Shimizu, H., and Suchi, T. A hypothesis on the etiology of adult T-cell leukemia/lymphoma. *Gann*, **72**, 684–691 (1981).
19. Tajima, K., Tominaga, S., Suchi, T., Kawagoe, T., Komoda, H., Hinuma, Y., Oda, T., and Fujita, K. Epidemiological analysis on distribution of antibody to adult T-cell leukemia-virus-associated antigen (ATLA): Possible horizontal transmission of adult T-cell leukemia virus. *Gann*, **73**, in press.
20. Takatsuki, K., Uchiyama, T., Sagawa, K., and Yodoi, J. Adult T-cell leukemia in Japan. *In* "Topics in Hematology," ed. S. Seno, F. Takaku, and S. Irino, pp. 73–77 (1976). Exerpta Medica, Amsterdam-Oxford.
21. The T- and B-cell Malignancy Study Group. Statistical analysis of immunologic, clinical and histopathologic data on lymphoid malignancies in Japan. *Jpn. J. Clin. Oncol.*, **11**, 15–38 (1981).
22. Uchiyama, T., Yodoi, J., Sagawa, K., Takatsuki, K., and Uchino, H. Adult T-cell leukemia in Japan. Clinical and hematologic features of 16 cases. *Blood*, **50**, 481–492 (1977).
23. Woke, P. A. and Konwinski, N. Insect transfer of labeled erythrocytes, with implications for circulating tumor cells. *J. Natl. Cancer Inst.*, **48**, 219–222 (1972).

ASSOCIATION OF A RETROVIRUS (ATLV) WITH ADULT T CELL LEUKEMIA: REVIEW OF SEROLOGIC STUDIES

Yorio HINUMA

Institute for Virus Research, Kyoto Univeristy*

Most of the serological studies which have been done on a human retrovirus (ATLV) detected in cultured cells of adult T-cell leukemia (ATL) patients from certain areas (mostly southwestern) of Japan, have been done by indirect immunofluorescence. ATLA (ATL-associated antigens), which was later confirmed to be specific for ATLV, was detected in ATL-related T-cell lines but not in other cell lines tested. For detection and titration of antibodies (IgG) to ATLA in human sera, an ATL cell line, MT-1, which contained a low percentage of ATLA positive cells was used. Anti-ATLA was detected in most patients with ATL and in a proportion (5–30%) of healthy adults in ATL(disease)-endemic areas, which correspond to ATLV (virus)-endemic areas. Frequency of seropositive individuals increased gradually with age reaching maximum (about 30%) at 40 years. A high incidence of anti-ATLA-positive individuals in families in an ATLV-endemic area was evident. From this serological observation, two main routes of natural transmission of ATLV were suspected. One was the route from mother to child and the other was husband to wife. Transmission of ATLV by blood transfusion was also suggested based on serological observation. Patients with cutaneous T-cell lymphoma/leukemia (mycosis fungoides and Sézary syndrome) in ATLV-non-endemic areas did not show development of anti-ATLA in their sera.

Adult T-cell leukemia (ATL), also called adult T-cell leukemia/lymphoma (ATLL) because of its leukemic lymphomatous nature, has been suspected to be caused by a virus ever since it was first described by Takatsuki *et al.* in 1977 (*15*) and confirmed by many Japanese investigators in 1980 (*14*) from the following reasons: 1) Human leukemia is probably similar to many leukemias in various animals, which are causally related to tumor viruses. 2) A striking feature of patients with ATL that is they mainly live in southwestern Japan, like patients with African Burkitt lymphoma, which is one of the few human tumors related to a tumor virus, Epstein-Barr virus.

We attempted to detect and isolate a virus causally related to ATL in 1980. In these studies, we found an antigen in an ATL cell line that reacted with sera of all patients with ATL, but not those of healthy adults in ATL-nonendemic areas, as shown by indirect immunofluorescence (*3*). We named this antigen ATL-associated antigen (ATLA) and found that is was related to type C retrovirus, which was detected in the same cell line. These facts strongly suggest a causal relationship between the

---

* Kawara-cho, Shogoin, Sakyo-ku, Kyoto 606, Japan (日沼賴夫).

retrovirus and ATL. Our studies eventually led to the biochemical characterization or a retrovirus in ATL-related cell lines, which we named ATL virus (ATLV) (18). From our results, we strongly suspected that ATLA was specific for ATLV.

ATLA and antibodies to ATLA have been used extensively in an indirect immunofluorescence test in diagnosis of ATL and studies on the epidemiology of ATL in Japan. This article reviews serological studies with this antigen/antibody system on the association of ATLV with ATL.

Determination of Antibodies to ATLA

1. Distinction of ATLA from non-specific staining

As described in a pevious paper (3), anti-ATLA positive human sera gave brilliant immunofluorescence in the cytoplasm of 1–5% of acetone-fixed cells of a ATL cell line, MT-1. The fact that only a small percentage of the MT-1 cells were ATLA-positive *per se* was useful for detection of ATLA-specific antibody in sera, since non-specific reactivities (mostly antibodies or reactants to cellular components), that reacted with almost all cells could be distinguished from anti-ATLA positive cells in a single visual field of stained preparations. The fluorescent ATLA-bearing cells were mononuclear cells or multinuclear giant cells, and the fluorescent antigens showed particulate features and often the shape of inclusion bodies and were localized in the cytoplasm, but not the nucleus. Sometimes a small percentage of the MT-1 cells showed non-specific staining with certain human sera, including anti-ATLA-positive and -negative sera, that differed from staining for ATLA. This non-specific fluorescence(s) was diffusely distributed in both the nucleus and cytoplasm unlike that of ATLA, and could be distinguished from ATLA-fluorescence even when it was present with ATLA-positive cells. The sera that reacted with this diffuse antigen in MT-1 cells also reacted with similar diffuse antigens in all 7 other human lymphoblastoid cell lines tested (one T-cell, 3 B-cell, and 2 non-T non-B lines). Thus it was not specifically related to ATLV or ATL cells.

2.   Immunoglobulin class of ATLA antibodies

The immunoglobulin classes of the antibody that reacted with ATLA were examined in 12 anti-ATLA-positive human sera (from 8 patients with ATL and 2 with other diseases and 2 healthy persons). Anti-ATLA was detected in only IgG, not in IgM, IgA or IgE (Hinuma et al., unpublished data).

3.   Difference between cytoplasmic and membrane antigens

The ATLA demonstrable in air-dried and acetone-fixed cells on glass should include the antigen in the cytoplasma and to also in the membrane to a lesser extend. However, even apparently peripherally localized antigen in fixed cells does not represent only membrane antigen, but rather mainly cytoplasmic antigen. For detection of membrane antigen on the cell surface, suspensions of living cells (or possibly cells lightly fixed with glutaraldehyde) should be stained by a membrane immunofluorescence procedure. In fact, in this way we demonstrated that ATLA-positive cells had cell surface antigen that reacted with anti-ATLA positive human sera. We named this antigen ATLMA (Chosa et al., unpublished data).

ATL-associated Antigen (ATLA)

1. ATLA-positive cells

In the first paper (*3*) on ATLA it was reported that in the indirect immunofluorescence reaction with certain human sera, antigen(s) was demonstrated in the cytoplasm of a few cells of a T-cell line, MT-1, derived from a patient with ATL. The antigen was named ATLA (ATL cell-associated antigen). No ATLA was detected in other human lymphoid cell lines, including six T-cell lines, seven B-cell lines, and four non-T non-B cell lines. The ATLA did not show cross antigenicity with that of any type of human oncogenic virus or one chicken herpesvirus (Marek's disease virus) or one monkey oncogenic herpesvirus (*Herpesvirus saimiri*). The proportion of ATLA-bearing cells was increased by a factor of more than 5 on culture in the presence of 5-iodo-2'-deoxyuridine (IUdR). Antibodies against ATLA in MT-1 cells were found in all 44 patients with ATL examined and in 32 of 40 patients with malignant T-cell lymphomas (most of them with diseases similar to ATL, except that no leukemic cells were detected in their peripheral blood). The antibodies were also detected in 26% of the healthy adults from ATL-endemic areas examined but in only a few of healthy adults from ATL-nonendemic areas examined. On electron microscopy, extracellular type C virus particles were detected in MT-1 cells cultured in the presence of IUdR. Hence, it was concluded that the type C retrovirus found in cultured MT-1 ATL cells is the most probable candidate virus for the antibody to ATLA and that ATLA is probably a virus-associated antigen. Soon after the finding of ATLA and retrovirus in MT-1 cell lines, we (*6*) demonstrated that 100% of the cells had ATLA in another ATL-related cell line, MT-2, which was established by co-culture of ATL cells from a female patient with normal human cord leukocytes from a male infant. Simultaneously, numerous type C retrovirus particles were detected by electron microscopy in the cells.

ATLA has been found not only in established long-term cultures of ATL cells, but also in short-term cultures of fresh leukemic cells of peripheral blood from ATL patients. ATLA was detectable in the fresh leukemic cells only after, but not before, their *in vitro* culture (*4*). Surprisingly ATLA as well as retrovirus particles was found in short-term cultures of peripheral leukocytes from anti-ATLA-positive healthy adults (*1, 7*). This finding shows that anti-ATLA positive individuals may be healthy carriers of ATLV. These findings suggest that replication of ATLV or formation of ATLA is mostly, but not entirely, suppressed *in vivo*, but that its suppression is released during *in vitro* culture.

2. Analysis of ATLA-related polypeptides

All these findings strongly suggested, but did not prove, that ATLA is specific for ATLV in these cells. Therefore further studies were undertaken to determine whether the ATLA is specific for ATLV (*16*). By use of sera from patients with ATL or healthy adults, in which anti-ATLA had been determined by indirect immunofluorescence, ATLA was analysed by a procedure of immunoprecipitation followed by SDS-polyacrylamide gel electrophoresis. For this, an ATLV-producer cell line, MT-2, was labeled with [^{35}S] methionine. All 12 anti-ATLA positive sera but none of the 8 anti-ATLA negative sera tested reacted specifically with 4 polypeptides with

molecular weights of 76,000, 53,000, 36,000, and 24,000 daltons. Furthermore, en-
richment of 3 polypeptides of 76,000, 43,000, and 28,000 daltons was observed on
reaction with anti-ATLA-positive sera. In control experiments using the ATLA-negative T-cell lines Motl-4 and HPB-ALL, none of these 7 polypeptides were precipitated
by reaction with anti-ATLA positive sera. All 6 anti-ATLA-positive sera tested were
shown .to react with a polypeptide of ATLV with a molecular weight of 24,000 (p24)
purified by sucrose density gradient centrifugation.

The fact that anti-ATLA-positive sera apparently precipitated only p24 of the
many viral structural polypeptides (p11, p14, p17, p24, and p45 at least) (*12*, *14*)
might be due to the very small quantity of labeled materials in purified virus fractions or to the very low levels of antibodies to other virus polypeptides in the sera.
Several questions remain to be answered: first, are p70, p53, and p28 actually viral
proteins or precursor polypeptides? In particular, is p70 a glycoprotein like gp70 of
other retrovirus, or a primary translational product that is later processed into smaller
polypeptides, like the polypeptides of other known retroviruses? Second, are the three
polypeptides (p76, p43, and p28) that show stronger reactivity with anti-ATLA-
positive sera than with anti-ATLA-negative sera really ATLA specific? Studies are
in progress on these questions and to obtain basic information for development of an
ATLV vaccine.

Antibodies to ATLA in Human Sera

1. Seroepidemiology of ATLV

As mentioned already, we found antibodies to ATLA (anti-ATLA) not only in
sera from ATL patients but also in those from healthy adults living in ATLA-endemic
areas in Japan (*3*). Then we made a nation-wide seroepidemiologic survey of ATLV,
detected as anti-ATLA (*5*).

The prevalence of ATLA antibody was determined in sera from adults of 40 years
old or over, since 40 years is the age at which the incidence of anti-ATLA is maximal.
These adults were healthy or had non-malignant diseases and were born and living in
15 different regions of Japan. High incidences (6 to 37%) of anti-ATLA-positive donors
were found in seven regions, one is northern Japan, and the other southwestern regions.
The presence of anti-ATLA in sera could the due to current or past infection with
ATLV. Indeed, our recent studies demonstrated that all the anti-ATLA-positive individuals, including both ATL patients and healthy donors, had ATLA bearing
(ATLV-carrying) T-cells in their peripheral blood (*1*, *4*). Hence, areas in which the
incidence of anti-ATLA-positive residents is high may be ATLV (virus)-endemic
areas, which correspond to ATL (disease)-endemic areas.

Examination of sera from healthy donors aged 6 to 80 years old ATLV-endemic
areas showed that the frequency of seropositive individuals increased gradually with
age, starting from a minimum (about 2%) at 6 to 10 years old and reaching a maximum
(about 30%) at 40 to 60 years old. However it is not clear yet why the incidence of
anti-ATLA gradually increases with age, specially in a relatively late period of life.

2. Familial incidence of anti-ATLA positive persons

Studies of the family trees of anti-ATLA-positive and -negative persons (Tajima *et al.*, unpublished data) showed a high incidence of anti-ATLA-positive individuals in individual families in an ATLV-endemic area. Several points were noticeable: Many women from families where most members were anti-ATLA-positive were married to men from ATLA-negative families and their children were ATLA-positive. Some children of ATLA-positive parents were anti-ATLA-positive but other children were anti-ATLA-negative. No children were anti-ATLA-positive in families in which both parents both were anti-ATLA-negative. There were few husband-positive/wife-negative couples, but husband-positive/wife-positive and husband-negative/wife-positive couples were fairly commonly. From these serological observations, two main routes of natural transmission of ATLV were suspected. One was the route from mother to child and other was horizontal, especially from husband to wife.

3. *Transfusion of anti-ATLA-positive blood*

Okochi *et al.* (unpublished data) observed that in 3 of 6 recipients of transfused blood containing formed elements from donors having ATLA antibody, anti-ATLA became demonstratable about one month or later after transfusion. This serologic result suggest transmission of ATLV by transfusion of lymphocytes contained in blood components, if the presence of anti-ATLA indicates persistent infection of ATLV. Sometimes anti-ATLA-positive adults were found in ATLV-nonendemic areas and it was evident that many of them had a history of blood transfusion in the past, suggesting ATLV transmission by transfusion.

The seroepidemiologic survey strongly suggested that ATLV may be found in a minority of residents in quite restricted regions of each island of Japan. This pattern may represent a relatively poor capacity of spread of ATLV among humans. This restriction of spread of virus does not resemble those of other highly contagious human viruses, such as entroviruses, myxoviruses, and herpesviruses, but resembles that of hepatitis B virus.

4. *Incidence of anti-ATLA in various diseases*

Almost all the 127 ATL patients in ATLV-endemic areas and all 15 ATL patients in ATLV-nonendemic areas tested were anti-ATLA-positive. The geometric mean titer (about 82) of anti-ATLA of ATL patients was higher than that (about 45) of healty subjects (5). In this study, two of the 142 patients with ATL were anti-ATLA-negative. In another study (13), two anti-ATLA-negative ATL patients were also found in ATLV-nonendemic areas. It will be interesting to clarify whether there are any differences in the clinical and hematological features of anti-ATLA-positive and -negative ATL patients. It is possible that certain ATL patients infected with ATLV do not develop detectable antibody to ATLV, because of either tolerance or insufficiency, or some other failure, of their immune response.

Of 8 adult patients with malignant T-cell lymphomas except ATL, mycosis fungoides, and Sézary syndrome, 6 had anti-ATLA. In many cases, malignant T-cell lympoma may change to leukemia during the course of the diesase. For this reason, ATL has been called ATLL. There are also certain adult malignant T-cell lymphomas distinct from ATLL, and most of them may by anti-ATLA-negative.

So-called cutaneous T-cell lymphoma/leukemias (CTCL) including mycosis fungoides and Sézary syndrome are known to be distributed throughout the world and not to be malignant. However, these diseases resemble ATL accompanied cutaneous affection in clinical and hematohistological features.

None of 12 CTCL patients (10 patients with mycosis fungoides and 2 with Sézray syndrome) in ATLV-nonendemic areas had anti-ATLA, suggesting that ATLV has no relation to CTCL. On the other hand, 6 of 9 patients with CTCL in ATL-endemic areas had anti-ATLA. This positive rate (66%) was much higher than that (about 25%) of ATLA antibody-positive adults in ATLV-endemic areas. Therefore, CTCL may be difficult to distinguish from anti-ATLA-positive ATL with cutaneous affection in ATL-endemic areas. This might lead to the higher incidence of anti-ATLA-positive CTCL patients, unlike in ATLV-nonendemic areas.

Thus ATLV may not in fact be related to CTCL, although Poiesz et al. (10, 11) considered that their retrovirus (HTLV) might be closely related to CTCL, because it was isolated from patients with CTCL. Very recently, Robert-Guroff et al. (12) reported that the sera of 6 of 7 patients with Japanese ATL had antibodies to HTLV isolated from Amerian patients with CTCL. However, they found it difficult to understand why antibodies to HTLV occur only rarely in patients with CTCL, from which HTLV was isolated, but very frequently in Japanese ATL patients. As a possible explanation, they suggested that the antibody-positive American CTCL might be of the same type as Japanese ATL. This problem must be examined by direct comparative studies not only on isolated Japanese ATLV and American HTLV, but also on Japanese and American CTCL and Japanese ATL. Robert-Guroff et al. also mentioned that none of the 39 healthy Japanese donors (whose ages were not mentioned) tested in an ATL-endemic area, Shikoku Island, had antibody to HTLV. This finding is different from our finding of a high incidence of anti-ATLA in adult donors in an ATL-endemic area, Uwajima in Shikoku. This discrepancy could be explained by selection of different areas of the island and different ages of blood donors for tests, if HTLV and ATLV are similar or identical.

CONCLUDING REMARKS

Henle and Henle's view (2) with slight modification is to that establish a link between a given virus and a specific malignancy four experimental approaches can be used:
1. Demonstration of viral genomes, viral antigens or viral particles in leukemic or lymphoma cells *in vivo* or in cultured neoplastic cells.
2. Transformation of normal blood cells by the retrovirus *in vitro*.
3. Induction of leukemia or lymphoma by the retrovirus in the homologous or a different animal species.
4. Detection of a broader spectrum and higher titers of virus-related antibodies in bearers of leukemia or lymphoma than in controls.

Henle and Henle reported this approach for studies of oncogenic herpesvirus (2). However, it can also be unequivocally applied to retroviruses. In agreement with their statement, each approach provides more or less significant evidence but none *per se* proves a causal relationship.

The first approach, the demonstration of proviral DNA of ATLV (*18*), ATLV antigens or particles (*3, 4, 6*) in fresh leukemic cells of peripheral blood of ATL patients or in cultures of ATL cells afforded strong evidence of an association.

According to the second approach, normal umbilical cord or adult peripheral lymphocytes were transformed by co-culture with the ATLV-carrier cell line, MT-2 (*8, 17*). Transformation by cell-free ATLV has not been achieved. Miyoshi *et al.* (*9*) reported transformation of normal lymphocytes of a Japanese monkey (*Macaca tuscata*) by co-culture with the MT-2 cell line.

Studies on the third approach, the induction of tumors or leukemia in experimental animals by infection with ATLV, are in progress.

Virus-related serological evidence, the fourth approach, is the main theme of this article. It was evident (*5*) that there were high incidences (more than 5%) of adults having antibodies to ATLV (anti-ATLA) in ATLV (virus)-endemic areas corresponding to ATL (disease)-endemic areas. Anti-ATLA was found in all but a few of more than 140 patients from ATL-endemic areas, but in only a few of those from ATL-nonendemic areas. The titer of anti-ATLA of ATL patients was about twice that of healthy donors. However, the antibodies against ATLV showed a broader spectrum in ATL patients than in healthy subject, because antibodies that form complexes with ATLV-associated antigens, which include ATLA and other ATLV-encoded antigens, have not been well characterized up to date. Further serological evidence is needed for definite proof of an eitological association of ATL with ATLV.

REFERENCES

1. Gotoh, Y., Sugamura, K., and Hinuma, Y. Healthy carriers of a human retrovirus, adult T-cell leukemia virus (ATLV): Demonstration by clonal culture of ATLV-carrying T-cell from peripheral blood. *Proc. Natl. Acad. Sci. U.S.*, **79**, 4780–4782 (1982).

2. Henle, W. and Henle, G. Comparison of immune responses and viral markers in herpesviruses-associated carcinomas: A review. *In* "Oncogenesis and Herpesviruses III," ed. G. de The', W. Henle, and F. Rapp, Part II, pp. 801–813 (1978). IARC, Lyon.

3. Hinuma, Y., Nagata, K., Hanaoka, M., Nakai, M., Matsumoto, T., Kinoshita, K., Shirakawa, S., and Miyoshi, I. Adult T-cell leukemia: Antigen in an ATL cell line and detection of antibodies to the antigen in human sera. *Proc. Natl. Acad. Sci. U.S.*, **78**, 6476–6480 (1981).

4. Hinuma, Y., Gotoh, Y., Sugamura, K., Nagata, K., Goto, T., Nakai, M., Kamada, N., Matsumoto, T., and Kinoshita, K. A retrovirus associated with human adult T-cell leukemia: *In vitro* activation. *Gann*, **73**, 341–344 (1982).

5. Hinuma, Y., Komoda, H., Chosa, T., Kondo, T., Kohakura, M., Takenaka, T., Kikuchi, M., Ichimaru, M., Yunoki, K., Sato, I., Matsuo, R., Takiuchi, Y., Uchino, H., and Hanaoka, M. Antibodies to adult T-cell leukemia virus-associated antigen (ATLA) in sera from patients with ATL and controls in Japan: A nation-wide seroepidemiologic study. *Int. J. Cancer*, **29**, 631–635 (1982).

6. Miyoshi, I., Kubonishi, I., Yoshimoto, S., Akagi, T., Ohtsuki, Y., Shiraishi, Y., Nagata, K., and Hinuma, Y. Detection of type C virus particles in a cord leukocytes and human leukemic T-cells. *Nature*, **296**, 770–771 (1981).

7. Miyoshi, I., Taguchi, H., H., Fujishita, M., Niiya, K., Kitagawa, T., Ohtsuki, Y., and Akagi, T. Asymptomatic type C virus carriers in the family of an adult T-cell leukemia patient. *Gann*, **73**, 339–340 (1982).

8. Miyoshi, I., Yoshimoto, S., Kubonishi, I., Taguchi, H., Shiraishi, Y., Ohtsuki, Y., and Akagi, T. Transformation of normal human cord lymphocytes by co-cultivation with lethally irradiated human T-cell line carrying type C virus particles. *Gann*, **72**, 997–998 (1981).

9. Miyoshi, I., Taguchi, H., Fujishita, M., Yoshimoto, S., Kubonishi, I., Ohtsuki, Y., Shiraishi, Y., and Akagi, T. Transformation of monkey lymphocytes with adult T-cell leukemia virus. *Lancet*, **i**, 1016 (1982).

10. Poiesz, B. J., Ruscetti, F. W., Gazdar, A. F., Bunn, P. A., Minna, J. D., and Gallo, R. G. Detection and isolation of type C retrovirus particles from fresh and cultured lymphocytes of a patient with cutaneous T-cell lymphoma. *Proc. Natl. Acad. Sci. U.S.*, **77**, 7415–7419 (1980).

11. Poiesz, B. J., Ruscetti, F. W., Reitz, M. S., Kalyanaraman, V. S., and Gallo, R. C. Isolation of a new type C retrovirus (HTLV) in primary uncultured cells of a patient with Sézary T-cell leukemia. *Nature*, **294**, 268–271 (1981).

12. Robert-Guroff, M., Nakao, Y., Notake, K., Ito, Y., Sliski, A., and Gallo, R. C. Natural antibodies to human retrovirus HTLV in a cluster of Japanese patients with adult T-cell leukemia. *Science*, **215**, 975–978 (1982).

13. Simoyama, M., Minato, K., Tobinai, K., Horikoshi, N., Ikuba, T., Deura, K., Nagatani, T., Ozaki, Y., Inada, N., Komoda, H., and Hinuma, Y. Anti-ATLA (antibody to the adult T-cell leukemia cell associated antigen) positive hematologic malignancies in Kanto District, Japan. *Jpn. J. Clin. Oncol.*, **12**, 109–116 (1982).

14. The T- and B-cell Malignancy Study Group. Statistical analysis of immunologic, clinical and histophathologic data on lymphoid malignancies in Japan. *Jpn. J. Clin. Oncol.*, **11**, 15–38 (1981).

15. Takatsuki, K., Uchiyama, T., Sagawa, K., and Yodoi, I. Adult T-cell leukemia in Japan. *In* "Topics in Hematology", ed. S. Seno, F. Takaku, and S. Irino, pp. 73–77 (1977). Excerpta Medica, Amsterdam.

16. Yamamoto, N. and Hinuma, Y. Antigens in an adult T-cell leukemia virus-producer cell line: Reactivity with human serum antibodies. *Int. J. Cancer*, in press.

17. Yamamoto, N., Okada, M., Koyanagi, Y., Kannagi, M., and Hinuma, Y. Transformation of human leukocytes by co-cultivation with an adult T-cell leukemia virus (ATLV) producer-cell line. *Science*, **217**, 737–739 (1982).

18. Yoshida, M., Miyoshi, I., and Hinuma, Y. Isolation and characterization of human adult T-cell leukemia and its implication in the disease. *Proc. Natl. Acad. Sci. U.S.*, **79**, 2031–2035 (1982).

TYPE C VIRUS-PRODUCING CELL LINES DERIVED FROM ADULT T CELL LEUKEMIA

Isao Miyoshi,*¹ Hirokuni Taguchi,*¹ Ichiro Kubonishi,*¹
Shizuo Yoshimoto,*¹ Yuji Ohtsuki,*² Yukimasa Shiraishi,*³
and Tadaatsu Akagi*²

*Departments of Medicine,*¹ *Pathology,*² *and Anatomy,*³
Kochi Medical School

We have established four unique cell lines, MT-1 to MT-4, by co-cultivation of adult T-cell leukemia (ATL) cells and human cord blood lymphocytes. All four cell lines possessed T-cell properties and lacked Epstein-Barr virus nuclear antigen. Chromosome analysis revealed MT-1 to be of ATL cell origin whereas at least two others, MT-2 and MT-3, were of cord lymphocyte origin. All these cell lines were found to be persistently infected with type C virus particles (ATLV) and positive for ATL-associated antigens (ATLA) which reacted specifically with sera from ATL patients. MT-2 was the highest producer of ATLV and MT-1 the lowest. The three cell lines tested, MT-1 to MT-3, were tumorigenic when transplanted into immunosuppressed newborn hamsters. Only the tumors produced with MT-3 were examined for virus and they were positive for ATLV and ATLA. Lymphoid cell lines with human chromosomes were readily recultured from MT-3-induced tumors.

Co-cultivation of human cord lymphocytes and lethally X-irradiated MT-2 cells gave rise to ATLV-producing cord T-cell lines. Cell-free ATLV, however, failed to transform cord lymphocytes. These findings strongly suggest that ATLV may be related to the etiology of ATL.

Adult T-cell leukemia (ATL) is a newly recognized disease which occurs endemically in southwestern Japan (*11, 12*). In 1978, we established an ATL cell line, MT-1, by cultivating ATL cells with feeder layers derived from human cord blood leukocytes (*3, 4*). Subsequently, the same co-culture procedure yielded three more cell lines. Chromosome analysis unexpectedly revealed that at least two of them, MT-2 and MT-3, were derived from cord lymphocytes (*6*). All four cell lines expressed T-cell markers and lacked Epstein-Barr virus nuclear antigen (EBNA). These four cell lines were later found to be persistently infected with type C virus particles (ATLV) and positive for ATL-associated antigens (ATLA) which reacted specifically with sera from ATL patients (*1, 5*).

Gallo and his associates (*9, 10*) at the National Cancer Institute also established two T-cell lines, with the use of T-cell growth factor, from patients with cutaneous

*¹, *², *³ Okō-cho, Nankoku-shi, Kochi 781-51, Japan (三好勇夫, 田口博国, 久保西一郎, 吉本静雄, 大朏祐治, 白石行正, 赤木忠厚).

T-cell lymphoma (mycosis fungoides and Sézary syndrome) and detected type C virus particles (HTLV) in both. These independent observations in the United States and Japan strongly suggest that type C virus is etiologically related to certain T-cell malignancies of man.

Establishment and Characteristics of ATLV-producing Cell Lines (Table I)

1. MT-1

The co-culture technique used for the establishment of MT-1 and characteristics of this cell line have been reported (3, 4). Briefly, ATL cells were co-cultured with feeder layers derived from human cord blood leukocytes for about 2 months, after which a continuous line of lymphoid cells was obtained. We used this technique with the hope of stimulating the growth of ATL cells by the feeder layers which usually had a limited life span in vitro. The donor was a 69-year-old patient and his ATL cells were co-cultured with cord leukocytes derived from a female infant. Chromosome analysis of MT-1 showed a male karyotype with a 14q+ chromosome and other complex structural abnormalities (4, 7). MT-1 cells produced serially transplantable lethal tumors in newborn hamsters treated with antilymphocyte serum (4). In 1981, a great discovery was made on MT-1 by Hinuma et al. (7); they found a few percent of ATLA-positive cells by indirect immunofluorescence and a small number of ATLV by electron microscopy. This observation gave an immediate impetus to the search for ATLV in the other ATL-related cell lines maintained in our laboratory.

2. MT-2

Since the MT-1 line was established from ATL cells by co-cultivating with feeder layers derived from human cord leukocytes, attempts were made to confirm this observation using the same co-culture technique. Co-cultivation of ATL cells from three

TABLE I. Cell Lines Derived by Co-culture of ATL Cells and Human Cord Leukocytes

	MT-1	MT-2	MT-3	MT-4
Patient	M. T.	S. O.	N. K.	A. I.
Age/sex	69/M	45/F	36/M	50/M
Culture of ATL cell	78-7-25	79-11-21	78-11-20	79-3-7
Infant/sex	F	M	M	M
Culture of cord cell	9-17	80-1-19	79-1-19	4-25
Co-culture	9-30	1-23	1-30	5-3
Subculture	11-30	3-16	4-8	6-17
Chromosome	14q+, −X, dup Yq	46,XY	46,XY	Polyploid, markers
E rosettes	85%	60%	34%	48%
Leu-1	98%	56%	85%	91%
OKI1	95%	100%	85%	92%
EBNA	0%	0%	0%	0%
ATLA	1-2%	100%	100%	85%
ATLV	+	╫	╫	╫
Xenograft	Yes	Yes	Yes	NT

The amount of ATLV is roughly estimated by electron microscopy. NT, not tested.

patients and cord leukocytes from three infants resulted in the establishment of three T-cell lines, MT-2 to MT-4, respectively. In the case of MT-2, a female patient's ATL cells were deliberately co-cultured with a male infant's cord leukocytes to make the identification of the established cell line easy. Chromosome analysis of MT-2 showed a normal male karyotype and its cord leukocyte origin (6). This was unexpected since no continuous culture line of T-cells was ever derived from human cord lymphocytes. The MT-2 line grew in suspension forming clumps of cells (Photo 1). Under the phase contrast microscope, MT-2 cells showed peculiar bulbous or hairy cytoplasmic projections (Photo 2). The cells were mostly immature lymphoid cells and mononuclear or multinuclear giant cells were often present (Photo 3). Almost 100% of the MT-2 cells showed brilliant ATLA staining in the cytoplasm when reacted with ATL patients' sera by indirect immunofluorescence (7) (Photo 4). Electron microscopy revealed a large number of ATLV in the extracellular spaces (Photos 5 and 6). ATLV measured about 80–150 nm in diameter and mostly had the morphology of mature type C virus particles. Immature or budding virus particles were rarely observed. These findings were reported elsewhere (5).

3. MT-3

The MT-3 line was established by co-cultivation of ATL cells from a male patient and cord leukocyte from a male infant. The origin of MT-3 was identified by comparison of karyotypes of the patient's ATL cells and MT-3 cells. The fresh ATL cells from the patient had chromosome abnormalities including a 14q+ marker as described previously (7), while the MT-3 line showed a normal male karyotype. Thus, it was considered that this cell line was derived from cord leukocytes, although its normal lymphocyte origin in the patient could not be completely excluded. MT-3 most closely resembled MT-2 not only in morphology but also in surface and antigen markers. In addition, MT-3 cells were almost 100% ATLA-positive and carried a moderate number of ATLV.

Heterotransplantation of MT-1 and MT-2 was performed before we knew about ATLV in these cell lines and the tumors produced in the heterologous hosts were not examined for ATLV. In a recent study, 1×10^7 MT-3 cells were implanted intraperitoneally into four newborn hamsters treated with antilymphocyte serum by the method described previously (4). After 2 weeks, two of them died apparently from tumor growth and the remaining two were sacrificed. At autopsy there were inguinal tumors and massive growth of mesenteric and retroperitoneal tumors with invasion of the neighboring organs (Photo 7). The histologic picture of these tumors was consistent with diffuse pleomorphic lymphoma (Photo 8). Invasive growth of cells was present in the liver (Photo 9) and genital organs and also a metastatic focus was found in the lung. The smears of tumor cell suspensions were immunofluorescently stained with ATL patients' sera and almost 100% of the cells were positive for ATLA (Photo 10). Electron microscopy of the tumors showed a moderate number of ATLV in the extracellular spaces (Photo 11). The tumors from two bearing-hamsters were recultured and a lymphoid cell line was readily established from each animal. Chromosome analysis of the recultured cell lines demonstrated a normal human male karyotype (Photo 12).

4. MT-4

The MT-4 line was similarly obtained by co-cultivation of ATL cells and human cord leukocytes. Chromosome analysis of MT-4 showed a polyploid constitution and marker chromosomes. Since the patient and infant whose leukocytes were co-cultured were both males and the patient's ATL cells were not cytogenetically studied, no conclusion could be reached as to the cell origin of MT-4. In other aspects, MT-4 resembled MT-2 and MT-3, although not all MT-4 cells were ATLA-positive and the number of ATLV was less than in MT-2 and MT-3.

Transformation of Human Cord Blood Lymphocytes by ATLV

As described above, co-cultivation of ATL cells and human cord leukocytes led to the establishment of four ATLV-producing T-cell lines. At least two of the four cell lines were shown to have originated from cord lymphocytes by chromosome analysis. This observation suggested that during co-culture of ATL cells and human cord leukocytes, ATLV or its genome was transmitted from ATL cells to cord T-cells and that the infected T-cells were transformed into ATLV-producers. In the following experiment to test the transforming ability of ATLV, we used the MT-2 line as the source of ATLV, because electron microscopic observation had shown that this cell line harbored a large number of ATLV.

Two methods of ATLV infection were used: one used cell-free filtrates of supernatant MT-2 culture fluids or of MT-2 culture materials subjected to three cycles of

TABLE II. Transformation of Normal Cord Lymphocytes with ATLV

	No. cord leukocyte samples	
	Cultured	Transformed
Untreated controls	2	0
Infected with MT-4 culture filtrates	4	0
Co-cultured with irradiated MT-2 cells	2	2

TABLE III. Cell Lines Derived from Cord Lymphocytes
by Co-culture with Irradiated MT-2 Cells

	Ok	Re
Infant/sex	F	F
Culture of cord cell	81-6-27	81-9-23
Radiation dose	6,000R	10,000R
Co-culture	7-8	10-3
Subculture	8-8	11-5
Chromosome	46,XX	46,XX
E rosettes	66%	55%
Leu-1	88%	95%
OKI1	92%	100%
EBNA	0%	0%
ATLA	100%	100%
ATLV	++	++

The amount of ATLV is roughly estimated by electron microscopy.

freezing and thawing, and the other used lethally X-irradiated MT-2 cells. Human cord lymphocytes separated by Ficoll-Conray gradient centrifugation were used as target cells of ATLV infection. Infection of cord lmphocytes with cell-free ATLV was carried out at 37°C for 2 hr and the cells were cultured in 35 mm Petri dishes using RPMI 1640 medium supplemented with 10% human cord serum, 10% fetal calf serum and antibiotics. Usually two Petri dishes containing 1×10^6 cells/ml were prepared for each cord blood sample. As shown in Table II, control cord leukocytes did not grow for more than 2 months. It was rather unexpected that all four cord leukocyte samples infected with cell-free ATLV failed to be transformed. In contrast, co-cultivation of cord lymphocytes and lethally irradiated MT-2 cells gave rise to a cord T-cell line in both of two cases (8). Table III shows two cell lines, Ok and Re, thus derived by the co-culture procedure. Cord leukocytes from female infants were first cultured at 1×10^6 cells/ml in two dishes, and 10–11 days later 1×10^6 lethally irradiated (6,000–10,000 R) MT-2 cells were added to each dish. After about one month of co-culture, the cells were first subcultured and have since been maintained in continuous culture. X-irradiated MT-2 cells cultured alone did not proliferate.

Both Ok and Re had a normal female karyotype distinct from the male karyotype of MT-2 used for co-culture. The growth pattern, morphology, and surface and antigen markers of both cell lines were almost identical to those of MT-2. Moreover, the two cell lines were almost 100% positive for ATLA when reacted with ATL patients' sera and found to carry a moderate number of ATLV by electron microscopy.

The *in vitro* transformation of human cord lymphocytes by ATLV is an important advance, because there has been no report of type C virus-induced human lymphocyte transformation. Studies now in progress indicate that human adult normal lymphocytes can also be transformed by the same co-culture method. In contrast to the B-cell transforming Epstein-Barr virus (2), ATLV appears to be a T-lymphotropic virus. Thus, it is now possible to transform both B- and T-cells from the same donor for comparative studies involving not only viral oncogenesis but also immunology and cytogenetics. At present, the failure of cell-free ATLV to transform normal human lymphocytes is difficult to explain; however, the results suggest that ATLV is transmissible by cell-to-cell contact or by cell-fusion.

Acknowledgments

This work was supported by Grants-in-Aid for Cancer Research from the Japanese Ministry of Education, Science and Culture and from the Japanese Foundation for Multidisciplinary Treatment of Cancer, and by a Princess Takamatsu Cancer Research Grant.

REFERENCES

1. Hinuma, Y., Nagata, K., Hanaoka, M., Nakai, M., Matsumoto, T., Kinoshita, K., Shirakawa, S., and Miyoshi, I. Adult T-cell leukemia: Antigen in an ATL cell line and detection of antibodies to the antigen in human sera. *Proc. Natl. Acad. Sci. U.S.*, **78**, 6476–6480 (1982).
2. Klein, G. The Epstein-Barr virus and neoplasia. *N. Engl. J. Med.*, **293**, 1353–1357 (1975).
3. Miyoshi, I., Kubonishi, I., Sumida, M., Hiraki, S., Tsubota, T., Kimura, I., Miyamoto, K., and Sato, J. A novel T-cell line derived from adult T-cell leukemia. *Gann*, **71**, 155–156 (1980).

4. Miyoshi, I., Kubonishi, I., Sumida, M., Yoshimoto, S., Hiraki, S., Tsubota, T., Kobashi, H., Lai, M., Tanaka, T., Kimura, I., Miyamoto, K., and Sato, J. Characteristics of a leukemic T-cell line derived from adult T-cell leukemia. *Jpn. J. Clin. Oncol.*, **9** (Suppl.), 485–494 (1979).

5. Miyoshi, I., Kubonishi, I., Yoshimoto, S., Akagi, T., Ohtsuki, Y., Shiraishi, Y., Nagata, K., and Hinuma, Y. Type C virus particles in a cord T-cell line derived by co-cultivating normal human cord leukocytes and human leukaemic T-cells. *Nature*, **294**, 770–771 (1981).

6. Miyoshi, I., Kubonishi, I., Yoshimoto, S., and Shiraishi, Y. A T-cell line derived from normal human cord leukocytes by co-culturing with human leukemic T-cells. *Gann*, **72**, 978–981 (1981).

7. Miyoshi, I., Miyamoto, K., Sumida, M., Nishihara, R., Lai, M., Yoshimoto, S., Sato, J., and Kimura, I. Chromosome 14q+ in adult T-cell leukemia. *Cancer Genet. Cytogenet.*, **3**, 251–259 (1981).

8. Miyoshi, I., Yoshimoto, S., Kubonishi, I., Taguchi, H., Shiraishi, Y., Ohtsuki, Y., and Akagi, T. Transformation of normal human cord lymphocytes by co-cultivation with a lethally irradiated human T-cell line carrying type C virus particles. *Gann*, **72**, 997–998 (1981).

9. Poiesz, B. J., Ruscetti, F. W., Gazdar, A. F., Bunn, P. A., Hinna, J. D., and Gallo, R. C. Detection and isolation of type C retrovirus particles from fresh and cultured lymphocytes of a patient with cutaneous T-cell lymphoma. *Proc. Natl. Acad. Sci. U.S.*, **77**, 7415–7419 (1980).

10. Poiesz, B. J., Ruscetti, F. W., Reitz, M. S., Kalyanaraman, V. S., and Gallo, R. A. Isolation of a new type C retrovirus (HTLV) in primary uncultured cells of a patient with Sézary T-cell leukaemia. *Nature*, **294**, 268–271 (1981).

11. The T- and B-cell Malignancy Study Group. Statistical analysis of immunologic, clinical and histopathologic data on lymphoid malignancies in Japan. *Jpn. J. Clin. Oncol.*, **11**, 15–38 (1981).

12. Uchiyama, T., Yodoi, J., Sagawa, K., Takatsuki, K., and Uchino, H. Adult T-cell leukemia: Clinical and hematologic features of 16 cases. *Blood*, **50**, 481–492 (1977).

EXPLANATION OF PHOTOS

PHOTO 1.   Phase contrast micrograph of MT-2 cells, showing clumps of cells in suspension.

PHOTO 2.   Phase contrast micrograph of MT-2 cells, showing bizarre cytoplasmic projections.

PHOTO 3.   Smear of MT-2 cells, showing primitive lymphoid cells and giant cells.

PHOTO 4.   Immunofluorescence micrograph of MT-2 cells, showing ATLA in the cytoplasm of all the cells.

PHOTOS 5 and 6.   Electron micrographs of MT-2 cells, showing many type C virus particles in the extracellular spaces. They are predominantly mature forms and show considerable variation in size. Virus particles budding from the cell membrane were rarely observed (arrow). (Photo 6 is reprinted from *Nature*, **294**, No. 5843, pp. 770–771 (1981))

PHOTO 7.   Hamster transplanted with MT-3 cells, showing inguinal and intra-abdominal tumors.

PHOTO 8.   Section of the tumor from hamster in Photo 6, showing a picture consistent with diffuse pleomorphic lymphoma.

PHOTO 9.   Section of the liver from hamster in Photo 6, showing invasive growth of cells.

PHOTO 10.   Immunofluorescence micrograph of the tumor cell smear from hamster in Photo 6, showing ATLA in all cells.

PHOTO 11.   Electron micrograph of the tumor from hamster in Photo 6, showing extracellular type C virus particles.

PHOTO 12.   Karyotype of the recultured cell line from hamster in Photo 6, showing a normal human male karyotype.

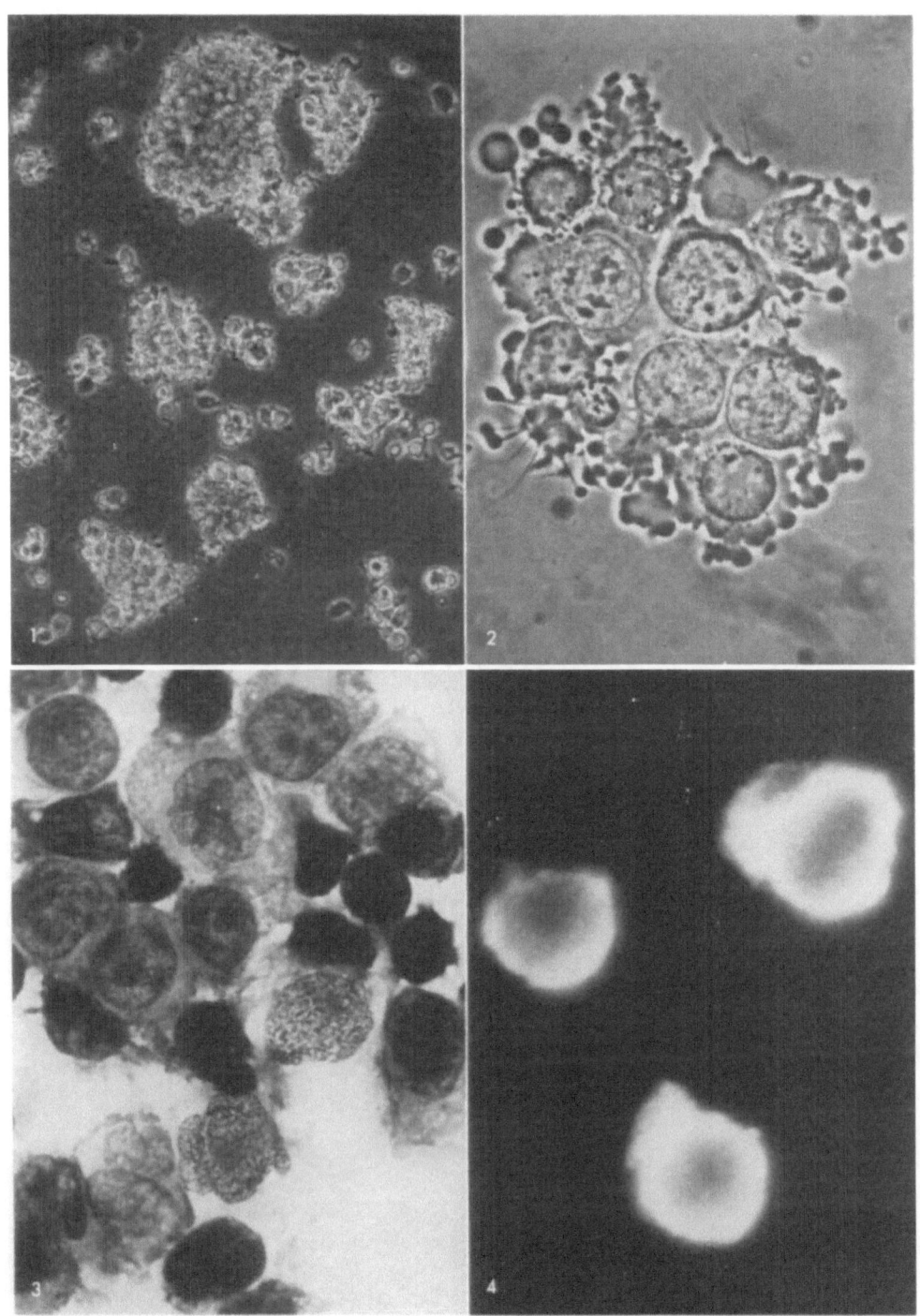

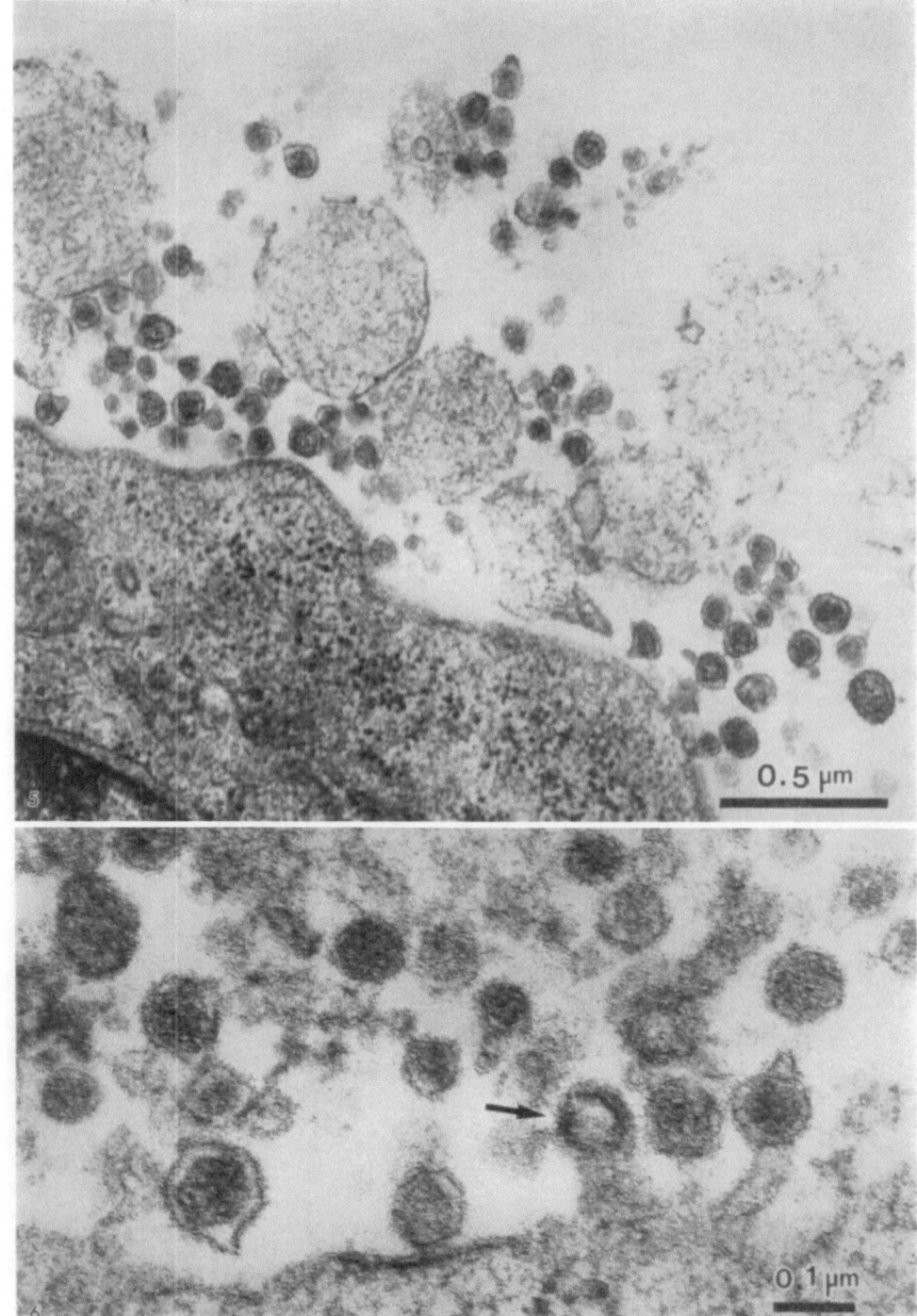

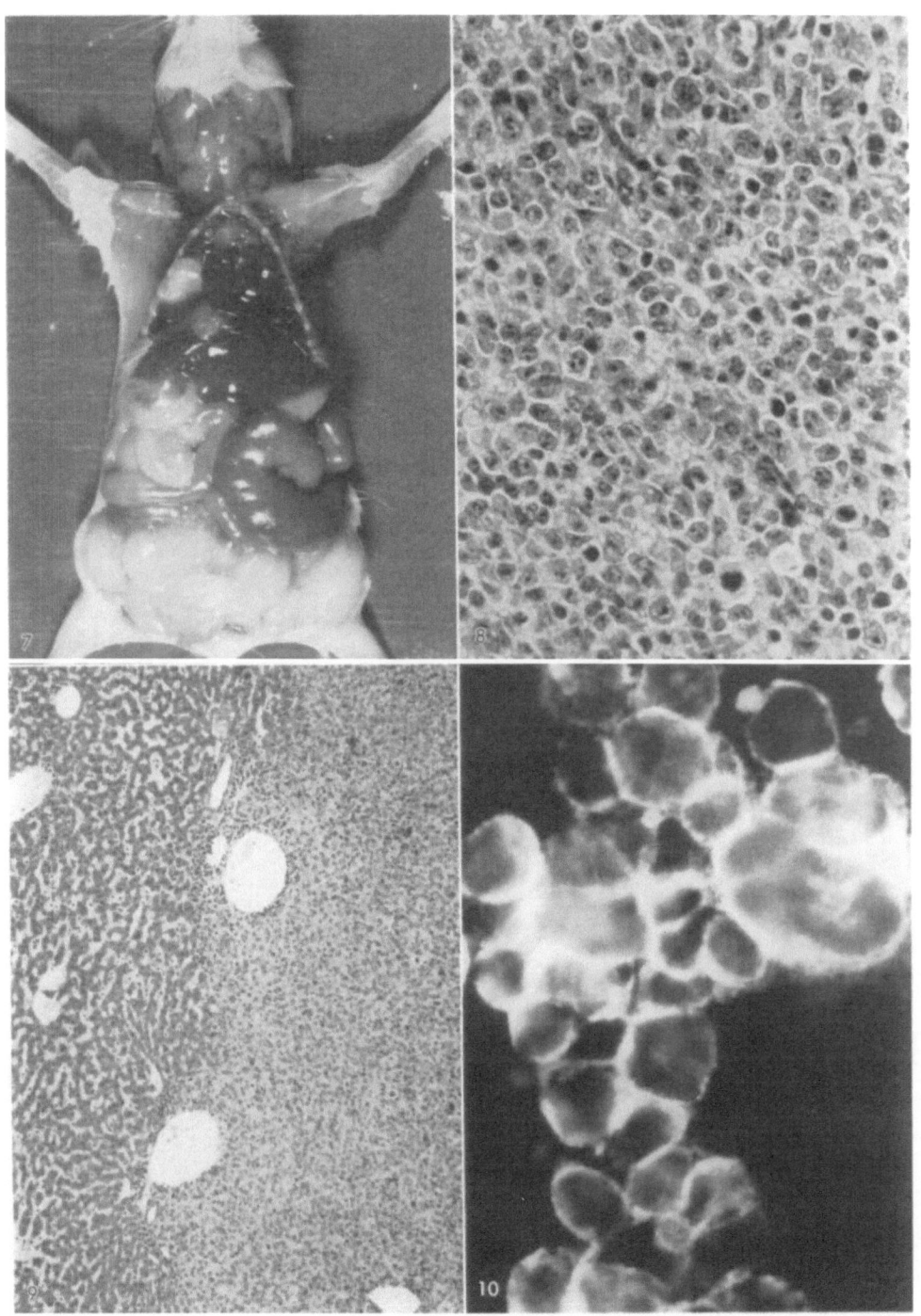

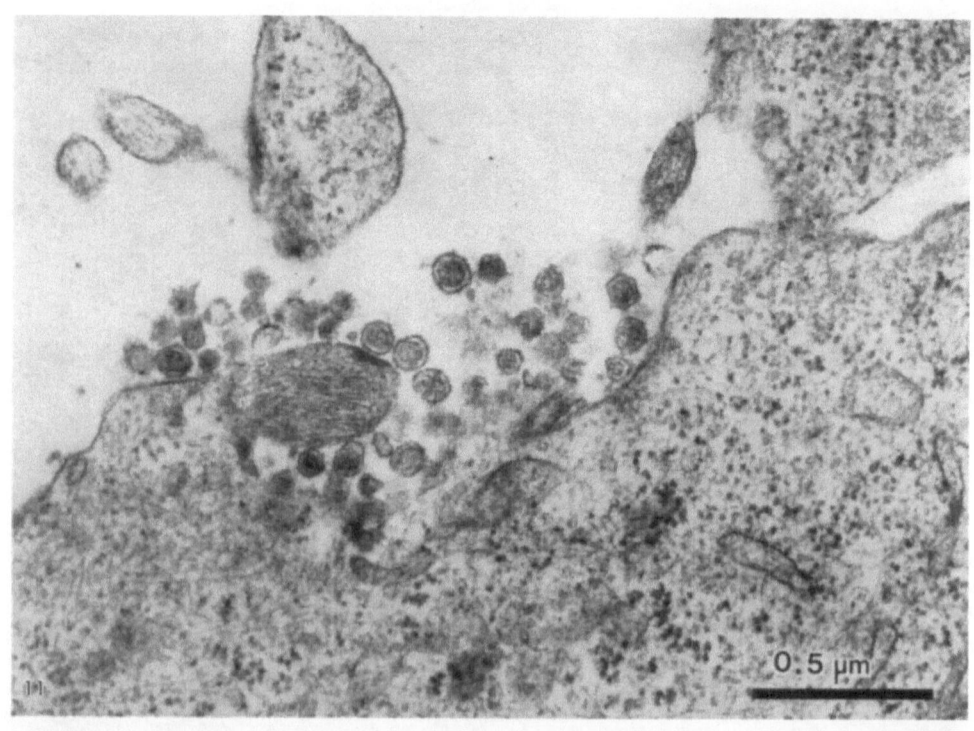

ISOLATION AND CHARACTERIZATION OF RETROVIRUS (ATLV) AND ITS ASSOCIATION WITH ADULT T CELL LEUKEMIA

Mitsuaki Yoshida,*1 Isao Miyoshi,*2 and Yorio Hinuma*3

*Department of Viral Oncology, Cancer Institute,*1 *Medicine, Kochi Medical School,*2 *and Institute for Virus Research, Kyoto University*3*

Human retrovirus, adult T-cell leukemia (ATL) virus (ATLV), was unequivocally demonstrated by biochemical techniques in cell lines from ATL. ATLV had (1) a density of 1.152–1.155 g/ml in sucrose gradient, (2) reverse transcriptase activity, (3) RNA, probably 35S species, as its genome, and (4) proteins with molecular weights of 11K, 14K, 17K, 24K, and 45K daltons. Furthermore, the proviral DNA of ATLV was detected as integrated forms in chromosomal DNA of cell lines derived from ATL-related cultures, but not in ATL-unrelated cells, indicating ATLV to be a non-endogenous virus. Close association of the ATLV with leukemia was suggested by the two findings that (a) all DNA preparations from fresh blood lymphocytes of ATL patients tested so far contained the integrated provirus DNA, but that it was not contained in those of normal adults, and (b) all three sera from ATL-patients reacted with p24 of ATLV. These observations strongly suggested that ATLV is involved in the leukemogenesis of leukemia.

Retroviruses have been isolated from many animal species such as chicken, mouse, rat, cat, cow, and monkey. Molecular analyses of these retroviruses have identified a number of transforming genes (*onc*) and have established that *onc* is the normal cell origin (*c-onc*), thus suggesting these cellular *onc* could be involved in general tumors. Therefore, if we had a human retrovirus, it was reasonably expected that it would provide very useful information and tools for studying the mechanisms of carcinogenesis in human. However, no well-established retrovirus of human origin was known until recently. R. Gallo and his colleagues (*10*) have recently reported the isolation and characterization of C-type retrovirus from cutaneous T-cell lymphoma and reported as HTLV.

We have tried to isolate the retrovirus from adult T-cell leukemia (ATL) in Japan (*13*). Recently, Hinuma *et al.* (*3*) found ATL-associated antigen(s), MT-1 and MT-2, cell lines, which were established by Miyoshi *et al.* (*7–9*) from peripheral leukemic cells of ATL patients after cocultivation with normal cord lymphocytes. Virus-like particles with C-type morphology were also found by electron microscopic study (*3, 8*). These observations suggested the presence and possible relation of C-type virus with ATL, and prompted us to isolate these particles and characterize them.

*1 Kami-Ikebukuro 1-37-1, Toshima-ku, Tokyo 170, Japan (吉田光昭).

*2 Okō-cho, Nankoku-shi, Kochi 781-51, Japan (三好勇夫).

*3 Kawara-cho, Shogoin, Sakyo-ku, Kyoto 606, Japan (日沼頼夫).

In this paper, we will describe the isolation and characterization of the retrovirus, ATL virus (ATLV), by biochemical techniques in two cell lines, MT-1 and MT-2. Furthermore, we present data indicating the close association of ATLV proviral DNA with human ATL. These pieces of direct evidence strongly suggest the involvement of the retrovirus, ATLV, in human leukemogenesis.

Characterization of the Retrovirus in the MT-1 and MT-2 Cells

The MT-2 cell line was established from the normal cord lymphocytes cocultivated with leukemic cells from ATL (8, 9) and the culture fluids of the MT-2 cells were used as a viral source. Virus particles were concentrated and purified from the cluture fluid and separated on a sucrose density gradient in essentially the same as avian sarcoma viruses (2, 16). The DNA polymerase activity of each fraction was measured using poly(A)-oligo(dT) and activity was detected in fractions with densities of 1.152–1.155 g/ml (Fig. 1a). Incorporation activity of ^{3}H-deoxy cytidine 5'-triphosphate (^{3}H-dCTP) into polymers was also detected at the same density without addition of the exogenous template (Fig. 1a). Since this activity was also detected in the presence of actinomycin D, which completely inhibits DNA-dependent polymerase, the polymerase activity seemed to be that of reverse transcriptase.

If this activity is reverse transcriptase associated with retrovirus particles, it should be associated with RNA and specific protein components. To demonstrate these, we added ^{3}H-uridine and ^{35}S-methionine separately to the MT-2 cell culture and carried out analysis as described above. ^{3}H-uridine incorporated into polymers was detected in the same fraction as polymerase activity, indicating the presence of RNA in these fractions (Fig. 1b). Proteins containing ^{35}S-methionine gave a peak at the same density as polymerase activity (Fig. 1c). Polyacrylamide gel electrophoresis of ^{35}S-methionine-labeled proteins gave two prominent bands with molecular weights of 24K and 45K daltons together with faintly labeled bands of 11K, 14K, and 17K (Fig. 1d). These bands were easily distinguished from cellular protein contaminants by their distribution at a density of 1.152–1.155 g/ml. Thus, it was concluded that the MT-2 cell line released retrovirus. This virus was named ATLV simply because it was isolated from ATL-cell lines. These molecular sizes of the proteins were very similar to those of human T-cell leukemia virus (HTLV) recently reported by Poiesz et al. (10).

Characterization of cDNA Prepared from ALTV

For characterization and further confirmation of ATLV, ^{32}P-cDNA$_{ATLV}$ was prepared by the endogenous reaction with detergent treated virions and analyzed. The cDNA$_{ATLV}$ hybridized nearly 90% to virion RNA with Crt$_{1/2}$ of 0.21 (Fig. 2). This Crt$_{1/2}$ value and the kinetics of the reaction were very similar to those obtained with Rous sarcoma virus (RSV) cDNA-RNA hybridization under the same conditions (M. Yoshida, unpublished data), indicating that the main fraction of cDNA$_{ATLV}$ was made from viral RNA contained in virions in a reasonably homogeneous state. Cellular RNA of MT-1 and MT-2 protected the cDNA from nuclease S1 digestion to nearly the same extent as virion RNA (Fig. 2), but cellular RNA of the human fibroblast cell

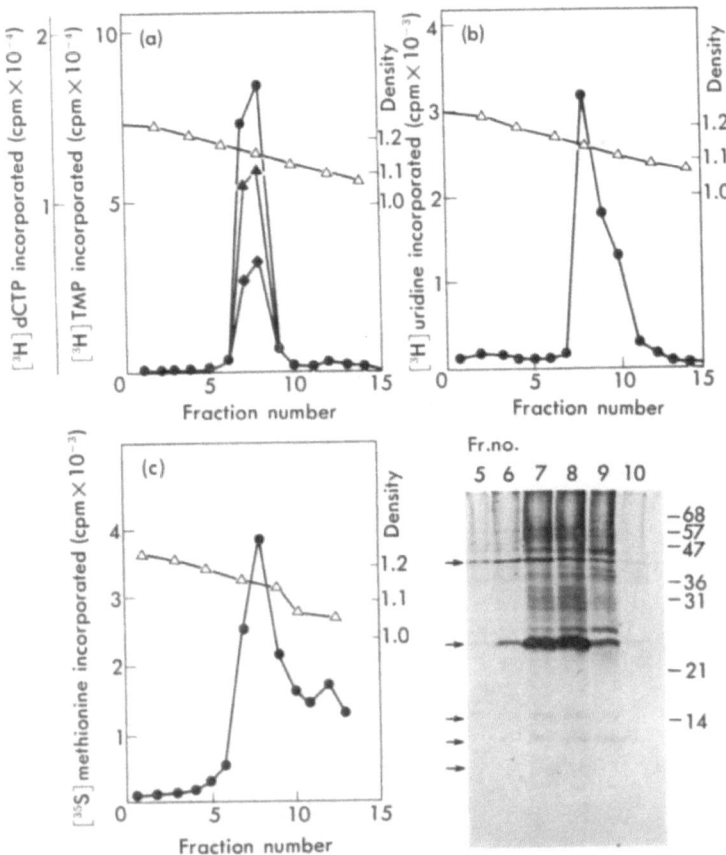

FIG. 1. DNA polymerase activities (a), RNA profile (b), and protein profiles (c and d) of concentrated ATLV particles released from MT-2 cells. Virus preparations were centrifuged on a gradient of 20–60% sucrose in an SW 41 rotor at 30,000 rpm for 18 hr and the gradient was collected in 14 or 15 tubes. $\triangle$ density determined by refractometry. (a) DNA polymerase activity was assayed in the presence of poly(A)-oligo(dT) with 10 mM $MgCl_2$ ($\bullet$) or absence of exogenous template with 3 mM $MgCl_2$ ($\blacktriangle$) or with 1 mM $MnCl_2$ ($\blacklozenge$). (b) MT-2 cells were incubated with ^{3}H-uridine and the labeled virus fractions were precipitated with 10% cold trichloro acetic acid (TCA) and counted. (c) Virus particles were labeled with ^{35}S-methionine and assayed as in Fig. 1b. (d) Portions of each fraction in Fig. 1c were treated with 0.1% sodium dodecyl sulfate (SDS) and analyzed by polyacrylamide gel electrophoresis (6). The dried gel was examined by autoradiography. The numbers on the top of lanes correspond to the fraction numbers in Fig. 1c.

line A204, unrelated to ATL, did not hybridize significantly. These findings clearly indicated that $cDNA_{ATLV}$ prepared from ATLV did not represent cellular RNA components such as rRNA or tRNA which are common to human cells.

To characterize the RNA in MT-1 and MT-2 cells, poly(A)-containing RNA were separated by agarose gel electrophoresis and transferred to diazobenzyloxymethyl (DBM) paper as described by Alwine et al. (1). As shown in Fig. 3, the main com-

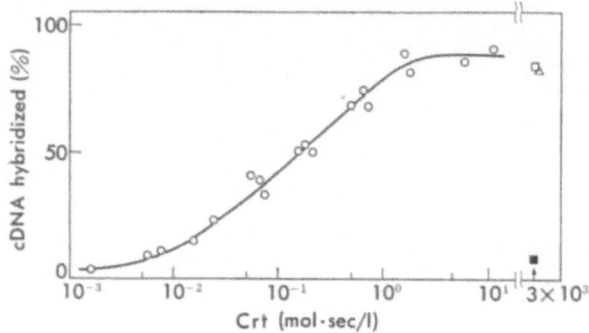

FIG. 2.   Hybridization of ^{32}P-cDNA$_{ATLV}$ with ATLV virion and cellular RNAs. ^{32}P-cDNA$_{ATLV}$ (5,000 cpm) was hybridized with various amounts of 30–70S virion RNA (○) or total cellular RNA from MT-1 (□), MT-2 (△), and A204 (■). Cellular RNA were extracted by the method of Weiss et al. (15).

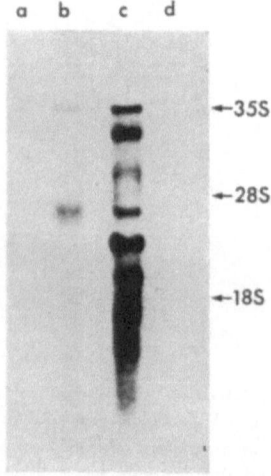

FIG. 3.   ATLV specific RNA in MT-1 and MT-2 cells. Poly(A)-containing RNA was selected with oligo(dT)-cellulose from total RNA of MT-1 cells (a), MT-1 cells treated with 50 μg/ml of IUDR for 24 hr (b), MT-2 cells (c), and A204 cells (d) and analyzed by northern transfer technique described by Alwine et al. (1). Hybridization with ^{32}P-cDNA$_{ATLV}$ was carried out as described by Alwine et al. (1).

ponent of MT-1 cells hybridized with cDNA$_{ATLV}$ was 35S RNA in addition to a component of about 26S, and the content of these RNAs was increased by treating the cells with 5-iodo-2′-deoxyuridine (IUDR). In MT-2 cells, 35S RNA was also detected, but several other smaller RNAs were observed as strong bands. Since the extent of maximum hybridization with MT-2 cellular RNA was almost the same as those with MT-1 and virion RNA (Fig. 2), it is reasonable to assume that these smaller RNA species contained sequences similar to 35S and 26S. However, it is still possible that these bands were detected by possible contaminant cDNA in cDNA$_{ATLV}$ preparation, thus further study is necessary to characterize them. In contrast to MT-1 and MT-2 cells, RNA from human sarcoma cell line A204 showed no detectable band. The presence of 35S RNA which was hybridizable to cDNA$_{ATLV}$ and was inducible with IUDR suggested that ATLV is a typical retrovirus containing 35S RNA as its genome and that cDNA$_{ATLV}$ was transcribed from the RNA.

ATLV Proviral DNA is Integrated into Chromosomal DNA of Cell Lines from ATL

Another requirement for retrovirus is that its genome should be integrated into the host chromosomal DNA during the replication. For demonstrating this, cellular high molecular weight DNA was carefully prepared from MT-1 and MT-2 cells and also from the human cell lines A204 and KB control. The high molecular weight DNA was digested with Eco RI or Bam HI and the digests were separated on agarose gel and transferred on to a nitrocellulose membrane by a modified method (17) of the Southern procedure (12) (Fig. 4). The DNAs of MT-1 and MT-2 cells gave several strong bands and some of them were larger than 10 kilobase pairs, which corresponded to the size of 35S RNA. These findings clearly demonstrated that the provirus DNA of ATLV is integrated into the chromosomal DNA of ATL-derived cell ines, probably as multicopies. In contrast to DNA of these cells, DNA of A204 and KB cells did not show strong bands. Very faint bands were visible after longer exposure in DNA of A204 and KB cells, however, it is unknown whether or not these bands represented shorter fragments of ATLV-related sequences, only partially homologous sequences, or ATLV-unrelated sequences detected with possible contaminant cDNA. In any case, it could be concluded that ATLV itself is not an endogenous virus widely distributed in human

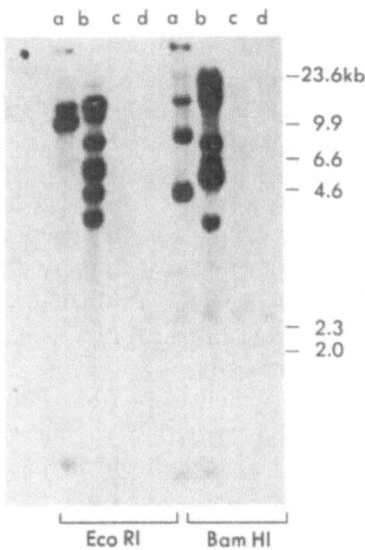

FIG. 4.   Detection of proviral DNA sequences of ATLV in MT-1 and MT-2 cell DNA. High molecular weight DNA extracted from MT-1 cells (a), MT-2 cells (b), A204 (c), and KB cells (d) was digested with Eco RI or Bam HI and analyzed by the Southern transfer technique (12). Hybridization with ^{32}P-cDNA$_{ATLV}$ was carried out as described in text.

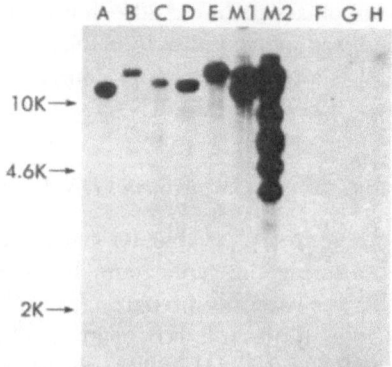

F<small>IG</small>. 5. Detection of proviral DNA of ATLV in leukemic cells from ATL patients. Total DNA was extracted from fresh lymphocytes in peripheral blood of ATL patients (A–E) and from those of healthy adults (F–H) and digested with Eco RI. The digests were analyzed as shown in Fig. 3. As positive controls MT-1 and MT-2 cell DNAs (M1 and M2) were also included.

cells. This conclusion was also supported by the finding that lymphocyte DNA from normal adults did not give any bands hybridizable with cDNA$_{ATLV}$ (see below: Fig. 5). Of course, the technique used in these experiments was not sensitive enough to exclude the possibility that small portions of the ATLV genome are contained in normal human DNA as discussed above.

Detection of ATLV Proviral DNA in Fresh Lymphocytes from ATL Patients

As shown above, the presence of the retrovirus ATLV was unequivocally demonstrated. To obtain more information of the association of ATLV with ATL, we tested for the presence of ATLV proviral DNA in cellular DNA fresh peripheral lymphocytes from ATL patients and from healthy adults. DNA was extracted from fresh lymphocytes from the peripheral blood of 5 patients with ATL, and analyzed by the Southern blotting procedure (*12*). As shown in Fig. 5, all five patients showed discrete positive bands indicating the presence of ATLV proviral DNA in their cellular DNA. The presence of only one band in each DNA with different sizes in different patients indicates variety in cellular sites of integration of ATLV proviral DNA. This finding was in agreement with the above conclusion that ATLV is not a widely distributed endogenous virus, but is acquired only locally.

DNA preparations of fresh lymphocytes from three healthy adults in a non-endemic area did not contain the proviral DNA sequences. This close association of ATLV proviral DNA with ATL suggested the involvement of ATL in leukemogenesis in human ATL.

DISCUSSION

Immunofluorescence studies have previously demonstrated ATL associated antigen(s), in cells in short-term cultures of peripheral lymphocytes, and the involvement of some viruses, possibly C-type virus, with ATL have been suggested (*3*). In this study, the retrovirus was unequivocally demonstrated in leukemic cell lines of ATL. The virus preparation from the MT-2 cell line (8) had the following properties: (1) Its density in a sucrose gradient was 1.152–1.155 g/ml. (2) It contained reverse transcriptase activity and the endogenous reaction was insensitive to actinomycin D. (3) It contained RNA labeled by ³H-uridine. (4) It contained specific proteins with molecular weights of 11K, 14K, 17K, 24K, and 45K daltons, the latter two being the main components labeled with ²²S-methionine.

Furthermore, cDNA prepared by the endogenous reaction of the detergent-treated virions hybridized to 35S RNA containing poly(A), which was inducible by IUDR treatment of MT-1 cells derived from leukemic cells of ATL; DNA sequences homologous with this cDNA were found in chromosomal DNA of MT-1 and MT-2 cell lines. All these observations fitted the requirements for retroviruses. From this study and the previous electron microscopic study (7, 9), this virus is concluded to be a C-type retrovirus, ATLV. The presence of 35S RNA containing poly(A), which was hybridizable with cDNA of ATLV and inducible by IUDR treatment of MT-1 cells, showed that ATLV is a typical retrovirus since all known lymphatic leukemia viruses of animal origin contain 35S RNA as their genome (14).

The molecular weight of the viral proteins and the effects of divalent cations on reverse transcriptase activity are very similar to those HTLV from T-cell lymphoblastoid cell lines derived from a cutaneous T-cell lymphoma, which were recently reported by Poiesz et al. (4, 10, 11). These results might suggest the similarity between

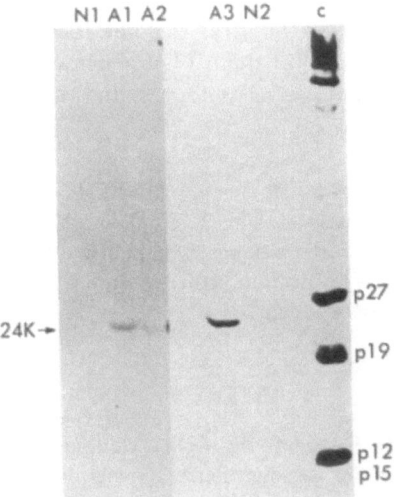

FIG. 6. Immunoprecipitation of ATLV protein of 24 K daltons by sera from patients with ATL. Virus particles labeled with ³⁵S-methionine (fraction No. 8 in Fig. 1c) were disrupted with RIPA buffer (10 mM Tris-HCl, pH 7.5, 150 mM NaCl, 1% sodium deoxycholate, 1% Triton X 100, 0.1% SDS) and treated with sera from patients with ATL (A1–A3) or from normal human adults (N1 and N2). The immunoprecipitates were isolated as described by Kessler (5) and analyzed on 10% polyacrylamide gel (6). Immunoprecipitate from chick cells transformed with Y73 sarcoma virus (18) was also subjected to electrophoresis as marked (c) and the molecular sizes are indicated.

ATLV and HTLV, however, we have no direct evidence on either difference or identity. The relationship between these two viruses would be an important subject to study since both were independently isolated from human leukemic T-cells of different areas.

Cell lines MT-1 and MT-2, derived from T-cells of ATL, contained the ATLV genome in their chromosomal DNA; other human cell lines unrelated to ATL did not contain the ATLV proviral DNA. These observations indicate that ATLV is not a typical endogenous virus widely distributed in human cells. However, DNA preparations from fresh peripheral lymphocytes of all five patients with ATL tested contained the ATLV proviral DNA. This finding strongly suggests that the ATLV is closely associated with human ATL. Furthermore, all three sera from ATL patients tested so far were shown to react with 24K viral protein of ATLV (Fig. 6). All sera from ATL patients including these three sera were previously shown to contain antibody against ATLA, indicating specific association of the antigen(s) with ATL (3). The finding in this paper clearly demonstrated that at least the 24K ATLV protein is one of the ATLA(s). Thus, in this work, association of ATLV protein and ATLV proviral DNA with ATL was demonstrated. This is direct evidence for the idea that the retrovirus ATLV is involved in the leukemogenesis of human leukemia.

It is noteworthy that only a single band of proviral DNA was obtained with each DNA of fresh lymphocytes from ATL patients and that the sizes varied in different patients. These results suggest that the cellular site of the integration of ATLV provirus differs, thus implying that ATLV is not a widely distributed endogenous virus but is acquired by locally. These findings and the endemic distribution of ATL indicate that the mode of transmission of the virus genome is a very important factor. More detailed studies on the distribution of the ATLV genome in Japanese people, especially in the endemic areas, are important for understanding the leukemogenesis of ATL.

Acknowledgments

The authors are grateful to Drs. H. Sugano and M. Hanaoka for discussion and encouragement during this work and also to Drs. T. Matsumoto, K. Kinoshita, and N. Kamada for supplying material. This work was partly supported by a Grant-in-Aid for Cancer Research from the Ministry of Education, Science and Culture and by a grant from the Ministry of Health and Welfare of Japan.

REFERENCES

1. Alwine, J. C., Kemp, D. J., and Stark, G. R. Methods for detection of specific RNAs in agarose gels by transfer to diazobenzyloxymethyl-paper and hybridization with DNA probes. *Proc. Natl. Acad. Sci. U.S.*, **74**, 5350–5354 (1977).
2. Duesberg, P. H., Robinson, H. L., Robinson, W. S., Huebner, R. J., and Turner, H. C. Proteins of Rous sarcoma virus. *Virology*, **36**, 73–86 (1968).
3. Hinuma, Y., Nagata, K., Hanaoka, M., Matsumoto, T., Kinoshita, K.-I., Shirakawa, S., and Miyoshi, I. Adult T-cell leukemia: Antigen in an ATL cell line and detection of antibodies to the antigen in human sera. *Proc. Natl. Acad. Sci. U.S.*, **78**, 6476–6480 (1981).
4. Kalyanaraman, V. S., Sarngadharan, M. G., Poiesz, B., Ruscetti, F. W., and Gallo, R. C. Immunological propertics of a type C retrovirus isolated from cultured human

T-lymphoma cells and comparison to other mammalian retroviruses. *J. Virol.*, **38**, 906–915 (1981).

5. Kessler, S. W. Ropia isolation of antigens from cells with a staphylococcal protein A-antibody adsorbent: Parameters of the interaction of antibody-antigen complexes with protein A. *J. Immunol.*, **115**, 1616–1624 (1975).

6. Laemmli, U. K. Cleavage of structural proteins during the assembly of the head of bacteriophage T4. *Nature*, **227**, 680–685 (1970).

7. Miyoshi, I., Kubonishi, I., Sumida, M., Hiraki, S., Tsubota, T., Kimura, I., Miyamoto, K., and Sato, J. A novel T-cell line derived from adult T-cell leukemia. *Gann*, **71**, 155–156 (1980).

8. Miyoshi, I., Kubonishi, I., Yoshimoto, S., Akagi, T., Ohtsuki, Y., Shiraishi, Y., Nagata, K., and Hinuma, Y. Type C virus particles in a cord T-cell line derived by co-cultivating normal human cord leukocytes and human leukemic T-cells. *Nature*, **294**, 770–771 (1981).

9. Miyoshi, I., Kubonishi, I., Yoshimoto, S., and Shiraishi, Y. A T-cell line derived from normal human cord leukocytes by co-culturing with human leukemic T-cells. *Gann*, **72**, 978–981 (1981).

10. Poiesz, B. J., Ruscetti, F., Gzdar, A. F., Bunn, P. A., Minna, J. D., and Gallo, R. C. Detection and isolation of type C retrovirus particles from fresh and cultured lymphocytes of a patient with cutaneous T-cell lymphoma. *Proc. Natl. Acad. Sci. U.S.*, **77**, 7415–7419 (1980).

11. Reitz, M., Poiesz, B. J., Ruscetti, F. W., and Gallo, R. C. Characterization and distribution of nucleic acid sequences of a novel type C retrovirus isolated from neoplastic human T lymphocytes. *Proc. Natl. Acad. Sci. U.S.*, **78**, 1887–1891 (1981).

12. Southern, E. M. Detection of specific sequences among DNA fragments separated by gel electrophoresis. *J. Mol. Biol.*, **98**, 503–517 (1975).

13. Uchiyama, T., Yodori, J., Sagawa, K., Takatsuki, K., and Uchino, H. Adult T-cell leukemia: clinical and hematologic features of 16 cases. *Blood*, **50**, 481–491 (1977).

14. Vogt, P. K. Genetics of RNA tumor viruses. *Compreh. Virol.*, **9**, 341–455 (1977).

15. Weiss, S. R., Varmus, H. E., and Bishop, J. M. The size and genetic composition of virus-specific RNAs in the cytoplasm of cells producing avian sarcoma-leukosis viruses. *Cell*, **12**, 983–992 (1977).

16. Yoshida, M., Yamashita, M., and Nomoto, A. Transformation-defective mutants of Rous sarcoma virus with longer sizes of genome RNA and their highly frequent occurrences. *J. Virol.*, **30**, 453–461 (1979).

17. Yoshida, M., Kawai, S., and Toyoshima, K. Uninfected avian cells contain structurally unrelated progenitors of avian sarcoma genes. *Nature*, **287**, 653–654 (1980).

18. Yoshida, M., Kawai, S., and Toyoshima, K. Genome structure of avian sarcoma virus Y73 and unique sequence coding for polyprotein p 90. *J. Virol.*, **38**, 430–437 (1981).

AUTHOR INDEX

SUBJECT INDEX